The Prostate

New Concepts and Developments

The Prostate
New Concepts and Developments

Edited by

Fouad K Habib

Department of Oncology
Prostate Research Group
The University of Edinburgh
Western General Hospital
Edinburgh
UK

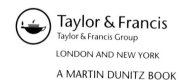

Taylor & Francis
Taylor & Francis Group

LONDON AND NEW YORK

A MARTIN DUNITZ BOOK

First published in the United Kingdom in 2004
by Taylor & Francis, an imprint of the Taylor & Francis Group, 11 New Fetter Lane, London EC4P 4EE

Tel.: +44 (0) 20 7583 9855
Fax.: +44 (0) 20 7842 2298
E-mail: info@dunitz.co.uk
Website: http://www.dunitz.co.uk

A CIP record for this book is available from the British Library.

Library of Congress Cataloging-in-Publication Data

Data available on application

ISBN 1 84184 140 4

Distributed in North and South America by

Taylor & Francis
2000 NW Corporate Blvd
Boca Raton, FL 33431, USA

Within Continental USA
Tel.: 800 272 7737; Fax.: 800 374 3401
Outside Continental USA
Tel.: 561 994 0555; Fax.: 561 361 6018
E-mail: orders@crcpress.com

Distributed in the rest of the world by
Thomson Publishing Services
Cheriton House
North Way
Andover, Hampshire SP10 5BE, UK
Tel.: +44 (0)1264 332424
E-mail: salesorder.tandf@thomsonpublishingservices.co.uk

Composition by J&L Composition, Filey, North Yorkshire, UK

Printed and bound in Spain by Grafos S.A. Arte Sobre Papel

Contents

Contributors

Merja H Ahonen
Medical School
University of Tampere
33014 Tampere
Finland

Georg Bartsch
Department of Urology
University of Innsbruck
Anichstrasse 35
A-6020 Innsbruck
Austria

Merja Bläuer
Medical School
University of Tampere
33014 Tampere
Finland

Leland WK Chung
Emory University
Molecular Urology and Therapeutics
 Program
Department of Urology
1365 Clifton Road
Atlanta GA 30322
USA

Fortunato Ciardiello
Cattedra di Oncologia Medica
Dipartimento di Endocrinologia e Oncologia
 Molecolare e Clinica
Universita di Napoli 'Federico II'
Via S Pansini 5
80131 Napoli
Italy

Zoran Culig
Department of Urology
University of Innsbruck
Anichstrasse 35
A-6020 Innsbruck
Austria

Olivier Cussenot
CeRePP-EA3104
Department d'Urologie
Universite Paris VII
Hospital Saint Louis
F-75475 Paris Cedex 10
France

Mustafa BA Djamgoz
Department of Biological Sciences
Sir Alexander Fleming Building
Imperial College of Science, Technology and
 Medicine
South Kensington
London SW7 2AZ
UK

Iris Eder
Department of Urology
University of Innsbruck
Anichstrasse 35
A-6020 Innsbruck
Austria

Masayuki Egawa
Emory University
Molecular Urology and Therapeutics Program
Department of Urology
1365 Clifton Road
Atlanta GA 30322
USA

Christopher S Foster
Department of Cellular and Molecular
  Pathology
University of Liverpool
Sixth Floor
Duncan Building
Daulby Street
Liverpool L69 3GA
UK

Cynthia J Girman
Department of Health Sciences Research
Section of Clinical Epidemiology
Mayo Clinic and Mayo Foundation
200 First Street SW
Rochester MN 55905
USA

Jan-Åke Gustafsson
Center for Biotechnology and Department of
  Medical Nutrition
Karolinska Institutet
Novum
SE-141 86 Huddinge
Sweden

Khaled S Hafez
Michigan Urology Center
University of Michigan
2916 Taubman Center
1500 E. Medical Center Drive
Ann Arbor MI 48109
USA

Fouad K Habib
Department of Oncology
Prostate Research Group
The University of Edinburgh
Western General Hospital
Crewe Road South
Edinburgh EH4 2XU
UK

Alfred Hobisch
Department of Urology
University of Innsbruck
Anichstrasse 35
A-6020 Innsbruck
Austria

Chia-Ling Hsieh
Emory University
Molecular Urology and Therapeutics Program
Department of Urology
1365 Clifton Road
Atlanta GA 30322
USA

Iveta Iotova
Department of Urology
University of Innsbruck
Anichstrasse 35
A-6020 Innsbruck
Austria

John Isaacs
Johns Hopkins Oncology Center
1650 Orleans Street
Baltimore MD 21231
USA

Steven J Jacobsen
Division of Epidemiology
Department of Health Sciences Research
Mayo Clinic College of Medicine
Harwick 6
Rochester MN 55905
USA

Vasilliki Karavana
Department of Cellular and Molecular
  Pathology
University of Liverpool
Sixth Floor
Duncan Building
Daulby Street
Liverpool L69 3GA
UK

Youqiang Ke
Department of Cellular and Molecular
  Pathology
University of Liverpool
Sixth Floor
Duncan Building
Daulby Street
Liverpool L69 3GA
UK

Helmut Klocker
Department of Urology
University of Innsbruck
Anichstrasse 35
A-6020 Innsbruck
Austria

Kenneth Koeneman
Department of Urology
University of Texas Southwestern
  Medical School
Dallas TX 75390
USA

Ilkka Laaksi
Medical School
University of Tampere
33014 Tampere
Finland

Menuhin I Lampe
Department of Urology
University Medical Center Nijmegen
Geert Grooteplein 10
6525 GA Nijmegen
The Netherlands

Andrew Law
Emory University
Molecular Urology and Therapeutics
  Program
Department of Urology
1365 Clifton Road
Atlanta GA 30322
USA

Michael M Lieber
Department of Urology
Mayo Clinic and Mayo Foundation
200 First Street SW
Rochester MN 55905
USA

Yan-Ru Lou
Department of Anatomy
Medical School
University of Tampere
33014 Tampere
Finland

Sari Mäkelä
Center for Nutrition and Toxicology
Hälsovägen 7–9, Huddinge
and
Department of Biosciences
Karolinska Institutet, Novum
141 57 Huddinge
Sweden

Nick M Makridakis
Institute for Genetic Medicine
Department of Biochemistry and Molecular
  Biology
University of Southern California
Keck School of Medicine
IGM240
2250 Alcazar Street
Los Angeles CA 90089
USA

Dieter Marmé
Institute of Molecular Oncology
Tumor Biology Center
Breisacher Str. 117
D-79106 Freiburg
Germany

Paula Martikainen
Department of Pathology
Tampere University Hospital
33521 Tampere
Finland

Shigeji Matsubara
Emory University
Molecular Urology and Therapeutics
 Program
Department of Urology
1365 Clifton Road
Atlanta GA 30322
USA

Susanna Miettinen
Medical School
University of Tampere
33014 Tampere
Finland

Peter FA Mulders
Department of Urology
University Medical Center Nijmegen
Geert Grooteplein 10
6525 GA Nijmegen
The Netherlands

Claudia Nessler-Manardi
Department of Urology
University of Innsbruck
Anichstrasse 35
A-6020 Innsbruck
Austria

Stefan Nilsson
KaroBio AB
Novum
S–141 86 Huddinge
Sweden

Egbert Oosterwijk
Department of Urology
University Medical Center Nijmegen
Geert Grooteplein 10
6525 GA Nijmegen
The Netherlands

Moon-Soo Park
Emory University
Molecular Urology and Therapeutics
 Program
Department of Urology
1365 Clifton Road
Atlanta GA 30322
USA

Pasi Pennanen
Medical School
University of Tampere
33014 Tampere
Finland

Sami Purmonen
Medical School
University of Tampere
33014 Tampere
Finland

Juergen KV Reichardt
Departments of Biochemistry and Molecular
 Biology and Preventive Medicine
Institute for Genetic Medicine
University of Southern California
Keck School of Medicine
IGM240
2250 Alcazar Street
Los Angeles CA 90089
USA

Hong Rhee
Emory University
Molecular Urology and Therapeutics
 Program
Department of Urology
1365 Clifton Road
Atlanta GA 30322
USA

Ronald K Ross
Norris Comprehensive Cancer Center
Department of Preventive Medicine
University of Southern California
Keck School of Medicine
IGM240
2250 Alcazar Street
Los Angeles CA 90089
USA

Martin G Sanda
Division of Urology
Beth Israel Deaconess Medical Center
Rabb Building, 4th Floor
330 Brookline Avenue
Boston MA 02215
USA

Heimo Syvälä
Medical School
University of Tampere
33014 Tampere
Finland

Giampaolo Tortora
Cattedra di Oncologia Medica
Dipartimento di Endocrinollgia e Oncologia
 Molecolare e Clinica
Universita di Napoli 'Federico II'
Via S Pansini 5
80131 Napoli
Italy

Pentti Tuohimaa
Medical School
University of Tampere and
Department of Clinical Chemistry
Tampere University Hospital
33014 Tempere
Finland

Annika Vienonen
Medical School
University of Tampere
33014 Tampere
Finland

Tapio Visakorpi
Institute of Medical Technology
University of Tampere and
Tampere University Hospital
33520 Tampere
Finland

Margaret Warner
Department of Medical Nutrition
Karolinska Institutet
Novum
SE-141 86 Huddinge
Sweden

Zhang Weihua
Department of Cancer Biology
Anderson Cancer Center
University of Texas
1515 Holcombe Boulevard
Houston TX 77030
USA

Michael G Wyllie
Urodoc Limited
Maryland
Ridgeway Road
Herne Village
Kent CT6 7LN
UK

Fan Yeung
Emory University
Molecular Urology and Therapeutics
 Program
Department of Urology
1365 Clifton Road
Atlanta GA 30322
USA

Timo Ylikomi
Medical School
University of Tampere and
Department of Clinical Chemistry
Tampere University Hospital
33014 Tampere
Finland

Haiyen E Zhau
Emory University
Molecular Urology and Therapeutics
 Program
Department of Urology
1365 Clifton Road
Atlanta GA 30322
USA

Preface

Recent years have witnessed major advances in our understanding of the pathogenesis of benign prostatic hyperplasia (BPH) and prostate cancer at both the molecular and cellular level. These developments were based essentially on fundamental research that as yet has not been substantially translated into clinical practice. Indeed, the speed of scientific development is difficult to follow, and it has become clear to the scientific community and the medical profession that both scientific discovery and technological advances leading to novel practices are occurring more quickly than can be assessed by either clinical trials or scientific evaluation. Nonetheless, important breakthroughs have also been made in the development of new treatments with significant implications for the management of prostate diseases.

This book brings together experts and specialists in the field. It covers a broad scientific background, from basic biology and regulatory mechanisms controlling abnormal growth and progression to metastasis to issues concerning the medical management of prostate diseases including gene therapy and immunotherapy. Internationally recognized experts have sum-marized their knowledge and provided an extensive up-to-date review covering a spectrum of topics as they relate to our understanding of the etiology, diagnosis, prognosis, and treatment of BPH and prostate cancer.

The contents of the book are largely based on a symposium held in Castres, France on March 21–23rd 2001. The meeting was sponsored by an individual grant from Pierre Fabre Medicament, which allowed cell and molecular biologists, epidemiologists and urologists from around the world to present their work and participate in discussions about the way forward. I am indeed indebted to all those who have contributed so widely to this book and wish to thank them for their excellent contributions, their time, knowledge, and patience.

Readers must recognize that research on the prostate is undergoing a major revolution in terms of our understanding of the disease processes of BPH and prostate cancer. This book is intended to inform and give guidance on the advances so far achieved and chart the future for more effective modalities in the diagnosis and prognosis of these diseases.

Fouad K. Habib

1 Natural history of benign prostatic hyperplasia

Steven J Jacobsen, Cynthia J Girman and Michael M Lieber

Introduction

Benign prostatic hyperplasia (BPH) and its related signs and symptoms (often referred to as prostatism) are extremely common among aging men, so much so that some have suggested that this condition is a natural concomitant of aging. In 1989, there were approximately 1.3 million office visits to physicians for BPH (Schappert 1993) and approximately 170 000 prostatectomies performed among inpatients in non-federal short-stay hospitals in the United States in 1992 (Xia *et al.* 1999). These numbers, however, pale in comparison with estimates based on the Agency for Health Care Policy and Research (AHCPR) Diagnostic and Treatment Guidelines for BPH (McConnell *et al.* 1994). Of the 22.5 million white men ages 50–79 years in the United States in 1990, we estimated that approximately 5.6 million would be expected to meet AHCPR guidelines criteria of American Urological Association Symptom Index (AUASI) >7 and peak urinary flow rate <15 ml/s for discussing treatment options for BPH (Jacobsen *et al.* 1995a). This demonstrates that (1) reliance upon utilization figures could drastically underestimate the burden of BPH and (2) that BPH is, indeed, very common in the population. Thus, it is somewhat surprising that so little is known about the natural history of BPH in the population.

This lack of knowledge about the natural history of BPH in the population setting hinders advances in primary, secondary and tertiary prevention. Without a solid understanding of the natural history of BPH, it may not be possible to interpret the results of clinical trials of effectiveness (Guess *et al.* 1995). Information on natural history helps to separate the effects of intervention from what might be expected in its absence. It is important to keep in mind that this information usually cannot be obtained in the context of a clinical trial for a number of reasons. Trials are usually conducted among patients drawn from a practice or group of practices in which referral patterns can severely alter the distribution of disease severity. Similarly, placebo and Hawthorne effects can alter behaviors and perceptions of benefits, creating a distorted picture. Thus, population-based studies of the natural history of BPH are essential to advance knowledge about treatment effectiveness and risk and prognostic factors.

One of the reasons that so little is known about the natural history of BPH may be related to the methods required to obtain a diagnosis. Technically, BPH is a histologic diagnosis based on an examination of a tissue specimen obtained during biopsy, surgery or autopsy. As the most common consequences of BPH are related to decrements in quality of life and not more dire, Institutional Review Boards are not likely to enthusiastically endorse a study requiring biopsy of large numbers of normal subjects. Even if approved, it is unlikely that subjects randomly sampled from the population would consent to such a protocol. Thus, autopsy studies provide some of the only data on the prevalence of histologically diagnosed BPH across the age spectrum. This approach gives limited insight into the incidence or progression of the disease, however, as histologic diagnoses do not always translate to clinical diseases. Because of this, investigators have turned to surrogate measures to assess BPH. In the following paragraphs, we discuss some of the surrogate measures that have been used, including clinical, physiologic, anatomic and biochemical measures. We then describe what has been learned about these measures in the community-setting.

Surrogate measures of BPH

Clinical measures of BPH (symptoms)

A number of investigators have suggested that clinical measures of BPH are the most important as these reflect the complaints of the patient. In response, there have been a number of scales developed to assess symptoms, whether in terms of frequency of occurrence, associated bother, impact on quality of life or interference with normal living activities. One of the most important advances was the development of the American Urological Association Symptom Index (AUASI) as a measure of BPH severity (Barry *et al*. 1992b). In a review of items from previously used scoring systems (Boyarsky *et al*. 1977; Fowler

et al. 1988; Madsen & Iversen 1983), an expert panel noted that some of the symptoms queried in these scales were probably not due to BPH and could be dropped and some important symptoms had not been assessed (e.g., weak urinary stream) and should be added. The resulting questions were then structured so that they could be answered on a self-administered questionnaire, instead of being filled out by a clinician. Subjects with clinical BPH were administered the pilot instrument along with a group of controls (without clinical BPH) from a general medical practice. Subjects were debriefed to highlight ambiguous or difficult questions and were reassessed 1 week later. The results of this pilot were assessed for test–retest reliability, self-reported difficulty, internal consistency, construct validity and criterion validity. This provided guidance for item reduction and the final instrument was tested in cases and controls.

This final instrument consisted of seven questions rated on a 0–5 scale. The test–retest reliability of the summary score was quite good, with an intraclass correlation of 0.93. Cronbach's alpha was 0.86, with none of the individual items demonstrating low correlations. The correlation with global bother score was 0.71 and the area under the receiver operator characteristic curve from the logistic regression was 0.85. In a pilot study of 27 patients undergoing treatment, 26 of the 27 subjects demonstrated a decrease in symptom score; 14 of the subjects reported a decrease of more than 7 points. In addition, the scale correlated well with self-administered versions of the Boyarsky, Madsen-Iversen and Maine Medical Assessment Program Symptom Scales (Barry *et al*. 1992a). Thus, the AUASI was shown to be a valid and reliable instrument for assessing the severity of symptoms commonly associated with BPH.

Since its publication in 1992, the AUASI has been used in many studies. For clinical practice, it plays a pivotal role in the Agency for Health Care Policy and Research Diagnostic and Treatment Guidelines for BPH (McConnell *et al*. 1994). After ruling out secondary causes of urinary symptoms, the assessment of symptom severity with the AUASI provides the decision node to consider further diagnostic workups or to consider treatment options. The International Consultation on Benign Prostatic Hyperplasia (Cockett *et al*. 1991, 1993) has recommended its use in studies to quantify the burden of BPH (as the International Prostate Symptom Score – IPSS), both for population studies and for clinical studies of treatment efficacy and effectiveness.

In addition to the AUASI, there are several other scales that are currently being used to assess BPH in epidemiologic and clinical studies. These include the Symptom Problem Index (SPI) (Barry *et al*. 1995), BPH Impact Index (BII) (Barry *et al*. 1995), and the BPH-Specific Interference with Activities Scale (BSIA) (Epstein *et al*. 1991, 1992). These measures are all highly correlated with the AUASI, but measure slightly different psychological constructs. For example, the SPI (Barry *et al*. 1995) queries the amount of bother associated with each of the seven symptoms queried in the AUASI. We examined the discrepancy between the SPI and AUASI (Jacobsen *et al*. 1993) to provide insight into health care-seeking behavior and acceptance of symptoms. The BSIA queries the amount of interference with seven normal day-to-day activities. We have used this scale to demonstrate the impact of symptomatic benign prostatic enlargement on a man's quality of life (Girman *et al*. 1994).

Physiologic measures of BPH (urinary flow rates)

An alternative means for identifying BPH through surrogate measures is by assessing lower urinary tract function. When BPH is present, pressure placed on the proximal urethra may cause a decrease in urinary flow during micturition. There are two primary methods by which lower urinary tract function is measured directly: pressure flow studies and uroflowmetry. A more indirect way to assess function is through measurement of post-void residual urine volume.

Pressure flow studies are invasive studies that simultaneously measure urinary flow rates, bladder pressure and abdominal pressure (Te & Kaplan 1998). Bladder pressure is measured by a transducer that is placed directly in the bladder, through either a urethral or suprapubic catheter. Abdominal pressure is measured by a transducer placed in the rectum. Flow rates are measured by a urometer, which assesses voided volume as a function of time. Nomograms have been developed to differentiate supra-vesicular from infra-vesicular causes of depressed flow rates on the basis of these measurements (Abrams & Griffiths, 1979). Thus, it is possible to determine which men have depressed flow rates due to bladder-related conditions such as neurologic conditions or impaired detrusor function. These studies do not, however, differentiate depressed flow rates due to BPH from those due to strictures.

A much less invasive technique for measuring lower urinary tract function is by measuring flow rates alone. This avoids the discomfort and potential complications (infection, acute urinary retention, strictures, etc.) of placing the pressure transducers in the bladder while providing a global assessment of urinary function. Standard measurements include voided volume, average flow rate (total volume/voiding time) and peak urinary flow rate (Qmax, the greatest flow/unit time), time to Qmax and voiding time. In general, Qmax increases with voided volume and this relationship stabilizes with voided volumes greater than 150 ml.

A third, but more indirect assessment of lower urinary tract function, is through measurement of post-void residual urine volume. As men become more and more obstructed, bladder emptying becomes less complete and residual volume increases. Residual volumes can be measured directly by catheterizing the bladder and measuring the urine volume. A less invasive method can be made by sonographically imaging the bladder. Estimates of the residual volume can be made by measuring the antero-posterior, transverse and inferior-superior dimensions of the residual urine in the bladder.

Anatomic measures of BPH (prostate volume)

A third surrogate means for identifying BPH is by assessing prostatic volume. The rationale for this is that with more BPH, the prostate tends to be larger. However, while all parts of the prostate can have BPH, those that are in closer proximity to the prostatic urethra are most likely to cause obstruction and symptoms. Measurement of prostate volume can be done by estimating the size during a digital rectal examination (DRE), during urethrocystoscopy or by imaging the prostate, either by ultrasound or magnetic resonance imaging.

A number of studies have assessed the accuracy and reliability of estimating prostate volume by DRE (Meyhoff & Hald 1978, Bissada et al. 1976, Meyhoff et al. 1981, Rahmouni et al. 1992, Roehrborn et al. 1997, Varenhorst et al. 1993). In general, the intra-observer reliability is good but the inter-observer reliability

is less so. There is also greater reliability among persons with greater experience in performing DREs. The accuracy, however, appears to vary with prostate size. In general, evaluators tend to be more accurate with smaller prostates, but tend to underestimate the volume of larger prostates. In a recent study, we have shown that the accuracy and precision of DRE in estimating prostatic volume can be increased with the use of a set of models (Roehrborn et al. 1997).

Estimates of prostatic volume can also be made during urethrocystoscopy. This procedure can also be used to estimate the length of the prostatic urethra and to identify bladder trabeculation, stones and diverticula. While this procedure plays a central role in urology practice for visualizing the lower urinary tract, it is not recommended as a diagnostic procedure in the AHCPR guidelines (McConnell et al. 1994) and is probably not useful in the community setting.

The reliability of estimating prostatic volume can be increased by imaging the prostate (Bates et al. 1996, Collins et al. 1995, Littrup et al. 1991, Watanabe et al. 1974). Transrectal sonographic imaging of the prostate is the most common means by which this is done. For this, the transducer is placed in the rectum and adjusted to identify the maximal transverse and antero-posterior dimensions. The transducer is then moved to identify the base of the bladder neck and inferior edge of the prostate (superior-inferior dimension). This method has been shown to produce more reliable results than identifying the superior aspect of the prostate (Collins et al. 1995). These three dimensions are then used to estimate prostate volume. Most typically, volume is estimated with the formula for a prolate ellipsoid. This formula has been shown to have a higher correlation with prostate volume than others, based on volumetric displacement of radical prostatectomy specimens (Terris & Stamey 1991).

In addition to assessing total prostatic volume, the sonographic image permits the estimation of central zone volume (Corica *et al.* 1999, Kaplan *et al.* 1995, Witjes *et al.* 1997). The image of the prostate reveals a central region that is hypo-echoic in comparison to the surrounding tissue. This region roughly corresponds to the transitional zone of the prostate. As this region is more prone to BPH and more directly impinges on the prostatic urethra, the size of this region may be more important to voiding function than total prostate volume. Measurement of the central zone is analogous to measuring total volume. The anatomic locations of the maximal dimensions are not necessarily the same, however. This makes retrospective assessments of central zone volume suspect. Magnetic resonance imaging (MRI) provides an alternative method for imaging the prostate (Williams *et al.* 1999). The images have greater precision than sonographic images, but the difference in cost and availability of machines make these less feasible.

In recent years, some investigators have suggested that non-invasive (sonographic) measurement of bladder wall thickness may provide insight into the presence of outlet obstruction (Manieri *et al.* 1998, Kojima *et al.* 1997). It has been suggested that this anatomic measure may be better in identifying bladder outlet obstruction than uroflowmetry – area under the receiver–operator characteristic curve of 0.86 versus 0.69 (Manieri *et al.* 1998). Computed tomography (CT) images have also been used to estimate bladder wall thickness (Schreyer *et al.* 2000). None of these technologies have been assessed in the community setting, however.

Biochemical measures of BPH (PSA)

BPH can also be assessed through the measurement of biochemical markers, primarily serum prostate specific antigen (PSA) levels. PSA is a 33-kDa serine protease produced by the epithelium of the prostate gland (Papsidero *et al.* 1981). Serum levels of PSA have been noted to be elevated in men with an enlarged prostate (Collins *et al.* 1993a, Oesterling *et al.* 1993, Stamey *et al.* 1987) and in men harboring prostate cancer (Oesterling 1991, Stamey *et al.* 1987). In men with enlarged prostates, elevated serum PSA levels have been assumed to be due to increased epithelial mass, whereas local tissue destruction and concomitant leakage of PSA into the systemic circulation are also thought to contribute to elevated serum levels of PSA in men with cancer (Brawer & Lange 1989). In the peripheral circulation, measurable PSA exists primarily in two forms: as a free, non-complexed form and complexed to alpha-1 antichymotrypsin. PSA also exists in a form complexed to alpha-2-macroglobulin (Lilja 1993, Lilja *et al.* 1991). The free form of PSA and PSA complexed to alpha-1 antichymotrypsin are both measurable by various commercial and research-based assays, whereas the PSA complexed to alpha-2-macroglobulin is not immunodetected by these assays (Christensson *et al.* 1990, Lilja 1993, Lilja *et al.* 1991, Sottrup-Jensen 1989, Zhou *et al.* 1993).

In recent years, it has been noted that concentrations of the free form of PSA are relatively higher in men with BPH than in men with prostate cancer (Lilja *et al.* 1991). Thus, both total serum PSA and serum free PSA may provide measures of prostatic growth or BPH (Carter *et al.*, 1992a).

In addition, it has been observed the PSA can also be identified in a 'clipped' form (Mikolajczyk *et al.* 2000), with cleavage at lysine 182. This form was identified in the transition zone of the prostate, and was elevated in transition zones with nodular hyperplasia as compared to 'normal'. This form of PSA, labeled as BPSA, can be identified with specific monoclonal antibodies (Wang *et al.* 2000), suggesting that it may be useful for identifying BPH, and in the presence of elevated total serum PSA levels, distinguishing prostate cancer from BPH. Further work needs to be done, however, as no studies have evaluated the measurement of BPSA in the community setting.

Problems with surrogate measures of BPH

Unfortunately, while each of these measures appears to capture some component of BPH, none is specific to BPH (McConnell *et al.* 1994). This lack of specificity is partly due to the effects of detrusor function on several of these measures. Impaired detrusor function, whether from intrinsic (e.g., changes associated with an aging bladder) or extrinsic causes (e.g., nerve damage from disease, surgery, injury or effect of medications) can lead to increased symptom severity and decreased urinary flow rates. In addition, other sources of outflow obstruction such as urethral strictures can lead to increased symptom severity and decreased urinary flow rates. Incontinence (Roberts *et al.* 1998) and prostatitis can lead to increased symptom scores while having little or nothing to do with BPH. While prostate volume may not be affected by any of these conditions, not all men with an enlarged prostate necessarily experience symptoms. Consequently, no one dimension appears to lend itself well for use as a diagnostic instrument for BPH in epidemiologic studies.

Community studies of the natural history of BPH

Despite the shortcomings of these surrogate measures of BPH, a number of investigators have judiciously used them to try to draw inference about the natural history of BPH. Unfortunately, many early studies tried to draw population inference from measurements made on clinical series of patients, in which the spectrum of disease differed from the population at large. More recently, however, it has been recognized that such an approach is not valid and there have been a number of population-based studies undertaken to draw more appropriate inference. In the following paragraphs, we highlight some of the findings from these studies and point to important unanswered questions.

Clinical measures of BPH

Recent studies have taken advantage of the AUASI (Barry *et al.* 1992b) and the closely related International Prostate Symptom Score (Cockett *et al.* 1991). A common thread among the findings is that the prevalence of moderate to severe symptoms as measured by the AUASI is fairly high. In an age-stratified random sample of the Olmsted County, Minnesota, USA population of men aged 40–79 years, we (Chute *et al.* 1993) reported that between 26 and 46% of men in the community had moderate to severe symptoms (AUASI >7). There was a strong age-related increase in symptom scores, with the mean score increasing about 0.8 per age year (Jacobsen *et al.*, 1995b). A similar age-related increase was recorded for a comparable study conducted in Scotland (Guess *et al.*, 1993), but symptom scores were, on average, lower than for the American men (Guess *et al.* 1993). Sagnier and others reported on the prevalence of moderate and severe symptoms in an age-stratified probability sample of men in France (Sagnier *et al.* 1994) and reports have also been generated from Japan (Tsukamoto *et al.* 1995), The Netherlands (Bosch *et al.* 1995), Spain (Chicharro-Molero *et al.* 1998, Hunter *et al.* 1996), United Kingdom (Trueman *et al.* 1999), Austria (Madersbacher *et al.* 1998), Korea (Lee *et al.* 1998), Singapore (Tan *et al.* 1997) and Wisconsin (Klein *et al.* 1999). While the absolute prevalence differs among studies, the similarity in age-related increase is quite striking. This suggests that there may be some cultural differences in reporting frequency of urinary symptoms, but that the age-related increase is consistent and parallels the monotonic age-related increase in prostate volume in autopsy studies (Berry *et al.* 1984).

These cross-sectional age-related increases, however, are not consistently found in the longitudinal follow-up of these cohorts. There is, in fact, a great deal of variability among individuals. After 1 year of follow-up, approximately 50% of Scottish men reported individual symptoms occurring at the same frequency as baseline (Garraway *et al.* 1993). Slightly more men reported worsening of individual symptoms (up to one-third of men), whereas approximately 20% reported considerable improvement. Among Olmsted County men (Jacobsen *et al.* 1996), we found, on average, a modest average annual increase in AUASI at 42 months follow-up (mean slope = 0.18 points/year, standard deviation = 1.22, $p<0.001$). The average annual change increased from 0.05/year among men in their forties at baseline, to 0.44/year among men in their sixties, leveling off for men in their seventies. This pattern is very similar to the sigmoid-shaped curve of the age-specific prevalence of BPH estimated by Berry *et al.*, but shaped

differently than the linear increases in prostate volume (Berry *et al.* 1984).

These differences raise questions about the true nature of changes in symptom severity across the lifespan. The difference between the cross-sectional and longitudinal estimate could be related to the baseline selection factors from the prevalence studies. In particular, the exclusion of men who had been treated for BPH would systematically eliminate those with the most severe disease. With longitudinal follow-up, some men would age into these more severely diseased categories. Therefore, it is not clear how much of the current discrepancy between cross-sectional and longitudinal findings is due to selection factors and whether or not these factors are continuing to influence estimates of age-related changes.

Physiologic measures of BPH

The overall high prevalence and age-related increase in lower urinary tract symptoms in the community has been reported for urinary flow rates as well. We reported community-based nomograms for peak and average urinary flow rates based on findings from the Olmsted County cohort (Girman *et al.* 1993). With a cutpoint of 15 ml/s for peak urinary flow rates, 24% of men aged 40–44 years are estimated to have impaired flow rates, compared to 69% for men aged 70 years and older. The more stringent cutpoint of 10 ml/s demonstrates a similar age-related increase, from 6% among men aged 40–44 years to 36% among older men. Diokno and others (Diokno *et al.* 1994) reported similar results from the volunteers of the Washtenaw County, Michigan study.

By contrast, we found that the annual change in peak urinary flow rates (Figure 1.1) differed across age groups (Roberts *et al.* 2000). Men in their forties at baseline experienced a 1.3%

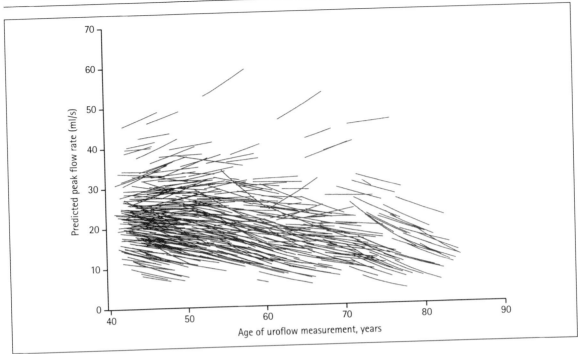

Figure 1.1
Predicted peak urinary flow rate based on mixed effects model by age at uroflow measurement (Roberts *et al.* 2000).

per year decline, whereas those in their seventies had a 6.5% per year decline. This differed from the cross-sectional results that suggested a consistent decline of 2% per year across all age groups. As with symptom severity, these differences raise questions about the true nature of changes in urinary flow rates across the lifespan. The difference between the cross-sectional and longitudinal estimates could be related to the baseline selection factors. However, the different pattern may be due to issues related to bladder function rather than the prostate, per se.

Anatomic measures of BPH

The high prevalence of prostatism as measured by symptoms or urinary flow rates is mirrored by measurements of prostate volume. A reanalysis of cross-sectional data from the Scottish cohort suggests that prostatic volume is strongly associated with age ($r = 0.44$, $p<0.001$) and that an extremely large percentage of men had a prostate volume >20 ml (88%) (Collins *et al.* 1993a). We previously reported similar results from the Olmsted County study (Oesterling *et al.* 1993). The cross-sectional regression analysis of prostate volume on subject age suggested that prostatic volume increased approximately 0.6% per year. Analysis of patterns of enlargement in BPH, however, suggests that this cross-sectional age-related increase is primarily in the adenomatous portion of the prostate (Collins *et al.* 1993b) and that the volume of the central, hypo-echoic region of the prostate is more closely associated with age than with total prostate volume (Bosch *et al.* 1994). Based on the baseline and 18-, 42- and 60-month follow-up examinations in the Olmsted County study, our mixed effects regression models (Figure 1.2)

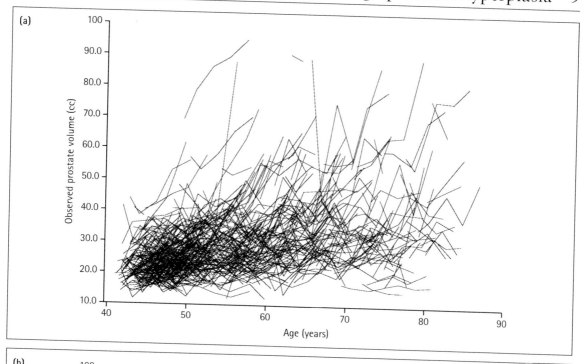

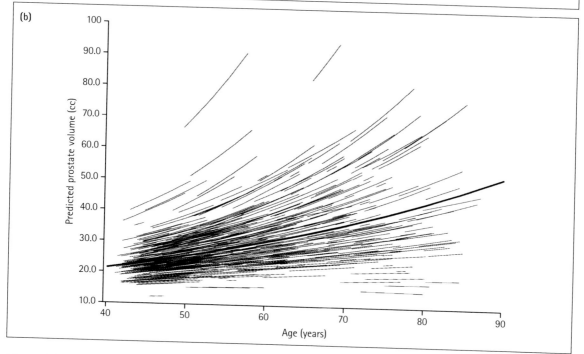

Figure 1.2

(a), plot of observed prostate volumes. Each line represents individual subject. *(b)*, plot of predicted prostate volumes as estimated by mixed effects regression model. Each line represents individual subject and thick line represents population average (Rhodes *et al.* 1999).

suggested that prostate volume increased about 1.6% per year on average (Rhodes *et al.* 1999). This did not vary by age, but was greater among men with larger prostates at baseline as compared to those with smaller prostates. This growth rate was greater than what was estimated from the baseline cross-sectional data (0.6% per year) but similar in shape to the autopsy-based estimates from Berry *et al.* (1984).

We have since used static images optimized for measuring total prostate volume to assess central zone volume (Corica *et al.* 1999). We found that central zone volume was more highly correlated with age than total prostate volume. This cross-sectional increase was, as for total prostate volume, an exponential increase at 2.3% per year and did not differ across ages.

As with symptom severity and flow rates, these differences across age groups raise questions about the true nature of changes in prostate growth rates across the lifespan. The difference between the cross-sectional and longitudinal estimate could be related to the baseline selection factors. Furthermore, there is no information on longitudinal central zone growth.

Correlation among surrogate measures of BPH

There have been a number of clinical studies suggesting no correlation amongst symptoms, flow rates and prostate size (Abrams & Feneley 1978, Barry *et al.* 1993, Christensen & Bruskewitz 1990, Graversen *et al.* 1989, Jensen *et al.* 1983, 1986). Most of these were based upon clinical series of patients in whom the spectrum of disease severity is likely limited, thereby damping any correlation amongst the variables. By contrast, population studies

conducted in Olmsted County, Scotland, The Netherlands and Japan have suggested correlations on the order of 0.2 for prostate volume and AUASI, -0.2 for prostate volume and peak urinary flow rate and -0.4 for peak urinary flow rate and AUASI (Bosch *et al.* 1994, Collins *et al.* 1993a, Oesterling *et al.* 1995, Girman *et al.* 1995). The three-dimensional surface plot from the Olmsted County study demonstrates these relationships (Figure 1.3).

While these data suggest some degree of relationship cross-sectionally, there are currently no data available describing the concomitant changes in these measures. Furthermore, as all of these cross-sectional measures could have been influenced by baseline selection factors, the observed relationships may not take into account some of the more extreme values.

Biochemical measures of BPH

There have been a number of cross-sectional studies that have examined the relationship between serum PSA level and age (Collins *et al.* 1993a, Gustafsson *et al.* 1998, Morgan *et al.* 1996, Oesterling *et al.* 1993, 1995, Weinrich *et al.* 1998). These studies have been conducted in clinical series, as well as convenience and population-based samples. Across nearly all studies, there is a strong age-dependent increase in serum PSA level in men without prostate cancer, although the magnitude of the relationship varies from study to study. This is important as serum levels of PSA increase with both BPH and prostate cancer and the risk of each of these, in turn, increases with age. Our cross-sectional findings from the baseline examination of the clinical subset of the Olmsted County Study (Oesterling *et al.* 1993) were the basis for age-specific reference ranges that are now in wide use. While these provide some adjustment for the prevalence of BPH, it

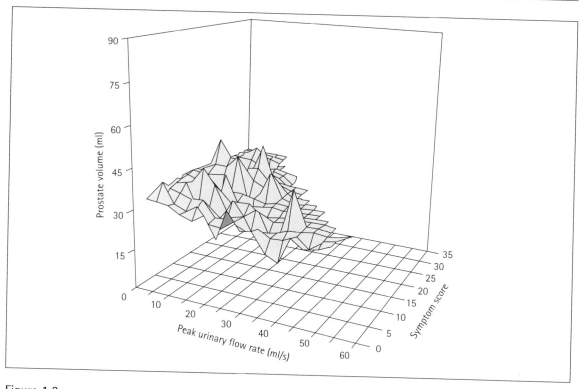

Figure 1.3
Three-dimensional gridded surface plot depicting relationship of prostate volume, peak urinary flow rate and AUA symptom index. Peaks in smoothed plot correspond to higher average levels of prostate volume for given levels of peak urinary flow rate and AUA symptom index, defined by x–y plane (Girman *et al.* 1995).

has been noted that the predictive value of serum PSA level for the detection of prostate cancer is markedly diminished among men with lower urinary tract symptoms (Carter *et al.* 1992a, 1992b, Meigs *et al.* 1996).

There are fewer data available on longitudinal changes in serum PSA level. Some studies have suggested that reference ranges could be based on either absolute or percentage increases of PSA. This may be problematic as these approaches produce drastically different results at the extremes of serum PSA levels. Cross-sectionally, the free form of serum PSA level appears to be more strongly correlated with age than total PSA. There are, however, very few data available on longitudinal changes in serum levels of free PSA (Pearson *et al.* 1996).

Long-term outcomes of BPH

As noted previously, BPH is a chronic progressive condition. Left untreated, there are a number of untoward sequelae that can occur (Meigs & Barry 1996). These include acute urinary retention (AUR), recurrent urinary tract infections, hydronephrosis and even renal failure. Unfortunately, most of the data available for these outcomes are based on clinical series from tertiary care centers where the mix of patients could greatly influence estimates of risk. In fact, published estimates of the 10-year cumulative incidence of AUR vary from 4% to as high as 73% (Barry 1990, Meigs & Barry 1996). With approximately 8000 person-years of follow-up in the Olmsted

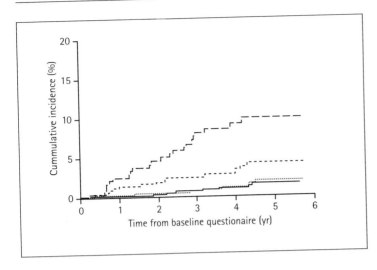

Figure 1.4
Plot of cumulative incidence of acute retention by years of follow-up since completion of baseline questionnaire. Different lines represent decades of age. Solid line represents ages 40–49, dotted line ages 50–59, medium dashed line ages 60–69 and large dashed line ages 70–79 (Jacobsen *et al.* 1997).

Table 1.1 Relative risk of acute urinary retention associated with baseline characteristics.

	Unadjusted		Adjusted*	
	Relative risk	*(95% CI†)*	*Relative risk*	*(95% CI)*
Age, years:				
40–49†	1.0		1.0	
50–59	1.2	(0.5–3.0)	0.9	(0.4–2.4)
60–69	3.0	(1.4–6.6)	2.1	(0.9–4.7)
70–79	7.8	(3.7–16.4)	4.8	(2.2–10.6)
AUASI:				
0–7†	1.0		1.0	
8+	3.2	(1.9–5.4)	2.3	(1.3–4.0)
Peak urinary flow rate (ml/s):				
Greater than 12†	1.0		1.0	
12 or less	3.9	(2.3–6.6)	2.1	(1.2–3.8)
Prostate volume (ml):‡				
30 or less†	1.0			
Greater than 30	3.0	(1.0–9.0)		

*Adjusted for age, AUA symptom index and peak urinary flow rate only.
†Reference category.
‡Adjusted estimates were not calculated due to the small sample size.

County Study, we identified 57 men who experienced AUR as documented in the community medical records (Jacobsen *et al.* 1997). This yielded a cumulative incidence rate of 6.8 per thousand person-years. There was a strong age-related increase in risk (Figure 1.4). In multivariable analyzes, baseline age, symptom severity and peak urinary flow rate were independently predictive of AUR (Table 1.1) but the number of events was too small to allow a multivariable assessment of prostate volume with these factors (there were 17 events in the clinical subset in whom prostate volume measurements were available). Similar estimates of risk were obtained from the Health Professionals Follow-up Study (Meigs *et al.* 1999).

Treatment for BPH

While not a naturally occurring long-term outcome, treatment of BPH can represent another hard measure of sequelae of disease. The Olmsted County Study provided estimates of the occurrence of treatment during follow-up of the cohort. During the first 10 458 person-years of follow-up, 167 men received treatment for BPH, including pharmacologic therapy ($N = 113$), minimally invasive surgical therapy ($N = 19$) and transurethral resection of the prostate (TURP, $N = 45$). The incidence of any treatment (Figure 1.5a) and TURP (Figure 1.5b) increased dramatically with age. Moreover, surrogate measures of BPH each independently predicted any treatment (Table

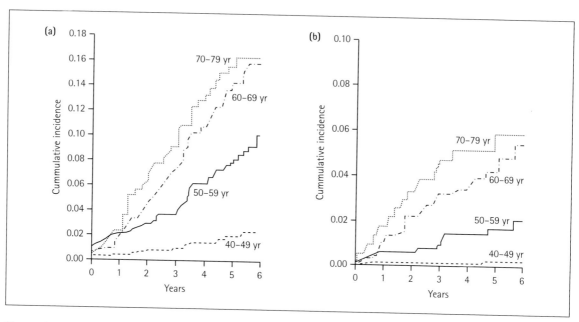

Figure 1.5
Cumulative incidence of BPH treatment *(a)* and transurethral prostatic resection *(b)* stratified by age at study entry. Curves represent Kaplan–Meier cumulative probability of any treatment (pharmacologic, minimally invasive or surgical) and of transurethral prostatic resection (Jacobsen *et al.* 1999).

1.2), after taking into account the strong age relationship. As with the findings on acute urinary retention, these data indicate that surrogate measures of BPH have predictive validity. However, unlike AUR, treatment decisions may have been influenced by measures made during the study.

Conclusions

These data, taken together, strongly support the notion that BPH is a chronic, progressive condition. The cross-sectional and longitudinal estimates of change in all surrogate measures substantiate this. There are, however,

Table 1.2 Association between baseline measures of lower urinary tract dysfunction and risk of any treatment during follow-up. The Olmsted County Study of Urinary Symptoms and Health Status among Men.

Baseline characteristic	Unadjusted*		Unadjusted (clinic cohort)[†]		Adjusted[‡]		Adjusted[§]	
	RR	95% CI	RR	95% CI	RR	95% CI	RR	95% CI
Age (years):								
40–49**	1.0		1.0		1.0		1.0	
50–59	4.5	2.6–7.9	5.1	1.5–17.9	3.3	0.9–12.0	4.2	1.2–14.8
60–69	8.4	4.8–14.5	10.8	3.2–37.0	3.7	1.0–14.0	4.0	1.1–14.8
70–79	9.4	5.2–16.9	10.1	2.8–36.9	3.2	0.8–12.7	3.1	0.8–12.3
Symptom severity:								
None/mild (=7)**	1.0		1.0		1.0		1.0	
Moderate/severe (>7)	4.8	3.5–6.7	8.4	4.0–17.5	5.3	2.5–11.1	5.6	2.6–11.9
Peak urinary flow rate (ml/s):								
>12**	1.0		1.0		1.0		1.0	
=12	3.8	2.8–5.1	5.2	2.9–9.6	2.7	1.4–5.3	2.8	1.4–5.5
Prostate volume (ml):								
=30**			1.0		1.0			
>30			4.2	2.2–8.2	2.3	1.1–4.7		
Serum PSA level (ng/ml):								
=1.4**			1.0				1.0	
>1.4			4.0	2.2–7.3			2.1	1.1–4.2

Association qualified as relative risk (RR), with associated 95% confidence interval (CI).
*Bivariate (crude) models based on entire cohort.
[†]Bivariate (crude) models based on subset randomly selected with clinical examination.
[‡]Multivariable models adjusting for all factors simultaneously, including prostate volume, based on subset with clinical examination.
[§]Multivariable models adjusting for all factors simultaneously, including serum PSA level, based on subset with clinical examination.
**Reference category.

differences in magnitude of the estimates of these changes across the various measures. Moreover, the rate of change differs across measures and between the cross-sectional and longitudinal estimates. Unfortunately, it is not yet clear how much of this is due to baseline selection factors, inherent to the differences between incident and prevalent measures, or due to differing study populations.

Secondly, these surrogate measures of BPH all appear to capture a component of the target disease. They have predictive validity for hard outcomes such as acute urinary retention and treatment. Moreover, these surrogate measures are probably better than surgery, per se, in defining BPH. Surgery as an outcome is limited, due to factors related to access to health care, care-seeking behavior and referral patterns. Provider preferences could also

have an impact on the use of surgery. In fact, the small area variability in TURP rates (Wennberg & Gittelsohn 1982) provided the foundation for studies investigating small area variations. As new technologies are incorporated into urologic practice, surgical rates appear to be declining (Figure 1.6) (Xia *et al.* 1999), with some shift towards minimally invasive therapies. Many of these are provided in the outpatient setting. These factors all make treatment a poor marker to define the presence of BPH for studies of etiology and outcome. The surrogate measures, however, do not represent a global solution as there is not a 1:1 correspondence with one another or with hard outcomes.

Finally, these data all suggest that these surrogate measures represent a continuum of disease severity and do not suggest a threshold

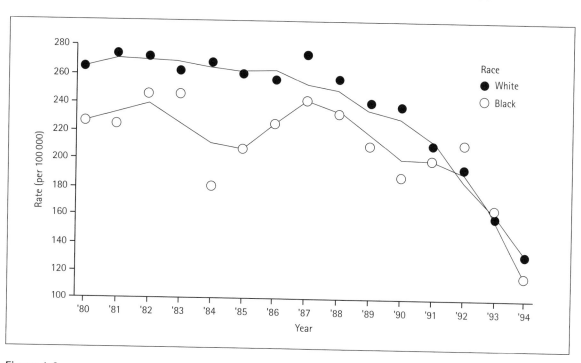

Figure 1.6
Annual age-adjusted discharge rate for prostatectomy, 1980–1994, by race. Data from National Hospital Discharge Survey (Xia *et al.* 1999).

affect. This suggests that the goal of arriving at an operational definition of BPH (yes/no) on the basis of these measures may not be appropriate. By contrast, studies of risk and prognostic factors could employ methods for quantitative traits based on these surrogate measures, and capitalize on the greater variability. However, this should not be done without regard to non-BPH related causes (Roberts 1999). Medical and surgical conditions responsible for changes in these surrogate markers should be taken into account. The use of these quantitative traits will permit studies to capitalize on rate of change in these surrogate measures as an outcome. While these are not available in most settings, studies are needed to determine the limitations of using cross-sectional measures as surrogate measures of rate of change.

In summary, much has been learned in recent years about the natural history of BPH. The availability of longitudinal data on surrogate measures of BPH should help the urological field to progress. Better studies of etiology and outcome can be undertaken by capitalizing on the spectrum of disease captured by these surrogate measures as quantitative traits. Through their association with these, lifestyle and constitutional factors may be identified for intervention or targeting therapeutic strategies.

Acknowledgement

The authors wish to acknowledge the staff in The Olmsted County Study for their efforts and for the continued support of subjects enrolled in the study. They also thank Ms. Sondra Buehler for her help with the preparation of this manuscript.

References

Abrams PH, Feneley RCL (1978) The significance of the symptoms associated with bladder outflow obstruction. *Urology* 33:171–174.

Abrams PH, Griffiths DJ (1979) The assessment of prostatic obstruction from urodynamic measurements and from residual urine. *Br J Urol* 51:129–134.

Barry MJ (1990) Epidemiology and natural history of benign prostatic hyperplasia. *Urol Clin North Am* 17:495–507.

Barry MJ, Cockett ATK, Holtgrewe HL, *et al.* (1993) Relationship of symptoms of prostatism to commonly used physiological and anatomical measures of the severity of benign prostatic hyperplasia. *J Urol* 150:351–358.

Barry MJ, Fowler FJ Jr, O'Leary MP, *et al.* (1992a) Correlation of the American Urological Association Symptom Index with self-administered versions of the Madsen-Iversen, Boyarsky and Maine Medical Assessment Program Symptom Indexes. *J Urol* 148:1558–1563.

Barry MJ, Fowler FJ Jr, O'Leary MP, *et al.* (1992b) The American Urological Association symptom index for benign prostatic hyperplasia. *J Urol* 148:1549–1557.

Barry MJ, Fowler FJ Jr, O'Leary MP, *et al.* (1995) Measuring disease-specific health status in men with benign prostatic hyperplasia. *Med Care* 33 (**Suppl**): AS145–AS155.

Bates TS, Reynard JM, Peters TJ, Gingell JC (1996) Determination of prostatic volume with transrectal ultrasound: A study of intra-observer and inter-observer variation. *J Urol* 155:1299–1300.

Berry SJ, Coffey DS, Walsh PC, Ewing LL (1984) The development of human benign prostatic hyperplasia with age. *J Urol* 132:474–479.

Bissada NK, Finkbeiner AE, Redman JF (1976) Accuracy of preoperative estimation of resection weight in transurethral prostatectomy. *J Urol* 116:201–202.

Bosch JLHR, Hip WCJ, Niemer AQHJ, *et al.* (1994) Parameters of prostate volume and shape in a community based population of men 55 to 74 years old. *J Urol* 152:1501–1505.

Bosch JLHR, Hop WCJ, Kirkels WJ, Schröder FH (1995) The International Prostate Symptom Score in a community-based sample of men between 55 and 74 years of age: Prevalence and correlation of symptoms with age, prostate volume, flow rate and residual urine volume. *Br J Urol* 75:622–630.

Boyarsky S, Jones G, Paulson DF, Prout GR Jr (1977) A new look at bladder neck obstruction by the Food and Drug Administration regulators: Guidelines for investigation of benign prostatic hypertrophy. *Trans Am Assoc Genito-Urin Surg* **68**:29–32.

Brawer MK, Lange PH (1989) Prostate specific antigen: its role in early detection, staging, and monitoring of prostatic carcinoma. *J Endourol* **3**:227–236.

Carter HB, Morrell CH, Pearson JD, *et al.* (1992a) Estimation of prostatic growth using serial prostate-specific antigen measurements in men with and without prostate disease. *Cancer Res* **52**: 3323–3328.

Carter HB, Pearson JD, Metter EJ, *et al.* (1992b) Longitudinal evaluation of prostate-specific antigen levels in men with and without prostate disease. *JAMA* **267**:2215–2220.

Chicharro-Molero JA, Burgos-Rodriguez R, Sanchez-Cruz JJ, *et al.* (1998) Prevalence of benign prostatic hyperplasia in Spanish men 40 years old or older. *J Urol* **159**:878–882.

Christensen MM, Bruskewitz RC (1990) Clinical manifestations of benign prostatic hyperplasia and indications for therapeutic intervention. *Urol Clin North Am* **17**:509–516.

Christensson A, Laurell CB, Lilja H (1990) Enzymatic activity of prostate-specific antigen and its reactions with extracellular serine proteinase inhibitors. *Eur J Biochem* **194**:755–763.

Chute CG, Panser LA, Girman CJ, *et al.* (1993) The prevalence of prostatism: a population-based survey of urinary symptoms. *J Urol* **150**:85–89.

Cockett ATK, Aso Y, Chatelain C, *et al.* (1991) *Proceedings of the 4th International Consultation on Benign Prostatic Hyperplasia (BPH)*. Channel Islands: Scientific Communication International Ltd.

Cockett ATK, Khoury S, Aso Y, *et al.* (1993) *Proceedings of The 2nd International Consultation on Benign Prostatic Hyperplasia (BPH)*. Channel Islands: Scientific Communication International Ltd.

Collins GN, Lee RJ, McKelvie GB, Rogers CAN, Hehir M (1993a) Relationship between prostate specific antigen, prostate volume and age in the benign prostate. *Br J Urol* **71**:445–450.

Collins GN, Lee RJ, Russell EB, Raab GM, Hehir M (1993b) Ultrasonically determined patterns of enlargement in benign prostatic hyperplasia. *Br J Urol* **71**:451–456.

Collins GN, Raab GM, Hehir M, King B, Garraway WM (1995) Reproducibility and observer variability of trans-rectal ultrasound measurements of prostatic volume. *Ultrasound Med Biol* **21**:1101–1105.

Corica FA, Jacobsen SJ, King BF, *et al.* (1999) Prostatic central zone volume, lower urinary tract symptom severity and peak urinary flow rates in community-dwelling men. *J Urol* **161**:831–834.

Diokno AC, Brown MB, Goldstein NG, Herzog AR (1994) Urinary flow rates and voiding pressures in elderly men living in a community. *J Urol* **151**:1550–1553.

Epstein RS, Deverka PA, Chute CG, *et al.* (1991) Urinary symptom and quality of life questions indicative of obstructive benign prostatic hyperplasia. Results of a pilot study. *Urol Suppl* **38**:20–26.

Epstein RS, Deverka PA, Chute CG, *et al.* (1992) Validation of a new quality of life questionnaire for benign prostatic hyperplasia. *J Clin Epidemiol* **45**:1431–1445.

Fowler FJ Jr, Wennberg JE, Timothy RP, *et al.* (1988) Symptom status and quality of life following prostatectomy. *JAMA* **259**:3018–3022.

Garraway WM, Armstrong C, Auld S, King D, Simpson RJ (1993) Follow-up of a cohort of men with untreated benign prostatic hyperplasia. *Eur Urol* **24**:313–318.

Girman CJ, Epstein RS, Jacobsen SJ, *et al.* (1994) Natural history of prostatism: Impact of urinary symptoms on quality of life in 2115 randomly selected community men. *Urology* **44**:825–831.

Girman CJ, Jacobsen SJ, Guess HA, *et al.* (1995) Natural history of prostatism: Relationship among symptoms, prostate volume and peak urinary flow rate. *J Urol* **153**:1510–1515.

Girman CJ, Panser LA, Chute CG, *et al.* (1993) Natural history of prostatism: Urinary flow rates in a community-based study. *J Urol* **150**:887–892.

Graversen PH, Gasser TC, Wasson JH, Hinman F Jr, Bruskewitz RC (1989) Controversies about indications for transurethral resection of the prostate. *J Urol* **141**:475–481.

Guess HA, Chute CG, Garraway WM, *et al.* (1993) Similar levels of urological symptoms have similar impact on Scottish and American men – although Scots report less symptoms. *J Urol* **150**:1701–1705.

Guess HA, Jacobsen SJ, Girman CJ, *et al.* (1995) The role of community-based longitudinal studies in evaluating treatment effects. Example: benign prostatic hyperplasia. *Med Care Suppl* **33**:AS26–AS35.

Gustafsson O, Mansour E, Norming U, *et al.* (1998) Prostate-specific antigen (PSA), PSA density and age-adjusted PSA reference values in screening for prostate cancer – a study of a randomly selected population of 2,400 men. *Scand J Urol Nephrol* **32**:373–377.

Hunter DJW, Berra-Unamuno A, Martin-Gordo A (1996) Prevalence of urinary symptoms and other urological conditions in Spanish men 50 years old or older. *J Urol* **155**:1965–1970.

Jacobsen SJ, Girman CJ, Guess HA, et al. (1993) Natural history of prostatism: Factors associated with discordance between frequency and bother of urinary symptoms. *Urology* **42**:663–671.

Jacobsen SJ, Girman CJ, Guess HA, Oesterling JE, Lieber MM (1995a) New diagnostic and treatment guidelines for benign prostatic hyperplasia: Potential impact in the United States. *Arch Intern Med* **155**:477–481.

Jacobsen SJ, Oesterling JE, Lieber MM (1995b) Community-based population studies on the natural history of prostatism. *Curr Opin Urol* 5:13–17.

Jacobsen SJ, Girman CJ, Guess HA, et al. (1996) Natural history of prostatism: Longitudinal changes in voiding symptoms in community-dwelling men. *J Urol* **155**: 595–600.

Jacobsen SJ, Jacobson DJ, Girman CJ, et al. (1997) Natural history of prostatism: Risk factors for acute urinary retention. *J Urol* **158**:481–487.

Jacobsen SJ, Jacobson DJ, Girman CJ, et al. (1999) Treatment for benign prostatic hyperplasia among community-dwelling men: The Olmsted County Study of Urinary Symptoms and Health Status among Men. *J Urol* **162**:1301–1306.

Jensen KM-E, Bruskewitz RC, Iversen P, Madsen PO (1983) Significance of prostatic weight in prostatism. *Urol Int* **38**:173–178.

Jensen KM-E, Jorgensen JB, Mogensen P, Bille-Brahe NE (1986) Some clinical aspects of uroflowmetry in elderly males: A population survey. *Scand J Urol Nephrol* **20**:93–99.

Kaplan SA, Te AE, Pressler LB, Olsson CA (1995) Transition zone index as a method of assessing benign prostatic hyperplasia: Correlation with symptoms, urine flow and detrusor pressure. *J Urol* **154**: 1764–1769.

Klein BE, Klein R, Lee KE, Bruskewitz RC (1999) Correlates of urinary symptom scores in men. *Am J Public Health* **89**:1745–1748.

Kojima M, Inui E, Ochiai A, et al. (1997) Noninvasive quantitative estimation of infravesical obstruction using ultrasonic measurement of bladder weight. *J Urol* **157**:476–479.

Lee E, Yoo KY, Kim Y, Shin Y, Lee C (1998) Prevalence of lower urinary tract symptoms in Korean men in a community-based study. *Eur Urol* **33**:17–21.

Lilja H (1993) Significance of different molecular forms of serum PSA. The free, noncomplexed form of PSA versus that complexed to alpha 1-antichymotrypsin. *Urol Clin North Am* **20**:681–686.

Lilja H, Christensson A, Dahlén W, et al. (1991) Prostate-specific antigen in serum occurs predominantly in complex with α_1-antichymotrypsin. *Clin Chem* **37**(9): 1618–1625.

Littrup PJ, Williams CR, Egglin TK, Kane RA (1991) Determination of prostate volume with transrectal US for cancer screening. Part II. Accuracy of in vitro and in vivo techniques [see comments]. *Radiology* **179**:49–53.

McConnell JD, Barry MJ, Bruskewitz RC, et al. (1994) *Benign Prostatic Hyperplasia: Diagnosis and Treatment. Clinical Practice Guideline, Number 8.* AHCPR Publication No. 94-0582. Agency for Health Care Policy and Research, Public Health Service, U.S. Department of Health and Human Services: Rockville, MD.

Madersbacher S, Haidinger G, Temml C, Schmidbauer CP (1998) Prevalence of lower urinary tract symptoms in Austria as assessed by an open survey of 2,096 men. *Eur Urol* **34**:136–141.

Madsen PO, Iversen P (1983) A point system for selecting operative candidates. In: Hinman, F, Jr, ed, *Benign Prostatic Hypertrophy* (Springer-Verlag: New York) 763–765.

Manieri C, Carter SS, Romano G, et al. (1998) The diagnosis of bladder outlet obstruction in men by ultrasound measurement of bladder wall thickness. *J Urol* **159**:761–765.

Meigs JB, Barry MJ (1996) Natural history of benign prostatic hyperplasia. In: Kirby R, McConnell J, Fitzpatrick J, Roehrborn C, Boyle P, eds, *Textbook of Benign Prostatic Hyperplasia* (Isis Medical Media Ltd: Oxford) 125–135.

Meigs JB, Barry MJ, Giovannucci E, et al. (1999) Incidence rates and risk factors for acute urinary retention: The Health Professionals Follow-up Study. *J Urol* **162**:376–382.

Meigs JB, Barry MJ, Oesterling JE, Jacobsen SJ (1996) Interpreting results of prostate-specific antigen testing for early detection of prostate cancer [see comments]. *J Gen Intern Med* **11**:505–512.

Meyhoff HH, Hald T (1978) Are doctors able to assess prostatic size? *Scand J Urol Nephrol* **12**:219–221.

Meyhoff HH, Ingemann L, Nordling J, Hald T (1981) Accuracy in preoperative estimation of prostatic size. A comparative evaluation of rectal palpation, intravenous pyelography, urethral closure pressure profile recording and cystourethroscopy. *Scand J Urol Nephrol* **15**:45–51.

Mikolajczyk SD, Millar LS, Wang TJ, *et al.* (2000) 'BPSA,' a specific molecular form of free prostate-specific antigen, is found predominantly in the transition zone of patients with nodular benign prostate hyperplasia. *Urology* **55**:41–45.

Morgan TE, Jacobsen SJ, McCarthy WF, *et al.* (1996) Age-specific reference ranges for prostate-specific antigen-based detection of prostate cancer in African American men. *N Engl J Med* **335**:304–310.

Oesterling JE (1991) Prostate specific antigen: A critical assessment of the most useful tumor marker for adenocarcinoma of the prostate. *J Urol* **145**: 907–923.

Oesterling JE, Jacobsen SJ, Chute CG, *et al.* (1993) Serum prostate-specific antigen in a community-based population of healthy men: Establishment of age-specific reference ranges. *JAMA* **270**:860–864.

Oesterling JE, Kumamoto Y, Tsukamoto T, *et al.* (1995) Serum prostate-specific antigen in a community-based population of healthy Japanese men: Lower values than for similarly aged white men. *Br J Urol* **75**:347–353.

Papsidero LD, Kuriyama M, Wang MC, *et al.* (1981) Prostate antigen: a marker for human prostate epithelial cells. *J Natl Cancer Inst* **66**:37–42.

Pearson JD, Luderer AA, Metter EJ, *et al.* (1996) Longitudinal analysis of serial measurements of free and total PSA among men with and without prostatic cancer. *Urology* **48**:4–9.

Rahmouni A, Yang A, Tempany CM, *et al.* (1992) Accuracy of in-vivo assessment of prostatic volume by MRI and transrectal ultrasonography. *J Comput Assist Tomogr* **16**:935–940.

Rhodes T, Girman CJ, Jacobsen SJ, *et al.* (1999) Longitudinal prostate growth rates during 5 years in randomly selected community men 40–79 years old. *J Urol* **161**:1174–1179.

Roberts RO (1999) Re: Alcohol consumption, cigarette smoking, and risk of benign prostatic hyperplasia. *Am J Epidemiol* **150**:321.

Roberts RO, Jacobsen SJ, Jacobson DJ, *et al.* (2000) Longitudinal changes in peak urinary flow rates in a community based cohort. *J Urol* **163**:107–113.

Roberts RO, Jacobsen SJ, Reilly T, Talley N, Lieber MM (1998) Natural history of prostatism: High American Urological Association Symptom scores among community-dwelling men and women with urinary incontinence. *Urology* **51**:213–219.

Roehrborn CG, Girman CJ, Rhodes T, *et al.* (1997) Correlation between prostate size estimated by digital rectal examination and measured by transrectal ultrasound. *Urology* **49**:548–557.

Sagnier P-P, Macfarlane G, Richard F, *et al.* (1994) Results of an epidemiological survey using a modified American Urological Association Symptom Index for benign prostatic hyperplasia in France. *J Urol* **151**:1266–1270.

Schappert SM (1993) *National Ambulatory Medical Care Survey: 1991 summary. Advance Data from Vital and Health Statistics; No 230* (National Center for Health Statistics: Hyattsville, Maryland).

Schreyer AG, Fielding JR, Warfield SK, *et al.* (2000) Virtual CT cystoscopy: color mapping of bladder wall thickness. *Invest Radiol* **35**:331–334.

Sottrup-Jensen L (1989) Alpha-macroglobulins: structure, shape, and mechanism of proteinase complex formation. *J Biol Chem* **264**:11539–11542.

Stamey TA, Yang N, Hay AR, *et al.* (1987) Prostate-specific antigen as a serum marker for adenocarcinoma of the prostate. *N Engl J Med* **317**: 909–916.

Tan HY, Choo WC, Archibald C, Esuvaranathan K (1997) A community based study of prostatic symptoms in Singapore [see comments]. *J Urol* **157**: 890–893.

Te AE, Kaplan SA (1998) Transurethral electrovaporization of the prostate. *Mayo Clin Proc* **73**:691–695.

Terris MK, Stamey TA (1991) Determination of prostate volume by transrectal ultrasound. J Urol **145**:984–987.

Trueman P, Hood SC, Nayak US, Mrazek MF (1999) Prevalence of lower urinary tract symptoms and self-reported diagnosed 'benign prostatic hyperplasia', and their effect on quality of life in a community-based survey of men in the UK. *BJU Int* **83**:410–415.

Tsukamoto T, Kumamoto Y, Masumori N, *et al.* (1995) Prevalence of prostatism in Japanese men in a community-based study with comparison to similar American study. *J Urol* **154**:391–395.

Varenhorst E, Berglund K, Löfman O, Pedersen K (1993) Inter-observer variation in assessment of the prostate by digital rectal examination. *Br J Urol* **72**:173–176.

Wang TJ, Slawin KM, Rittenhouse HG, Millar LS, Mikolajczyk SD (2000) Benign prostatic hyperplasia-associated prostate-specific antigen (BPSA) shows unique immunoreactivity with anti-PSA monoclonal antibodies. *Eur J Biochem* **267**:4040–4045.

Watanabe H, Igari D, Tanahashi Y, Harada K, Saito M (1974) Measurements of size and weight of prostate by means of transrectal ultrasonotomography. *Tohoku J Exp Med* **114**:277–285.

Weinrich MC, Jacobsen SJ, Weinrich SP, *et al.* (1998) Reference ranges for serum prostate-specific antigen (PSA) in Black and White men without cancer. *Urology* **52**:967–973.

Wennberg J, Gittelsohn A (1982) Variations in medical care among small areas. *Sci Am* **246**:120–134.

Williams AM, Simon I, Landis PK, *et al.* (1999) Prostatic growth rate determined from MRI data: age-related longitudinal changes. *J Androl* **20**:474–480.

Witjes WP, Aarnink RG, Ezz-el-Din K, *et al.* (1997) The correlation between prostate volume, transition zone volume, transition zone index and clinical and urodynamic investigations in patients with lower urinary tract symptoms. *Br J Urol* **80**:84–90.

Xia Z, Roberts RO, Schottenfeld D, Lieber MM, Jacobsen SJ (1999) Trends in prostatectomy for benign prostatic hyperplasia among black and white men in the United States: 1980 to 1994. Urology **53**:1154–1159.

Zhou AM, Tewari PC, Bluestein BI, Caldwell GW, Larsen FL (1993) Multiple forms of prostate-specific antigen in serum: differences in immunorecognition by monoclonal and polyclonal assays [see comments]. *Clin Chem* **39**:2483–2491.

2 Cellular and molecular mechanisms that modulate prostate cancer metastasis

Christopher S Foster, Vasilliki Karavana, Youqiang Ke and Mustafa BA Djamgoz

Introduction

There is now little doubt that the majority of human cancers are caused by specific somatic mutations within the genome. However, it remains possible that this is not the sole route by which a cell develops the potential to become malignant, and there remains a small amount of controversy as to whether or not epigenetic switching of a non-mutational type might be sufficient to initiate some malignancies. The theory of somatic mutation begins with the classic experiments of Harris (1965) when the seminal cell-hybridization experiments were performed to determine how malignancy was inherited when cells of differing phenotype were fused. These studies were developed, particularly by Weinberg (1981), and led to Knudsen's 'two-hit hypothesis' (1971, 2001). In contrast, the epigenetic switching theory, enshrined in the experiments of Illmensee & Mintz (1976), seeks to explain the initiation of malignancy on the basis of altered phenotypic regulation, without invoking genetic mutation as an initiating event, and irrespective of whether genetic structural modifications occur at some later time as a consequence of instability invoked by the initiation of malignant transformation.

The origin(s) of metastases, rather than of the primary neoplasm, raises a second group of problems. Again, the two contrasting theories of somatic mutation and genetic switching may be invoked. With respect to metastases, there is now compelling evidence that somatic mutation is not required to initiate or to promote the process and that altered phenotypic/homeostatic regulation is sufficient to account for the metastatic process. The essence of metastatic dissemination is that neoplastic cells gain access to the vascular space (either blood or lymphatic) and become relocated to regions of the body that are discontiguous with the site of origin. The cellular attributes required of the metastatic phenotype are now well recognized. While there is no philosophical necessity to invoke the so-called 'metastasis genes' there is a requirement to express particular genes that will endow cells with the attributes required of them to become successfully metastatic. Broadly, these may be considered as the two groups of enhanced expression of metastasis-promoting genes and decreased expression of metastasis-suppressing genes.

Current inability to distinguish aggressive from non-aggressive forms of prostate cancer, while it remains confined to the gland, is a fundamental problem in the management of the disease. Lack of diagnostic ability is the single most important factor in the dilemma of deciding the most appropriate treatment for each individual patient (Foster *et al.* 1999, 2000). Consequently, there is an urgent need to develop new methods: (i) to improve early diagnosis, leading to a realistic prognostic assessment; (ii) to facilitate the decision-making process regarding possible surgery; and (iii) to develop new therapies to combat prostate cancer.

Identification of genes regulating metastasis

Essentially, there are three approaches to the ultimate identification of genes that regulate the metastatic process: (i) directly through DNA analysis; (ii) by a reverse approach through RNA expression; and (iii) indirectly from expressed proteins. Subsequent *in-vivo* testing of the identified genes in an appropriate animal model is the ultimate test of the behavioral properties of a particular gene sequence. Comparative analysis of the DNA contained within two cells of contrasting metastatic ability is unlikely to yield the identity of individual metastasis-promoting genes. Rather, enzymatic disaggregation of the genome of a cell type having clear metastatic properties and subsequent analysis of the released fragments by *in-vivo* assay is a powerful technique for identification of those DNA sequences to promote the metastatic phenotype. This approach has been successfully employed by Ke *et al.* (1999a,b) who applied the technique to the Dunning model of rat prostate cancer and identified metastasis-promoting gene sequences derived from the Dunning cell line, when these were transfected into the Rama-3322 (rat mammary) recipient benign cell line. The principle of this technique is that the genome of the original metastatic cells is partially cleaved using Hind III to yield DNA fragments in the range 500 kb to 5 mb. These fragments are then ligated with syn-

thetic linkers that have been engineered to contain particular restriction enzyme cleavage sites. Thereafter, the original genomic DNA fragments derived from the partially cleaved genome may be identified and manipulated through the particular properties of the linking fragments. Since sites *Not-1* and *Sfi-1* are highly infrequent within the human genome (frequencies of the order 5×10^{-5} bases and 5×10^{-7} bases, respectively), subsequent use of these enzymes will release DNA fragments without appreciable damage to the intervening genes. Thereafter, the Hind III fragments of the genomic DNA, flanked by their synthetic linkers may then be cloned into a suitable vector for amplification or transfer into appropriate recipient cells for *in-vivo* assessment.

RNA analysis

The concept of RNA differential display was first introduced by Liang & Pardee (1992). Since it is the spectrum of expressed proteins that defines the phenotype of a particular cell, comparative analysis of genotypically equivalent metastatic and non-metastatic cells is likely to identify those proteins responsible for the two distinct phenotypes. Briefly, total RNA is extracted from cells using a conventional protocol and used to synthesize double-stranded DNA. The synthesized DS DNA is then cleaved using a restriction enzyme with a four-base recognition sequence (e.g. Tau-2) and the fragments ligated to a suitable promoting sequence. The 3′-fragments are then separated and amplified by polymerase chain reaction (PCR), incorporating ^{32}S into the reaction mixture. The amplified fragments are then displayed on a sequencing gel to identify those fragments differentially expressed between the two cell phenotypes. Different bands may then be cut-out and verified by Northern blot analysis or by *in-situ* hybridization onto appropriate tissue sections.

The technique of systematic differential display (SDD) devised by Ke *et al*. (1999a,b) is a powerful refinement of the basic differential display approach. Most of the biological and molecular markers related to the metastatic phenotype of prostate cancer have been identified through the methods based on the analysis of differential gene expression at the mRNA (or cDNA) level. It is possible that some of the genes expressed at higher levels in malignant cells are candidates as oncogenes, whereas some of those expressed in higher levels in benign cells are candidates as tumor suppressor genes. Identification of the genes differentially expressed between benign and malignant phenotype is only a small part of the work in searching for and determining the metastasis-related genes. However, this part of the work is an essential first step, which may provide a pool of a large number of candidate genes for further analyzes, which will lead to the ultimate identification and isolation of the possible metastasis promoting- or suppressing-genes. Although many different methods are used to analyze differentially expressed genes, the majority of currently available techniques may be classified into two types: the hybridization-based techniques and PCR-based techniques.

The most basic form of hybridization-based methods for analysis of genes differentially expressed is subtractive hybridization, developed by Wieland *et al*. (1990) and Rubenstein *et al*. (1990). Subtractive hybridization may be used for isolating mRNA species present in one (tester) population but absent in another (driver) population. By subtractive hybridization, a large excess of driver is used to remove sequences common to a biotinylated tester, enriching the target species that is unique to the tester. Through combination with a suppression PCR procedure, a suppression subtractive hybridization approach had been developed to improve the efficiency of subtractive hybridization.

Gene chip hybridization arrays, also known as microarray and/or high-density oligonucleotide arrays, is a powerful technique that may be used to analyze the expression profiles of thousands of genes and to assess the genes differentially expressed on a global scale (Schena *et al*. 1995, DeRisi *et al*. 1996). The general approach for hybridization arrays is to immobilize several thousand gene-specific sequences (probes) on a solid-state matrix, such as nylon membranes, glass microscope slides or silicon/ceramic chips. The immobilized sequences are then queried through hybridization with labeled copies of cDNA sequences from biological or pathological samples (targets). The underlying principle is that the greater the expression of a gene, the greater amount of labeled target, and hence, the greater the amount of output signal. Thus, the differential expression of a gene in different targets may be assessed by comparing the intensities of the output hybridization signals (Freeman *et al*. 2000).

PCR-based techniques used to analyze the differential expression of genes include series analysis of gene expression (SAGE) and differential display. SAGE was a method designed for the quantitative cataloging and comparison of expressed genes in samples of mRNAs from different sources. In SAGE, each gene transcript is uniquely represented by a short nucleotide sequence tag isolated from a defined position within the transcript. Efficient analysis of the transcripts in a serial manner may be performed by sequencing multiple tags within a single clone obtained through short tag concatenation. Thus, the relative expression status of a gene may be determined by the frequency of appearance of its representative sequence tag. Genes differentially expressed between benign and malignant tissues may be identified by comparing the relative expression status of each gene in the two different mRNA sources.

A number of import genes related to the metastatic phenotype of prostate cancer, such as KAI-1 (Dong *et al*. 1995) and thymosin β15 (Bao *et al*. 1996), were discovered by using a differential display method. This PCR-based method remains the most wildly employed method for identification of novel genes differentially expressed between benign and malignant cells. The concept of RNA differential display (or RNA finger-printing) was introduced by Liang & Pardee (1992) and Welsh *et al*. (1992) and involves reverse transcription of the mRNAs with oligo-dT primers anchored to the beginning of the poly(A) tail followed by a PCR reaction in the presence of a second primer that is arbitrary in sequence. The amplified cDNA sub-populations of 3′ termini of mRNAs, defined by the primer pair, are distributed on a DNA sequencing gel. By changing the primer combinations, a large number of mRNA species from different cellular sources may be visualized and compared simultaneously. This will allow genes differentially expressed to be identified and recovered from the sequencing gel.

Differential display is a valuable method for identifying differentially expressed genes. Since the first publication of this technique, it quickly became one of the most popular methods adopted worldwide. Despite its popularity, the usefulness of the original differential display approach had been limited by the random nature of its arbitrary primers. Frequently encountered problems in the original differential display protocol include high false-positive rates, repeated amplification of abundant mRNA species by different primer combina-

tions and that individual bands in a sequencing gel may contain more than one molecule. Since the original differential display protocol, efforts have been made to improve its vitality and effectiveness. More than 20 alternative methods have been devised to analyze genes differentially expressed. Some of the methods have greatly improved, or extended, the usefulness of the original protocol (Ivanova & Belyavsky 1995, Kato 1995, Prashar & Weissman 1996, Matz *et al*. 1997). Recently, systematic differential display (SDD) was developed to assess the entire spectrum of genes expressed differentially between benign and malignant cells (Ke *et al*. 1999a,b). Later, a novel molecular approach, named complete comparison of gene expression (CCGE), was developed to assess all genes differentially expressed by analysing cDNA fragments within or near to the protein-coding region in a systematic manner (Ke *et al*. 1999a).

The most significant improvement on the original differential display technique is the recent establishment of microquantity differential display (MDD) (Jing *et al*. 2000a). In this technique, summarized in Figure 2.1, double-stranded cDNA transcribed from mRNA is fragmented with two five-base recognition Type IIS restriction enzymes (Step 1), and ligated to a mixture of four short DNA adapters (Step 2). The 3′-terminal cDNA fragments are selectively amplified by suppression PCR (Step 3). By extending the fragments by two more bases, and using all possible permutations of the 3′-ends of both primers from P2 and anchor primer groups, the entire cDNA fragments may be divided into 192 subsets, amplified by PCR, separated and compared in denaturing gels (Step 4) in a systematic manner. Similar to SDD, those Type IIS enzymes generating a random one-base overhang at a precise distance away from their recognition sites were chosen to digest the cDNA to

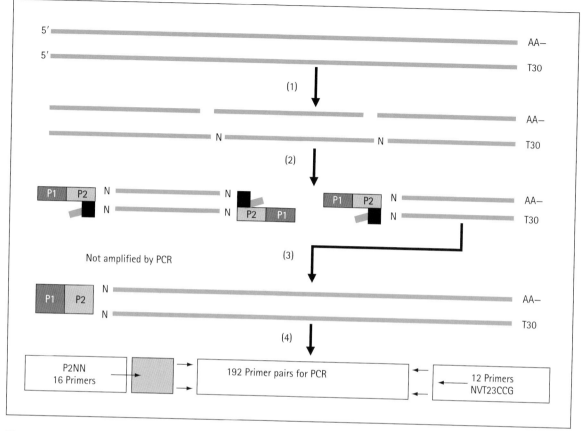

Figure 2.1

Schematic illustration of the detailed procedures of the microquantity differential display (MDD) approach. B = T, G, or C. V = C, G, or A. N = A, T, G, or C. M = G, C, A, or T. In Step 1, the double-stranded cDNA is digested with two five-base recognition, class IIS restriction endonucleases to generate cDNA fragments with a random one-base overhang. In Step 2, the cDNA fragments are 'tagged' by a mixture of four short DNA adapters, each consisting of a 'pseudo-double stranded' DNA, with the longer strand containing an outer (P1) and an inner (P2) primer sequence for polymerase chain reaction (PCR). Each of these adapters also has a random one-base over-hang (A, T, C, or G) through the shorter stand at its double-stranded end, which complements the overhangs at the end of the cDNA fragments. In Step 3, the 3'-cDNA fragments are amplified by PCR, using the primer pairs of P1 (positive strand) included in the adapter, and 5'-T30-3' (negative strand hybridizing to the poly A sequence) used originally for RNA transcription. In Step 4, the products from Step 3 are used as a template pool to perform further PCR, using the inner primers P2 and the anchor primers 5'-GCCT23VN-3'. By extending two more base and using all possible permutations of the 2 bases at their 3' ends, 16 (4^2) primers (P2NN) may be derived from the P2 primer group, and 12 primers (5'-GCCT23VN-3') may be derived from the anchor primer group. This yields a total of (16 × 12) 192 possible primer combinations for amplification, and hence the entire cDNA fragments may be selectively divided into 192 subsets for PCR. Each subset of cDNA fragments amplified by PCR may be separated by electrophoresis in a denaturing polyacrylamide gel. The entire genes differentially expressed may be identified in a systematic manner by comparing the intensities of the cDNA bands.

avoid symmetrical recognition sequences being included in the inner primer (P2) and to minimize the number of adapters needed to tag the resulting fragments. Digestion by two five-base-recognition Type IIS enzymes ensures that every cDNA species in the population is likely to be digested and that the sizes of the resulting fragments are within the suitable size range for separation in a typical sequence gel. Although all cDNA fragments generated in Step 1 may be tagged by the 'pseudo-double-stranded' adapters, either at one or at both ends at Step 2, the adapters are constructed in such a way that only the 3'-terminal cDNA fragment of each molecule is selectively amplified by PCR in Step 3. Other cDNA fragments are not amplified, since the P1 primer does not have a complementary sequence on the opposite strand of the templates. Through this nested PCR, a sufficient quantity of cDNA is obtained for further analysis in Step 4. The 3'-terminal cDNA fragments, representing the entire cDNA population, are then amplified by a further round of PCR, using the positive strand primer P2 included in the adapter and the negative strand hybrid anchor primer at the poly-A end.

By extending two more bases, a maximum of 16 (4^2) primers may be derived from the P2 primer group to synthesize the positive strand of the cDNA. Similarly, by utilizing all permutations of the two-anchor bases, a maximum of 12 (3×4) primers may be derived from the anchor primer group for synthesis of the negative cDNA strand. Altogether, 192 primer combinations (12×16) may be formed for PCR. Thus, the entire 3'-cDNA fragments may be divided into a total of 192 subsets and amplified in a systematic manner. In addition, through the nested PCR in Step 3, a sufficient quantity of cDNA may be obtained as a template pool for further analyzes in Step 4. It is this nested PCR step that may greatly increase

sensitivity and should enable MDD to be conducted with a very small quantity of starting RNA, such as that extracted from cells microdissected from small pathological lesions.

Recent identification of two new markers involved in the metastatic phenotype of prostate cancer (Jing *et al.* 2000b, 2001, 2002) are typical examples of differential display analysis to distinguish metastasis-related genes from a pool of selected candidates. To distinguish metastasis-related genes from the vast majority of functional genes whose expression is not related to cancer, a strategy comprising several steps of 'subtractive selections' was employed. By excluding genes not fulfilling each selection criterion, those genes whose biological activity is involved in malignant progression of prostate cancer are eventually determined from the last remaining candidates. In the first round of the selection, the entire cDNA species expressed differentially between a benign and a malignant prostate cell line was systematically assessed by recently developed differential expression analyzes (Ke *et al.* 1999a, 1999b, Jing *et al.* 2000a). In the second round of selection, the cDNA fragments selected from the first round were used as probes to screen a wider range of benign and malignant cell lines by Northern and slot-blot analysis to reduce the number of candidates. In the third round of selection, *in-situ* hybridization detected expression of candidate mRNAs in a large number of benign and malignant prostate tissues to exclude further mRNAs from the remaining candidates. Only those genes that exhibited significant differences in their expression levels between benign and malignant tissues were subjected to the final selection round in which full-length candidate cDNAs were been transfected into cell models appropriate for assaying malignant activities of genes. After testing in the *in-vitro* invasiveness of the transfectants, whether or not the candidate genes are promoters or suppressors for malignant progression was eventually determined by their ability to promote or suppress the tumorigenicity of the DNA recipient cells *in vivo*. These subtractive selection procedures led to the successful characterization of a metastasis-inducing gene (c-FABP) and a tumor suppressor gene in prostate cancer (Jing *et al.* 2000b, 2002). Subtractive selection has provided an ideal general strategy with which to select the phenotype-related genes from the vast number of candidates obtained from differential expression analysis.

Protein analysis

Irrespective of the genetic complement of a cell, or of the transcribed messenger RNA, the ultimate functional determinants of the phenotypic characteristics of a cell are the proteins. A variety of different methods are currently available with which to identify proteins having particular functions – whether enzymatic, adhesion (ligand-binding) or transportation (relocation or electrical). Electrophysiological analysis of prostatic epithelial cells of the metastatic phenotype confirmed the presence of ion channels previously reported only in electrically excitable tissues (Grimes *et al.* 1995). This finding posed the question as to the functional relevance of these channels in prostate cancer, particularly emergence of the metastatic phenotype. Analysis of the electrochemical characteristics of these channels confirmed the current–voltage relationships to be identical with equivalent channels identified in neuromuscular tissues, including inhibition by specific toxins.

Ion channels

Ion channels are proteins embedded in the plasma membrane; some are present also in the membranes of intracellular organelles. The channels open in response to a number of gating stimuli, including change in membrane potential, binding of a chemical or tension in the membrane. Open ion channels allow passive flow of the permeable ion(s) at a rate of some 10^7 ions/s in single-file mode. The associated changes in the intracellular ion concentrations and/or the membrane potential, which is equivalent to some 10^7 V/m, play a crucial role in a range of cellular functions from motility and enzyme activity to gene expression. It is not surprising, therefore, that defects in ion channel expression and/or functioning may lead to a wide variety of diseases, such as cystic fibrosis, angina pectoris, hyperkalemic periodic paralysis, epilepsy and migraine. On the whole, there are two broad categories of ion channel defects – those resulting from mutations in the underlying genes and transcriptional channelopathies. The latter are 'epigenetic' and involve abnormal cellular expression of a gene which, otherwise, has a normal sequence.

Voltage-gated Na^+ (VGS) currents and/or increased expression of voltage-gated Na^+ channel (VGSC) mRNA has been found in several different cancer cell types, suggesting that VGSC expression/upregulation may be a widely conserved mechanism involved in the metastatic spread of numerous cancers (Figure 2.2). A growing body of evidence suggests that VGSC activity plays a critical role in prostate cancer cell invasion (Grimes *et al.* 1995, Laniado *et al.* 1997, Smith *et al.* 1998a). The molecular identity of VGSC has been attributed to a combination of VGSC types, the predominant subtype being the tetrodotoxin-sensitive (TTX-S) $Na^+v1.7$ (Diss *et al.* 2001).

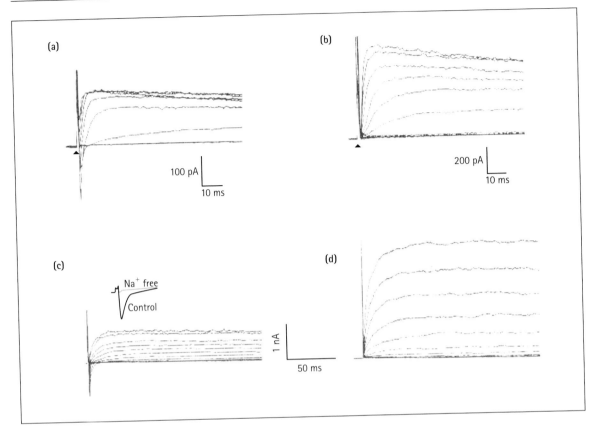

Figure 2.2
Patch-clamp recording of voltage-gated membrane ion currents in rat (a and b) and human (c and d) prostate cancer cell lines. a and c, strongly metastatic MAT-LyLu and PC-3 cells, respectively. b and d, weakly metastatic AT-2 and LNCaP cells, respectively. In both rat and human, there is an inward Na^+ current present (downward-going current traces) in the strongly metastatic cells. *Inset.* Recording showing disappearance of the inward current in Na^+-free solution (c). In the weakly metastatic cells, an Na^+ current is absent, but there is a large, outward K^+ current (upward-going current traces). Holding potentials, -90 mV. Arrowheads indicate application of clamp voltages (shown only in a and b). Modified from Grimes *et al.* (1995) (a and b) and Laniado *et al.* (1997) (c and d).

Accordingly, blockage of VGSC currents in human and rat prostate cancer cell lines, following application of TTX, significantly reduced their invasive potential. A subsequent study on seven rat and four human prostate cancer cell lines, combining flow cytometry and invasion assay techniques, extended this to show a positive correlation between the proportion of cells expressing VGSC protein and their invasive ability (Smith *et al.* 1998) (Figure 2.3). This study also revealed a basal level of VGSC protein expression in weakly metastatic cells, including LNCaP and AT-2 cell lines, which was apparently undetected by electrophysiology.

At present, the mechanisms responsible for the high level of VGSC expression in strongly metastatic prostate cancer cells are not known. Signalling mechanisms upstream of the VGSC gene may be responsible for upregulating

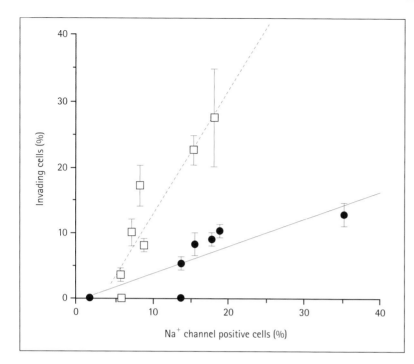

Figure 2.3
Relationship between invasiveness (Matrigel assays) and voltage-gated Na⁺ channel protein expression levels in two groups of prostate cancer cells. Both data sets (means ± standard errors) are expressed as percentages. Open symbols/dotted line, Dunning rat prostate cancer cell lines. Closed symbols/solid line, human RAMA37 cell lines transfected with rat prostate cancer cDNA. A highly significant linear correlation was observed in both cases. Modified from Smith *et al.* (1998).

VGSC expression. Furthermore, the external environment could influence VGSC expression or upregulation during the metastatic cascade. The plasma membrane not only protects the integrity and homeostatic balance of the cell by acting as a physiochemical barrier but also it allows the selective permeability of substances. Communication with the external environment is made possible by specific proteins on the cell membrane, integral or peripheral, having a variety of function including facilitation of transport, receptor signalling and attachment to the substrate in association with the cytoskeleton.

Voltage-gated Na⁺ channels in strongly metastatic prostate cancer cells

Using electrophysiological ('patch-clamp') recording initially to detect individual cells' minute electrical signals in a comparative cellular approach, it has been shown that strongly metastatic prostate cancer cells from both human and rat (PC-3 cells and MAT-LyLu, respectively) express voltage-gated Na⁺ channels (VGSCs) that would allow influx of Na⁺ into cells. In contrast, no VGSC activity was detected in corresponding weakly metastatic (AT-2 and LNProstate cancer) cells. Furthermore, the strongly metastatic cells had significantly smaller outward K⁺ currents and relatively depolarized resting potentials. Taken together, these characteristics would render the strongly metastatic prostate cancer cells potentially 'excitable'. A parallel of this situation has also been seen *in vivo* by immunohistochemical labelling of VGSC protein with a pan-VGSC antibody (Stewart *et al.* 1999). Thus, in histological sections of clinical human prostate, a low level of VGSC protein expression was apparent in benign prostatic hyperplasia and low-grade PIN (prostatic intraepithelial neoplasia), and this was significantly increased and maintained in high-grade PIN and *in-situ* malignancy.

Molecular nature of prostate cancer VGSC

Pharmacological characterization of the prostate cancer VGSC first suggested that the Na^+ current could be half-blocked by about 20 nmol tetrodotoxin (TTX) (Grimes & Djamgoz, 1998). This implied that the VGSC belonged to the TTX-sensitive (TTX-S) class of VGSCs. The molecular nature of the 'culprit' VGSC was determined by a combination of degenerate screening and semiquantitative PCR analyzes, and revealed that the predominant VGSC subtype in prostate cancer cells (of both rat and human origin) is $Na_v1.7$, consistent with the TTX-S nature of the channel pharmacology. These experiments also showed (1) that a basal, low level of channel mRNA was present in the weakly metastatic cells and (2) that a number of other minor VGSC mRNAs were also expressed (in both cell types). Interestingly, $Na_v1.7$ is the peripheral nerve channel, which, in humans, was originally cloned from a neuroendocrine tumor (Klugbauer *et al.* 1995). Thus, it would appear that the low level of $Na_v1.7$ mRNA expressed in the weakly metastatic cells is upregulated some 1000-fold in the strongly metastatic phenotype, in accordance with an epigenetic transformation. Significantly, the $Na_v1.7$ VGSC in prostate cancer was expressed in the *neonatal* rather than the *adult* form, consistent with the dedifferentiated nature of the cells.

Role of VGSC in cellular behavior involved in the metastatic cascade

Blocking VGSC activity *in vitro* with TTX produced a variety of cellular effects, consistent with the channel accelerating the metastatic process. The cellular behaviors enhanced by VGSC activity include morphological development/process extension (Fraser *et al.* 1999), lateral motility (Fraser *et al.* 1998, 2001), gal-vanotaxis (directional movement in small dc electric field) (Djamgoz *et al.* 2001), secretion (Mycielska *et al.* 2001, 2003), gene expression (Stewart & Djamgoz 2001, Stewart *et al.* 2001) and transverse 'Matrigel' invasion. The role of VGSC in galvanotaxis is particularly interesting since it would imply that the transepithelial potential (of around -10 mV in rat, lumen-side negative (Szatkowski *et al.* 2000)) that could be expected in the prostate gland could influence the directional migration of metastatic cells during early local invasion. Furthermore, the transepithelial potential itself, and the ionic mechanisms generating it, are themselves potential targets for suppressing the metastatic tendency in prostate cancer. In a recent independent study, Abdul & Hossein (2001) have shown that VGSC blocker anticonvulsant drugs (e.g. phenytoin) reduced PSA release from human prostate cancer cells, indicating strongly that the findings concerning VGSC expression/activity could have clinical application (Djamgoz *et al.* 2001).

Regulation of VGSC expression by hormones and growth factors

At present, the mechanism(s) upstream of VGSC expression in prostate cancer is/are not known. Importantly, however, there is considerable evidence that VGSC activity/expression is highly dynamic and may be controlled by steroid hormones, including androgen (Zakon 1998). This is interesting since it is well known that androgen depletion may suppress prostate cancer for some time (approximately 2 years), but once androgen independence sets in, prostate cancer may be lethal within some months (Feldman & Feldman 2001). Growth factors have also been suggested to be involved in prostate cancer progression (Barton *et al.* 2001). In the context of VGSC expression, an interesting candidate is nerve growth factor

(NGF) which, outside the nervous system, is expressed in the prostate gland at the highest level in the body. Importantly, in PC12 cells, even brief exposure to NGF may lead to significant upregulation of $Na_v1.7$ VGSC expression (Toledo-Aral *et al.* 1995). It is not known if a similar situation exists in the prostate. An interesting possibility would be if VGSC activity controlled NGF release and a circular positive feedback cycle operated and steadily enhanced metastasis, as follows:

VGSC upregulation $\rightarrow$ NGF release $\rightarrow$ VGSC upregulation $\rightarrow \ldots \rightarrow$ metastatic progression

The electrophysiological approach to prostate cancer has led to a novel concept in which the metastatic behavior of prostate cancer cells is associated with the 'excitability' of their membranes, consistent with the hyperactive behavior of strongly metastatic cells. The working hypothesis is that upregulation of functional VGSC expression enhances the cells' metastatic ability by potentiating key cellular behaviors integral to the metastatic cascade in prostate cancer. Accordingly, VGSC (in particular, $Na_v1.7$) expression is a novel prognostic marker of prostate cancer. Furthermore, since VGSC activity would appear to have a direct potentiating role in metastatic cell behavior, it may be possible to treat metastatic prostate cancer by exploiting a variety of clinically accepted VGSC modulators (Clare *et al.* 2000).

Growth factors

In addition to the widely accepted paradigm of androgen-governed prostate growth, growth factors exert a fundamental influence on the phenotypic differentiation and proliferation of prostate cancer cells. Androgenic stimulation

of fibroblast growth factor 7 (FGF7/KGF) receptors in the stroma contribute to prostatic epithelial growth (Planz *et al.* 2001) while growth factors such as plasma insulin-like growth factor Type 1 (IGF-1) are associated with increased risk of prostate cancer (Chan *et al.* 1998). The prominent role of growth factors appears to reside in prostate cancer progression where, in the absence of androgen, cells acquired survival pathways to proliferate. IGFs and EGFs are thought to play an important role in supporting tumor growth following relapse from androgen ablation (Foster *et al.* 1998). Similarly, NGF (Geldof *et al.* 1997) and FGF-7 could stimulate invasiveness of prostate cancer cells (Ropiquet *et al.* 1999). Autocrine release of growth factors is a common feature of some cells, such as keratinocytes involving NGF and TrkA receptors (Pincelli & Marconi 2000). In cancer, autocrine loops involving secretion of TGF-α and epidermal growth factor receptor (EGFr) activation have been found in prostate cancer (Sporn & Todaro 1980) and other adenocarcinomas (Hsieh *et al.* 2000). Additional autocrine loops include the IGF receptor (IGFr) in prostate cancer (Figueroa *et al.* 1995).

Prostatic stroma has been implicated in various aspects of the cancer progression (Condon & Bosland 1999, Rowley 1998). Olumi *et al.* (1999) demonstrated fibroblasts from prostate carcinomas, but not normal prostate, to stimulate growth of normal prostate cells, leading to the onset of cancer. This suggested the ability of unknown factors secreted from transformed cells to act upon normal cells and to induce malignancy. In addition, stromal cells of cancerous prostatic tissues contain platelet-derived endothelial growth factor and were suggested to promote prostate cancer angiogenesis. Expression of specific growth factor receptors is thought to provide a selective advantage whereby metastases may be formed at secondary sites where the respective ligands are available. For example, chemokine receptors present in cancer cells permit their preferential metastasis to bone where chemokines are being released (Muller *et al.* 2001). Djakiew *et al.* (1993) showed prostate cancer cell stimulation in response to secreted proteins from stromal cells, suggesting that metastasis could occur by chemotaxis to distant sites. Festuccia *et al.* (2000) demonstrated that prostate cancer cells respond to osteoblast-derived TGF-β1 by producing proteases, believed to be responsible for their invasion of bone.

EGF, TGF-α, amphiregulin, heparin-binding EGF (HB-EGF), betacellulin and epiregulin comprise a group of structurally and functionally related growth regulatory proteins that may bind EGFr (Riese *et al.* 1996). They are characterized by a six-cysteine consensus motif that forms three intramolecular disulphide bonds crucial for receptor binding. EGF is a 6 kDa polypeptide composed of 53 amino acids and is highly expressed in the prostate (Elson *et al.*, 1984). EGF plays a critical role in the proliferation, differentiation and maturation of prostate cells (Chen *et al.* 1996b). EGFr is composed of a single polypeptide chain that is highly N-glycosylated in the external domain (Carpenter & Cohen 1990) and its biological properties are subject to modulation by altered glycosyl transferase activities characteristic of malignant cells (Foster 1990). The extracellular region comprises four subdomains with particular ligand-binding roles being attributed to subdomains I and III. Upon ligand binding (critical on correct glycosylation), EGFr dimerizes and this is critical for conversion to the high-affinity binding state as well as for autophosphorylation (Downward *et al.* 1984) or activation of tyrosine kinase activity (Spaargaren *et al.* 1991). Homodimers, as well as various combinations of heterodimers, are formed, depending on the relative levels of the

four receptors, as well as the activating ligand (Sherrill & Kyte 1996).

Heterodimerization provides a complex and ultimately a flexible role in signalling (Graus-Porta *et al.* 1997). Unlike EGFr, kinase-deficient ErbB-3 cannot interact with adaptor proteins or Cbl proto-oncogene, but may associate with adaptors *Shc* and *Grb7* (Fedi *et al.* 1994). Although EGF activates EGFr/ErbB-3 or EGF/ErbB-4 heteromers, ErbB-2 is crucial for EGF binding. Therefore, it was suggested that heteromerization is a dynamic process, involving possibly EGF and ErbB-2 heteromerization in the first instance, followed by the dissociation of ErbB-2 and its replacement with ErbB-3 or ErbB-4. Such heterodimers may form when only one member of the pair binds its ligand (Sako *et al.* 2000). EGFr is also postulated to act as an adhesion protein and to affect actin filament organization (Are *et al.* 2001) and, in this activity, interacting with fascin to organize/stabilize actin bundles at the time of cell migration, including metastasis.

EGFr, along with other receptor tyrosine kinases (RTKs), is involved in transactivation, defined as the pathway of G-protein-coupled receptor (GPCR)-mediated mitogen-activated protein kinase (MAPK) activation. EGFr transactivation was first suggested to be independent of EGFr ligands, based on the rapid onset of tyrosine phosphorylation in the absence of EGFr ligands (Daub *et al.* 1996) and may be mediated by HB-EGF. HB-EGF is a member of the EGF family and is synthesized as a transmembrane precursor that is proteolytically processed into the mature, soluble growth factor. Prenzel *et al.* (1999) showed that in response to GPCR agonists (e.g. endothelin, thrombin, carbachol, lysophosphatidic acid and tetradecanoylphorbol-13-acetate), activation of GPCR leads to release of G-protein subunits that allows metalloproteinase (MMP) cleavage of pro-HB-EGF, releasing free HB-

EGF to subsequently bind EGFr, thus leading to EGFr homodimerization and autophosphorylation. EGFrvIII is the most common deletion variant of EGFr (801 bp deletion in the external domain) found in prostate cancer (Olapade-Olaopa *et al.* 2000). It lacks binding ability and possesses constitutive kinase activity equivalent to that of activated wild-type EGFr, although downstream signalling is different, including decreased *Ras* and mitogen-activating protein (MAP) activities (Moscatello *et al.* 1996). In addition to association of EGFr with ErbB-2 and ErbB-3, demonstrated in several different cancers, over-expression of EGFr has been correlated with tumor progression and is an indicator of poor prognosis in some cancers (Ma *et al.* 1998, Kim & Muller, 1999). Prostate cancer appears more complicated, with some studies reporting no difference in EGFr expression during cancer progression (Toning *et al.* 2000), some showing no correlation (Ibrahim *et al.* 1993, Robertson *et al.* 1994, Maddy *et al.* 1989), while others a positive correlation (MacDonald & Habib 1992, Turkeri *et al.* 1994, Glynne-Jones *et al.* 1996, Kumar *et al.* 1998).

Growth factors and associated signalling pathways are able to modulate voltage-gated ion channels. Binding of RTKs by growth factors (NGF and FGF) upregulates voltage-gated calcium channels (VGCCs) through *Ras* signalling (Lei *et al.* 1998, Katsuki *et al.* 1998). In addition, VGCC may be upregulated through the *Src* signalling pathway (Wijetunge *et al.* 1995, 2000), stimulated by IGF-1 (Bence-Hanulec *et al.* 2000) and PDGF. Conversely, regulation of VGSC by growth factors such as NGF, EGF and FGF-3 is independent of *Ras* signalling (Fanger *et al.* 1993, Hilbom *et al.* 1997, Choi *et al.* 2001), while VGSC enhancement by PDGF involves the *Src* family of non-receptor tyrosine kinases including *Yes* and

Fyn (Fanger *et al.* 1997). Furthermore, NGF upregulation of Na^+ 1.7 in prostatic PC-12 cells is mediated via PLC-γ signalling.

Ca^{2+} signalling pathways

Calcium ions (Ca^{2+}) play a key role in transmembrane activity and are important second messengers involved in intracellular signalling, giving rise to a variety of cellular effects, including gene transcription, differentiation, proliferation and apoptosis (Mellstrom & Naranjo 2001, Berridge 1997). Intracellular Ca^{2+} is involved in cell motility. Entry of Ca^{2+} into cells occurs via one or more channels, classified according to their activation mechanism, and including voltage-gated Ca^{2+} channels (VGCCs), receptor-operated Ca^{2+} channels (ROCCs) and store-operated Ca^{2+} channels (SOCCs). Both VGCCs and ROCCs have only short open times, while SOCCs provide a more sustained influx. Elementary events, leading to rapid elevation of intracellular Ca^{2+}, result from the opening of a small group of intracellular channels, while complex 'global' Ca^{2+} signals (such as intracellular Ca^{2+} oscillations and waves) arise from concomitant Ca^{2+} signals from a large population of intracellular stores (Berridge 1997). Thus, the diverse signalling mechanisms of Ca^{2+} control a range of cellular processes. Ca^{2+} homeostasis and intracellular signalling may be important in cancer, since tumor cells possess altered signalling response to factors that regulate growth, differentiation, migration and apoptosis. For example, binding of chemokine CXCLI2 to its receptor (CXCR4) triggers an intracellular Ca^{2+} signalling event and the directed migration of ovarian cancer cells. Carboxyamidotriazole (CAT), an inhibitor of ROCC and arachidonic acid release, inhibits malignant proliferation and invasion of breast cancer (Lambert *et al.* 1997) and prostate cancer (Wasilenko *et al.* 1996). Phase II clinical trials for the treatment of androgen-independent prostate cancer are already occurring (Bauer *et al.* 1999).

VGCC are structurally similar to voltage-gated Na^+ channels (Tanabe *et al.* 1987). The basic structure comprises a pore-forming α_1-subunit, supplemented with auxiliary subunits. The multiple subtypes of VGCC, designated as T, L, N, P, Q, and R, are classified according to functional channel characteristics or molecular sequences (Dolphin 1995). Ca^{2+} influx through VGCCs contributes to cellular activities such as exocytosis, excitation–contraction coupling, synaptic plasticity, gating of other ion channels, gene expression, growth and apoptosis. ROCC are a structurally and functionally diverse group that open directly in response to ligand binding and include nicotinic receptors, GABA receptors (GABAA and GABAc), cationic glutamate receptors (e.g. N-methyl-D-aspartate receptor and kainate receptors) and ATP receptors (North 1996, Le Novere & Changeux 1999). Different ROCCs are activated by a wide range of agonists that include ATP, serotonin, glutamate and acetylcholine. SOCCs are activated in response to depletion of intracellular Ca^{2+} stores, possibly through the mechanism of 'conformation coupling' in which conformational change of intracellular Ca^{2+} stores open SOCCs, allowing the influx of extracellular Ca^{2+}. This mechanism usually involves inositol 1,4,5-trisphosphate ($InsP_3$) stimulation of Ca^{2+} release from Ca^{2+} stores, such as the endoplasmic reticulum, leading to an initial increase in intracellular Ca^{2+} followed by a positive feedback of Ca^{2+}, stimulating further Ca^{2+} release (Clapham 1995). Involvement of Ca^{2+} mobilization in cell proliferation has been shown by studies on smooth muscle and prostate cancer cells (Haverstick *et al.* 2000) in which store-

operated release of Ca^{2+}, as well as the subsequent increase in intracellular (Ca^{2+}) via SOCCs stimulate an apoptotic response in the weakly metastatic LNCaP cells (Wertz & Dixit 2000).

Na^+–Ca^{2+} exchangers couple bidirectional movement, dependent on ionic gradient, of one Ca^{2+} in exchange for three Na^+, and is an essential component of Ca^{2+} signaling in several epithelial tissues (He *et al.* 1998, Kofuji *et al.* 1992). The Na^+–Ca^{2+} exchanger is also present in cancer cells and responds to extracellular Ca^{2+} concentrations. The calcium-sensing receptor (CaR) is a G-protein-coupled receptor, mutations of which have been shown to contribute to inherited disorders of Ca^{2+} homeostasis. CaR has been detected in breast cancer and is suggested to be involved in osteolytic metastases by the secretion of parathyroid hormone-related peptide (Sanders *et al.* 2000). There are three groups of Ca^{2+} binding proteins (CaBPs): EF hand motif-containing proteins, Ca^{2+} storage proteins and Ca^{2+}/phospholipid binding proteins (Niki *et al.* 1996). All have the ability to bind Ca^{2+} and potentially may buffer intracellular (Ca^{2+}).

Ca^{2+} binding – protein p9Ka

Protein p9Ka (S100A4) was identified by Barraclough & Rudland (1994), by subtractive hybridization, as a gene product expressed in carcinomas of the human breast, but not in normal breast epithelium. It appears to be expressed at high levels by all metastatic epithelial cells, including the prostate. The S100 protein family constitutes a large subgroup of CaBP of EF-hand motif, and is composed of at least 16 different members displaying 25–65% identity at the amino acid level. The EF-hand protein, which is able to bind one Ca^{2+}, normally exists in pairs, and has been shown to regulate protein phosphorylation, ATPase and cytoskeleton (Donato 2001); there is also a recent suggestion of its involvement in the downregulation of E-cadherin (Kimura *et al.* 2000). In particular, p9Ka has been closely associated with metastasis in cancers of breast (Wang *et al.* 2000) and prostate (Ke *et al.* 1997). S100A4 proteins are activated by a conformational change upon Ca^{2+} binding that allows interaction with target proteins (e.g. non-muscle tropomyosin and myosin) *via* hydrophobic domains. The best characterized EF-hand protein is calmodulin, which is the receiver of rapid transient Ca^{2+} fluxes. Calreticulin and calsequestrin are intracellular storage proteins that have a high affinity for Ca^{2+} and act in the endoplasmic reticulum and sarcoplasmic reticulum, respectively.

Two types of intracellular Ca^{2+} channels currently recognized are the inositol triphosphate receptor ($InsP_3R$) and the iyanodine receptor (RyRs); they have many structural and physiological similarities (Taylor & Traynor 1995). $InsP_3Rs$ are a functionally diverse group, comprising at least three different isoforms, and are capable of forming heteromers (Taylor *et al.* 1999). In addition to being activated by $InsP_3$, $InsP_3R$ are modulated by Ca^{2+}. While InP_3Rs are widely expressed across mammalian tissues, RyRs are mainly found in excitable cells. The endogenous ligand for RyR is the cyclic ADP ribose.

Proteins expressed embryologically – fascin

Immunohistochemical analysis of proteins expressed by prostatic epithelium from normal embryonic development through normal tissue structure to neoplasia and metastatic cancer is a powerful tool for identifying proteins that are functionally relevant to the malignant and metastatic processes. During embryonic development, fascin is expressed from the time the earliest epithelial buds emerge from the rudimentary urethra and penetrate the nascent prostatic stroma (Figure 2.4). Within the epithelium of the developing prostate; expression of fascin is related to the migratory epithelial cells, and hence occurs at the tips of the buds penetrating the stroma. Those epithelial cells that have become static relative to the underlying stroma during the process of morphogenesis no longer express fascin in the normal, non-neoplastic, prostate; fascin is not expressed either in the luminal or basal layers of the epithelium. However, neo-expression of this protein is prominent in malignant prostatic epithelium.

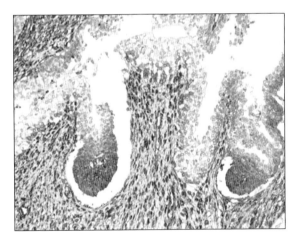

Figure 2.4
Fetal human prostate gland (22 weeks post-implantation) in which epithelial buds penetrating the surrounding stroma express fascin at their tips – but not by those cells that are no longer migrating and have started to undergo differentiation. The majority of stromal cells also express fascin at this stage – emphasizing their migratory phenotype during prostatic organogenesis (magnification ×200).

Glycosyl transferase activities

Many cellular proteins, particularly those directed towards plasma membranes, are glycoproteins. The attached sugar sequences are assembled onto nascent protein backbones in a highly organized and stochastic manner through the cisternae of the Golgi apparatus. This environment is highly regulated with respect to pH and ionic content. A pH gradient is strictly maintained from *cis-* to *trans-* cisternae, ranging from approximately 8.6 to 3.5, respectively. Embedded within the walls of the cisternae are the glycosyl transferase enzymes. The physical distribution of the enzymes, together with the pH gradient across the Golgi apparatus and the concentrations of free divalent cations within the individual cisternae, create a highly organized spectrum of glycosyl transferase activities. Potentially, individual glycosyl transferase with differing specific activities but similar substrate specificities compete to elaborate different oligosaccharide structures. Maintenance of the intracisternal environments, with respect to pH and divalent cations, is of crucial importance in determining the relative activities of these competing enzymes and hence of the structures subsequently elaborated onto a particular oligosaccharide substrate structure. Previously, it was believed that alterations in glycoprotein oligosaccharide structure characteristic of all epithelial malignancies was due to the presence of novel or abnormal glycosyl transferase enzymes. However, purification and characterization of a number of glycosyl transferase enzymes, particularly those synthesized from their cloned genes, has confirmed that, in all instances examined, both the genes and the resultant enzymes are structurally unaltered. In contrast, perturbation of the intracisternal environment, whether of the pH gradient or the divalent cation concentrations, is sufficient to reset the relative activity of competing glycosyl transferase enzymes such that abnormal structures are synthesized and that these become substrates for enzymes not commonly active in the normal epithelial cells. Hence, modulation of intracisternal homeostasis in malignancy produces an epigenetic switch that may profoundly influence the intracellular trafficking of glycoproteins normally directed to the plasma membranes where they might function as ligand receptors or transducers of other information between the intracellular and external environments (Figure 2.5).

Protein kinase C isoenzymes

Protein kinase C (PKC) is a family of serine/threonine kinases which play a major role in transmembrane signal transduction pathways and which regulate cell proliferation (Lord & Pongracz 1995), differentiation (Clemens *et al.* 1992), cell-to-cell interaction (Freed 1989), secretion (Lord & Ashcroft

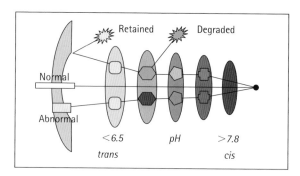

Figure 2.5
Schematic emphasizing the potential routes of trafficking of glycoproteins through the Golgi apparatus with respect to the pH gradient across the cisternae. A shift in intracisternal pH results in a change in the actual (and relative) activity of the constituent glycosyltransferase enzymes, resulting in aberrant glycosylation and an alteration in the trafficking routes of individual glycoproteins.

1984), cytoskeletal function (Owen *et al.* 1996), gene transcription (Berry & Nishizuka 1990) and apoptosis. Activation of PKC by phorbol esters has shown dose-dependent inhibition of cell proliferation and induction of apoptosis. Bryostatin-1, an alternative PKC activator, induces apoptosis with associated reduction of Bcl-2 expression and increased p53 protein expression (Mohammed, 1995). It has become apparent that individual PKC isoenzymes have discrete functions, specificity being generated by activation of co-factors, downregulation following activation, subcellular location and substrate specificity. PKC's α and δ appear to be crucial for cell differentiation, whereas PKCβ is involved in proliferation (Murray *et al.* 1993) and apoptosis (MacFarlane & Manzel 1994). PKCε has been suggested to act as an oncogene in rat fibroblasts (Cacace *et al.* 1993) and increase proliferation, while PKCζ appears to be lost as tumors become more aggressive (Powell *et al.* 1994). Cornford *et al.* (1999) showed that as PKCβ is lost from early prostate cancers PKCε expression is reciprocally increased and proposed that this imbalance in PKC expression helps to explain malignant growth of prostatic epithelium. It has recently been established that inhibiting total PKC prevents proliferation of prostate cells *in vitro* (Sosnowski *et al.* 1997). Rusnak & Lazo (1996) suggested that, in DU-145 cells, this may occur through specific downregulation of PKCε. However, it is known that PKCs may also regulate heat shock protein (hsp 70) production in the same cell line (Lee *et al.* 1994). In intact prostatic tissues, hsp 70 expression is also downregulated in prostate cancer (Cornford *et al.* 2000). At present, this complex field remains in a state of flux since few of the reported data have been independently confirmed and the exact roles of these various factors remain to be elucidated.

PKC isoenzymes have been proposed to have a role in carcinogenesis, because of their central role in regulating critical intracellular pathways, and have been implicated in metastatic development (Herbert 1993) and in chemotherapy-associated multidrug resistance (Blobe *et al.* 1993). Interest in the role of PKC in prostate cancer was stimulated when it was shown that PKC activity was vital for androgen-independent prostate cells (Krongrad & Bai 1994), whereas in androgen-sensitive cell lines PKC activity appears to cause apoptosis (Young *et al.* 1994). Powell *et al.* (1996) suggested that activation of PKCα is a critical point in the apoptosis pathway in the androgen-sensitive LNProstate cancer cell line and that lack of PKCα in androgen-independent PC-3 and Du 145 prostate cell lines may explain these lines resistance to apoptosis. Conversely, Lamm *et al.* (1997) showed that a reduction in PKCα causes growth impairment in PC-3 cells, while Liu *et al.* (1994) showed that activation of PKCα is associated with increased invasiveness in Dunning R3327 rat prostate adenocarcinoma cells. Other isoenzymes involved in prostate cancer include PKCε, whose downregulation appears to prevent apoptosis, and PKCζ overexpression (Figure 2.6) which decreases invasive and metastatic potential (Powell *et al.* 1996b).

Heat shock proteins

Heat shock proteins (hsps), comprise one of the most conserved groups of proteins throughout evolution. Although first identified in response to thermal stress, these proteins may be induced by a wide range of exogenous stimuli, which include oxidative injury, heavy metal toxicity, growth nutrient deprivation and inflammation. Hsps are classified into five predominant families of the low-molecular-weight proteins together with the four groups

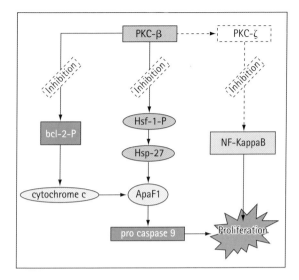

Figure 2.6
Schematic relating activation of PKCβ with the anti-apoptotic actions of Bcl-2 and hsp-27 with NF-kappaB. Loss of PKCβ early in prostatic neoplasia results in inhibition of apoptosis, with the consequence that potentially malignant cell clones are able to expand. Even if PKCβ activity is later restored, as occurs in a proportion of invasive malignant prostatic carcinomas, its activity is insufficient to restore an effective level of apoptosis to those cells.

known as hsp65, hsp70, hsp90 and hsp100, according to their relative molecular masses. Each family comprises several individual members having similar molecular weights but different patterns of induction and tissue expression. In addition to functioning as stress proteins, some hsps are normal cellular proteins expressed under non-stressed conditions and in a cell cycle-dependent manner. Some hsps are chaperonins of nascent proteins and have well-defined roles as regulators of protein folding, translocation, protein–protein interaction and prevention of inappropriate protein aggregation under normal conditions as well as in response to stress. In neoplasia, hsps have been implicated in multidrug resistance (Ciocca *et al.* 1993), in regulating apoptosis

and as modulators of p53 function (Levine *et al.* 1991).

hsp27, a member of the low-molecular-weight family, is constitutively expressed at low levels in the cytosol of most human cells (Lindquist & Craig 1988). Within a short time interval of exposure to appropriate stress, hsp27 becomes phosphorylated and, at the same time, transfers from the soluble to the insoluble protein compartment of the cell and translocates from cytoplasm to within or around the nucleus. Phosphorylation of hsp27 occurs at specific serine residues (Landry *et al.* 1992) through interaction with a specific kinase which may be activated by several different signal transduction mechanisms. It is currently believed that phosphorylation is a key regulator of hsp27 function and its contribution to cell survival following a stress insult (Benndorf *et al.* 1994).

Cornford *et al.* (2000) demonstrated that all control non-neoplastic prostatic tissues contained positive staining for hsp27 and that expression of hsp27 in BPH tissues occurred with a similar frequency to the controls so that no qualitative or quantitative differences in staining were identified. However, with respect to early malignancy (pT_{1-2}), there was a highly significant ($p < 0.0001$) decrease in expression of hsp27 such that the neoplastic components in 84% did not express this protein. However, expression of hsp27 by adjacent non-neoplastic epithelial components was indistinguishable from that found in the control normal and BPH tissues. Of the invasive prostate cancers (pT_{3-4} N_x M_0), 43% were positive with hsp27 protein expressed as fine granules distributed throughout the cytoplasm of the malignant cells in different regions of their invasive components. This distribution was highly significant ($p < 0.0001$). Although there was an appreciable correlation between hsp27 expression by each invasive carcinoma and its

Gleason grade ($p < 0.04$), the more outstanding finding was the relationship between semi-quantitative assessment of the level of hsp27 expressed and tumor behavior such that hsp27 expression became independently powerful at predicting clinical outcome. As a potential marker of early prostatic neoplasia, expression of hsp27 appears to offer independent objective information as to the regions of epithelium that are becoming phenotypically unstable while remaining morphologically unremarkable.

In control non-neoplastic tissues, hsp60 expression within the epithelial compartment varied from negative to strong. Although the distribution of this protein was also cytoplasmic, the appearance of the stained protein was coarsely granular, in distinction to that seen for hsps 27 and 70. An appreciable amount of epithelium in all BPH tissues expressed hsp60. Characteristically, the appearance of the coarse granular cytoplasmic deposits of protein in the cancer cells appeared more numerous and intense than in the non-neoplastic component of the corresponding malignant specimen. In regions of high-grade PIN, expression of hsp60 was elevated when compared to BPH or to normal control tissues. In 24 of 25 (96%) radical prostatectomies and 83 of 95 (87%) morphologically advanced invasive prostate cancers, hsp60 expression was strong when compared to non-neoplastic tissues ($p < 0.0001$). However, no association was apparent between semiquantitative assessment of the level of hsp60 expression and Gleason grade in either the early or the advanced cancers.

In all control normal tissues, hsp70 protein was expressed to a variable extent. Characteristically, staining was uniformly cytoplasmic and varied from diffusely non-granular to finely granular. In 12% of BPH tissues, no staining of the epithelium was identified. Neither the *in-situ* neoplasia nor the invasive malignant component in 16% of radical prostatectomies and 32% of advanced invasive carcinomas expressed hsp70. This finding was of only moderate statistical significance ($p < 0.005$) with respect to the control normal tissues. Immunohistochemical expression of this protein by invasive prostate cancer cells was generally less intense, although of the same character (i.e. uniform and finely granular) as in the non-malignant epithelium. No association was found between intensity of staining and Gleason grade in either the early or advanced cancers, so that some Gleason grade 5 carcinomas experienced this protein very strongly.

Conclusions

The *metastatic* phenotype of prostate cancer is promoted by specific cellular processes, in contrast to those that initiate or maintain the *neoplastic* phenotype (Foster and Abel 1992). A third group of cellular changes that occur in prostate cancer are epiphenomena that do not contribute to either neoplasia or to metastasis. Identification of metastasis-promoting events is currently hampered by lack of knowledge concerning the very earliest that occur in prostatic neoplasia. However, isolation of individual cellular proteins, and their expression in non-neoplastic cell lines, strongly suggests that the three processes of neoplasia, metastasis and epiphenomena are functionally distinct. All the evidence accumulated thus far suggests that promotion of metastasis involves inappropriate or abnormal expression of cellular proteins otherwise found in normal cells. Furthermore, the proteins involved in those processes (e.g. ion channel activity, glycosylation, hsp or PKC regulation of apoptosis, etc.)

are of normal structure and function. While some of these proteins may be of fetal type (e.g. ion channel isoforms), and not usually expressed in adult cells, none are from mutated genes such that they are of abnormal structure or function (Figure 2.7).

There is no question that, in the final analysis, activation of the genes encoding the

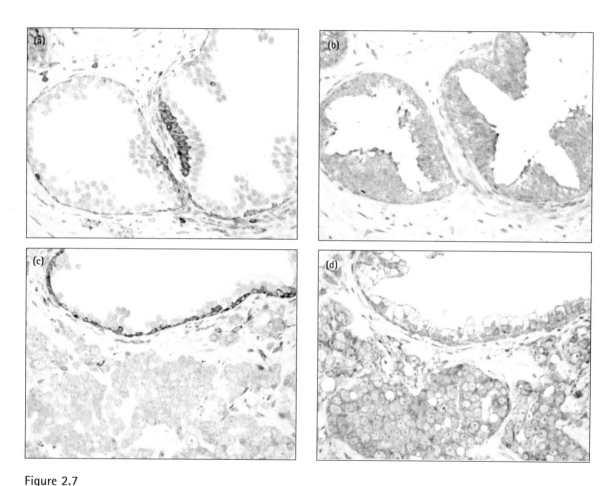

Figure 2.7

(a) Focus of prostatic basal cells in benign hyperplasia expressing high levels of anti-apoptotic Bcl-2 and hence protected from apoptosis. A thin rim of normal basal epithelial cells is evident surrounding the glands. Luminal epithelial cells, despite their abnormal appearance with large nucleoli, are not protected. (b) Adjacent tissue section stained for proapoptotic bax, confirming low-level expression of this protein in the luminal cells, but with minimal amounts in the focus of basal cells strongly expressing Bcl-2. (c) Portion of a benign prostatic gland in which basal cells (but not luminal cells) strongly express Bcl-2. Adjacent invasive prostatic adenocarcinoma (Gleason pattern 5) is unstained, indicating that these cells are not protected from apoptosis, despite their morphological appearance. (d) Tissue section adjacent to that in (c) in which normal basal cells do not express bax – confirming their protected status. However, the carcinoma cells express moderate amounts of bax, also suggesting that these cells are unlikely to be protected and hence subject to apoptosis. Clinically, the carcinoma illustrated in (c) and (d) behaved less aggressively than might have been expected from its appearance (magnification ×350).

proteins responsible for promoting metastases occurs at the DNA level. Such activation may be compensatory in response to events that distort or silence (possibly by mutation, deletion, etc.) normal genes, as a part of the malignant process. Alternatively, differential methylation, as a non-mutating regulatory process, might promote altered expression of genes that are normally silent. Ongoing studies are revealing how DNA methylation and chromatin structure are intimately linked such that methylation 'anomalies' are causal in tumorigenesis (Robertson 2001). Functionally, DNA methyltransferases appear to be components of large complexes actively involved in transcriptional control and chromatin structure modulation. It remains to be demonstrated whether, in prostate cancer, DNA methylation is a common mechanism responsible for suppression of proteins such as the MHC determinants (Sharp *et al.* 1992, Lu *et al.* 1998), RARbeta2 (Nakayama *et al.* 2001) or E-cadherin (Li *et al.* 2001). Alternatively, these proteins may become downregulated through other mechanisms of gene regulation and modulation since alterations in their structure have not been reported until very late stages of prostate cancer.

Finally, if the hypothesis is correct that metastasis is a consequence of altered homeostasis (in the general sense of the word) rather than a result of structural changes in particular genes, then the likelihood of regulating the process, therapeutically, becomes simultaneously easier and more challenging! Whereas correction of a structural genetic abnormality within an intact tissue is an unlikely prospect, at least within the foreseeable future, corrective modulation of intracellular homeostatic mechanisms is distinctly feasible. The challenge will be to develop the specificity to modulate the malignant cells without affecting normal tissues – *plus ça change!*

References

Abdul M, Hossein N (2001). Inhibition by anticonvulsants of prostate-specific antigen and interleukin-6 secretion by human prostate cancer cells. *Anticancer Res* 21:2045–2048.

Are A, Pinaev O, Burova E, Lindberg U (2001) Attachment of A-43 1 cells on immobilized antibodies to the EGF receptor promotes cell spreading and reorganization of the microfilament system. *Cell Motil Cytoskeleton* 48:24–36.

Bao L, Loda M, Janmay PA, *et al.* (1996) Thymosin β15: A novel regulator of tumor cell motility upregulated in metastatic prostate cancer. *Nature Medicine* 2:1322–1328.

Barraclough R, Rudland PS (1994) The S-100-related calcium-binding protein, p9Ka, and metastasis in rodent and human mammary cells. *Eur J Cancer* 30:1570–1576.

Barton J, Blackledge G, Wakeling A (2001) Growth factors and their receptors: New targets for prostate cancer therapy. *Urology* 58 (suppl 2A): 114–122.

Bauer KS, Figg WD, Hamilton SM, *et al.* (1999) A pharmacokinetically guided Phase II study of carboxyamido-triazole in androgen-independent prostate cancer. *Cancer Res* 5:2324–2329.

Bence-Hanulec KK, Marshall J, Blair LA (2000) Potentiation of neuronal L calcium channels by IGF-1 requires phosphorylation of the alpha subunit on a specific tyrosine residue. *Neuron* 27:121–131.

Benndorf R, Hayess K, Ryazantsev S, *et al.* (1994) Phosphorylation and supramolecular organization of murine small heat shock protein HSP25 abolish its actin polymerization-inhibiting activity. *J Biol Chem* 269:20780–20784.

Berridge MJ (1997) Elementary and global aspects of calcium signalling. *J Physiol* 499:291–306.

Berry N, Nishizuka Y (1990) Protein kinase C and T cell activation. *Eur J Biochem* 189:205–214.

Blobe GC, Sachs CW, Khan WA, *et al.* (1993) Selective regulation of expression of protein kinase C (PKC) isoenzyme in multidrug resistant MCF-7 cells – functional significance of enhanced expression of PKC-alpha. *J Biol Chem* 268:658–664.

Cacace AM, Guadagno SN, Krauss RS, Fabbro D, Weinstein IB (1993) The epsilon isoform of protein kinase C is an oncogene when overexpressed in rat fibroblasts. *Oncogene* 8:2095–2104.

Carpenter O, Cohen S (1990) Epidermal growth factor. *J Biol Chem* 265:7709–7712.

Chan JM, Stampfer MI, Oiovannucci E, *et al.* (1998) Plasma insulin-like growth factor-I and prostate cancer risk: a prospective study. *Science* 279:563–566.

Chen P, Xie H, Wells A (1996) Mitogenic signaling from the egf receptor is attenuated by a phospholipase C-gamma/protein kinase C feedback mechanism. *Mol Biol Cell* 7:871–881.

Choi DY, Toledo-Arai J, Lin HY, *et al.* (2001) Fibroblast growth factor receptor 3 induces gene expression primarily through Ras-independent signal transduction pathways. *J Biol Chem* 276:5116–5122.

Ciocca DR, Clark GM, Tandon AK, *et al.* (1993) Heat shock protein hsp70 in patients with axillary lymph node-negative breast cancer: prognostic implications. *J Nat Cancer Inst* 85:570–574.

Clapham DE (1995) Calcium signaling. *Cell* 80: 259–268.

Clare JJ, Tate SN, Nobbs M, Romanos MA (2000) Voltage-gated sodium channels as therapeutic targets. *Drug Development Trends* 5:506–520.

Clemens MJ, Trayner I, Meneya J (1992) The role of protein kinase C isoenzymes in the regulation of cell proliferation and differentiation. *J Cell Sci* 103:881–887.

Condon MS, Bosland MC (1999) The role of stromal cells in prostate cancer development and progression. *In Vivo* 13:61–65.

Cornford PA, Dodson AR, Parsons KF, *et al.* (2000) Heat shock protein (HSP) expression independently predicts clinical outcome in prostate cancer. *Cancer Res* 60: 7099–7105.

Cornford PA, Evans JD, Dodson AR, *et al.* Protein kinase C (PKC) isoenzyme patterns characteristically modulated in early prostate cancer. *Am J Pathol* 154: 137–144.

Daub H, Weiss FU, Wallasch C, Ullrich A (1996) Role of transactivation of the EGF receptor in signalling by 0-protein-coupled receptors. *Nature* 379:557–560.

DeRisi J, Penland L, Brown PO, *et al.* (1996) Use of a cDNA microarray to analyse gene expression patterns in human cancer. *Nature Genetics* 14:457–460.

Diss JK, Archer SN, Hirano I, Fraser SP, Djamgoz MB (2001) Expression profiles of voltage-gated Na$^+$ channel alpha-subunit genes in rat and human prostate cancer cell lines. *Prostate* 48:165–178.

Djakiew D, Pilug BR, Delsite R, *et al.* (1993) Chemotaxis and chemokinesis of human prostate tumor cell lines in response to human prostate stromal cell secretory proteins containing a nerve growth factor-like protein. *Cancer Res* 53:1416–1420.

Djamgoz MBA (2001). Excitability of prostate cancer cells – A new concept in the pathophysiology of metastatic disease. *Br J Cancer* 85 (suppl.1): 8.

Djamgoz MBA, Mycielska ME, Madeja Z, Fraser SP, Korohoda W (2001). Directional movement of rat prostate cancer cells in direct-current electric field: Involvement of voltage-gated Na$^+$ channel activity. *J Cell Sci* 114: 2697–2705.

Dolphin AC (1995) Voltage-dependent calcium channels and their modulation by neurotransmitters and G proteins. *Exp Physiol* 80:1–36.

Donato R (2001) S 100: a multigenic family of calcium-modulated proteins of the EF hand type with intracellular and extracellular functional roles. *Int J Biochem Cell Biol* 33:637–668.

Dong JT, Lamb PW, Rinkerschaeffer CW, *et al.* (1995) A metastasis suppressor gene for prostate-cancer on human-chromosome 11p11.2. *Science* 286: 884–886.

Downward J, Parker P, Waterfield MD (1984) Autophosphorylation sites on the epidermal growth factor receptor. *Nature* 311:483–485.

Elson SD, Browne CA, Thorburn GD (1984) Identification of epidermal growth factor-like activity in human male reproductive tissues and fluids. *J Clin Endocrinol Metab* 58:589–594.

Fanger OR, Erhardt P, Cooper GM, Maue RA (1993) ras-independent induction of rat brain type II sodium channel expression in nerve growth factor-treated PC12 cells. *J Neurochem* 61:1977–1980.

Fanger OR, Vaillancourt RR, Heasley LE, *et al.* (1997) Analysis of mutant platelet-derived growth factor receptors expressed in PC 12 cells identifies signals governing sodium channel induction during neuronal differentiation. *Mol Cell Biol* 17:89–99.

Fedi P, Pierce SF, di Fiore PP, Kraus MH (1994) Efficient coupling with phosphatidylinositol 3-kinase, but not phospholipase C gamma or GTPase-activating protein, distinguishes ErbB-3 signaling from that of other ErbB/EOFR family members. *Mol Cell Biol* 14:492–500.

Feldman BJ, Feldman D (2001). The development of androgen-independent prostate cancer. *Nat Rev Cancer* 1:34–45.

Festuccia C, Angelucci A, Gravina GL, *et al.* (2000) Osteoblast-derived TGF-beta1 modulates matrix degrading protease expression and activity in prostate cancer cells. *Int J Cancer* 86:888.

Figueroa JA, Lee AV, Jackson JO, Yee D (1995) Proliferation of cultured human prostate cancer cells is inhibited by insulin-like growth factor (IOF) binding protein-1: evidence for an IOF-II autocrine growth loop. *J Clin Endocrinol Metab* **80**:3476–3482.

Foster CS (1990) Processing of N-linked oligosaccharide glycoproteins in human tumours. *Br J Cancer* **62** (suppl. 10):57–63.

Foster CS, Abel PD (1992) Clinical and molecular techniques for diagnosis and monitoring prostatic cancer. *Human Pathol* **23**:395–401.

Foster CS, Bostwick DG, Bonkhoff H, *et al.* (2000) Cellular and molecular pathology of prostate cancer precursors. *Scand J Nephrol* Suppl. **205**:19–43.

Foster CS, Cornford P, Forsyth L, Djamgoz MBA, Ke Y (1999) The cellular and molecular basis of prostate cancer. *BJU Int* **83**:171–194.

Foster BA, Kaplan PJ, Greenberg NM (1998) Peptide growth factors and prostate cancer: new models, new opportunities. *Cancer Metastasis Rev* **17**:317–324.

Fraser SP, Ding Y, Liu A, Foster CS, Djamgoz MBA (1999). Tetrodotoxin suppresses morphological enhancement of the metastatic MAT-LyLu rat prostate cancer cell line. *Cell Tissue Res* **295**:505–512.

Fraser SP, Salvador V, Djamgoz MBA (1998). Voltage-gated Na$^+$ channel activity contributes to rodent prostate cancer cell migration in vitro. *J Physiol* **513P**:131P.

Fraser SP, Salvador V, Manning E, *et al.* (2003). Contribution of functional voltage-gated Na$^+$ channel expression to cell behaviours involved in the metastatic cascade in rat prostate cancer: II. Lateral motility. *J Cell Physiol* **195**:479–487.

Freed E (1989) A novel intergrin beta subunit is associated with the vitronectin receptor alpha-subunit (alpha-v) in a human osteosarcoma cell line and is a substrate for protein kinase C. *EMBO J* **8**: 2955–2965.

Freeman WM, Robertson DJ, Vrana KE (2000) Fundamentals of DNA hybridization arrays for gene expression analysis. *Biotechniques* **29**: 1042–1055.

Geldof AA, De Kleijn MA, Rao BR, Newling DW (1997) Nerve growth factor stimulates in vitro invasive capacity of DU145 human prostatic cancer cells. *J Cancer Res Clin Oncol* **123**:107–112.

Glynne-Jones E, Goddard L, Harper ME (1996) Comparative analysis of mRNA and protein expression for epidermal growth factor receptor and ligands relative to the proliferation index in human prostate tissue. *Hum Pathol* **27**:688–694.

Graus-Porta D, Beerli RR, Daly JM, Hynes NE (1997) ErbB-2, the preferred heterodimerization partner of all ErbB receptors, is a mediator of lateral signaling. *EMBO J* **16**:1647–1655.

Grimes JA, Djamgoz MBA (1998). Electrophysiological characterization of voltage-activated Na$^+$ current expressed in the highly metastatic MAT-LyLu cell line of rat prostate cancer. *J Cell Physiol* **175**:50–58.

Grimes JA, Fraser SP, Stephens GJ, *et al.* (1995). Differential expression of voltage-activated Na$^+$ currents in two prostatic tumour cell lines: contribution to invasiveness in vitro. *FEBS Letters* **369**: 290–294.

Harris H (1965) Behaviour of differentiated nuclei in heterokaryons of animal cells from different species. *Nature* **206**:583–588.

Haverstick DM, Heady TN, Macdonald TL, Gray LS (2000) Inhibition of human prostate cancer proliferation in vitro and in a mouse model by a compound synthesized to block Ca^{2-} entry. *Cancer Res* **60**:1002–1008.

He S, Ruknudin A, Bambrick LL, Lederer WJ, Schulze DH (1998) Isoform-specific regulation of the Na/Ca^{2+} exchanger in rat astrocytes and neurons by PKA. *J Neurosci* **18**:4833–4841.

Herbert JM (1993) Protein kinase C: a key factor in the regulation of tumor cell adhesion to the endothelium. *Biochem Pharmacol* **45**:527–537.

Hilborn MD, Rane SG, Pollock JD (1997) EGF in combination with depolarization or cAMP produces morphological but not physiological differentiation in PC12 cells. *J Neurosci Res* **47**:16–26.

Hsieh ET, Shepherd FA, Tsao MS (2000) Co-expression of epidermal growth factor receptor and transforming growth factor-alpha is independent of ras mutations in lung adenocarcinoma. *Lung Cancer* **29**:151–157.

Ibrahim GK, Kerns BJ, MacDonald JA, *et al.* (1993) Differential immunoreactivity of epidermal growth factor receptor in benign, dysplastic and malignant prostatic tissues. *J Urol* **149**:170–173.

Illmensee K, Mintz B (1976) Totipotency and normal differentiation of single teratocarcinoma cells cloned by injection into blastocysts. *Proc Natl Acad Sci* **73**:549–553.

Ivanova NB, Belyavsky AV (1995) Identification of genes differentially-expressed by restriction endonuclease-based gene expression fingerprinting. *Nucleic Acids Res* **23**:2954–2958.

Jing C, Beesley C, Foster CS, *et al.* (2001) Human cutaneous fatty acid-binding protein induces metastasis through up-regulating the expression of vascular endothelial growth factor gene in the Rama 37 model. *Cancer Res* **61**:4357–4364.

Jing C, Rudland PS, Foster CS, Ke YQ (2000a) Microquantity differential display: A strategy for a systematic analysis of differential gene expression with a small quantity of starting RNA. *Anal Biochem* **287**:334–337.

Jing C, Beesley C, Foster CS, *et al.* (2000b) Identification of human cutaneous fatty acid-binding protein as a metastasis-inducer. *Cancer Res* **60**: 2390–2398.

Kato K (1995) Description of the entire mRNA population by a 3′ end cDNA fragment generated by class IIS restriction enzymes. *Nucleic Acids Res* **23**:3685–3690.

Katsuki H, Shitaka Y, Saito H, Matsuki N (1998) A potential role of Ras-mediated signal transduction for the enhancement of depolarization-induced Ca²⁺ responses in hippocampal neurons by basic fibroblast growth factor. *Brain Res Dev Brain Res* **111**:169–176.

Ke Y, Jing C, Barraclough R, Smith P, Davies MP, Foster CS (1997) Elevated expression of calcium-binding protein p9Ka is associated with increasing malignant characteristics of rat prostate carcinoma cells. *Int J Cancer* **71**:832–837.

Ke YQ, Rudland PS, Jing C, Smith P, Foster CS (1999a) Systematic differential display: a strategy for a complete assessment of differential gene expression. *Anal Biochem* **269**:201–204.

Ke YQ, Jing C, Rudland PS, Smith P, Foster CS (1999b) Systematic comparison of gene expression through analysis of cDNA fragments within or near to the protein-coding region. *Nucleic Acids Res* **27**:912–914.

Kim H, Muller WJ (1999) The role of the epidermal growth factor receptor family in mammary tumorigenesis and metastasis. *Exp Cell Res* **253**:78–87.

Kimura K, Endo Y, Yonemura Y, *et al.* (2000) Clinical significance of 51 00A4 and E-cadherin-related adhesion molecules in non-small cell lung cancer. *Int J Oncol* **16**:1125–1131.

Klugbauer N, Lacinova N, Flockerzi V, Hofman F (1995) Structure and functional expression of a new member of the tetrodotoxin-sensitive voltage-activated sodium channel family from neuroendocrine cells. *EMBO J* **14**:1084–1090.

Knudsen AG (1971) Mutation and cancer: statistical study of retinoblastoma. *Proc Natl Acad Sci USA* **68**:820–832.

Knudsen AG (2001) Two genetic hits (more or less) to cancer. *Nature Rev Cancer* **1**:157–162.

Kofuji P, Hadley RW, Kieval RS, Lederer WJ, and Schuize DH (1992) Expression of the NatCa²⁺ exchanger in diverse tissues: a study using the cloned human cardiac Na/Ca²⁺ exchanger. *Am J Physiol* **263**:C1241–C1249.

Krongrad A, Bai G (1994) c-fos promoter insensitivity to phorbol ester and possible role of protein kinase C in androgen-independent cancer cells. *Cancer Res* **54**:203–210.

Kumar VL, Majumder PK, Gujral S, Kumar V (1998) Comparative analysis of epidermal growth factor receptor mRNA levels in normal, benign hyperplastic and carcinomatous prostate. *Cancer Lett* **134**:177–180.

Lambert PA, Somers KD, Kohn EC, Perry PR (1997) Antiproliferative and anti-invasive effects of carboxyamido-triazole on breast cancer cell lines. *Surgery* **122**:372–378.

Lamm ML, Long DD, Goodwin SM, Lee C (1997) Transforming growth factor beta 1 inhibits membrane association of protein kinase C alpha in a human prostate cancer cell line, PC3. *Endocrinology* **138**:4657–4664.

Landry J, Lambert H, Zhou M, *et al.* (1992) Human HSP27 is phosphorylated as serines 78 and serines 82 by heat shock and mitogen-activated kinases that recognize the same amino acid motif as S6 kinase II. *J Biol Chem* **267**:794–803.

Laniado ME, Lalani E-N, Fraser SP, *et al.* (1997). Expression and functional analysis of voltage-activated Na⁺ channels in human prostate cancer cell lines and their contribution to invasion in vitro. *Am J Pathol* **150**:1213–1221.

Le Novere N, Changeux JP (1999) The ligand gated ion channel database. *Nucleic Acids Res* **27**:340–342.

Lee YJ, Berns CM, Erdos G, Carry PM (1994) Effectiveness of isoquinolinesulfonamides on heat shock gene expression during heating at 41 °C in human carcinoma lines. *Biochem Biophys Res Commun* **199**:714–719.

Lei S, Dryden WF, Smith PA (1998) Involvement of Ras/MAP kinase in the regulation of Ca²⁺ channels in adult bullfrog sympathetic neurons by nerve growth factor. *J Neurophysiol* **80**:1352–1361.

Levine AJ, Momand J, Finlay CA (1991) The p53 tumor suppressor gene. *Nature* **351**:453–456.

Li LC, Zhao H, Nakajima K, *et al.* (2001) Methylation of the E-cadherin gene promoter correlates with progression of prostate cancer. *J Urol* **166**:705–709.

Liang P, Pardee AB (1992) Differential display of eukaryotic messenger RNA by means of the polymerase chain reaction. *Science* **257**:967–971.

Lindquist S, Craig EA (1988) The heat shock proteins. *Annu Rev Gen* **22**:631–677.

Liu B, Maher RJ, Hanun YA, Porter AT, Honn KV (1994) 12(S)-HETE enhancement of prostate tumor cell invasion: selective role of PKC alpha. *J Nat Canad Inst* **86**:1145–1151.

Lord JM, Ashcroft SJH (1984) Identification and characterisation of Ca^{2+}-phospholipid-dependent protein kinase in rat islets and hamster beta cells. *Biochem J* **219**:547–551.

Lord JM, Pongracz J (1995) Protein kinase C: a family of isoenzymes with distinct roles in pathogenesis. *J Clin Pathol: Mol Pathol* **48**:57–64.

Lu Q-L, Abel PD, Foster C, Lalani EN (1996) *bcl*–2: Role in epithelial differentiation and oncogenesis. *Human Pathol* **27**:102–110.

Ma L, Gauville C, Berthois Y, *et al.* (1998) Role of epidermal-growth-factor receptor in tumor progression in transformed human mammary epithelial cells. *Int J Cancer* **78**:112–119.

MacDonald A, Habib FK (1992) Divergent responses to epidermal growth factor in hormone sensitive and insensitive human prostate cancer cell lines. *Br J Cancer* **65**:177–182.

MacFarlane DE, Manzel L (1994) Activation of beta-isoenzyme of protein kinase C (PKC beta) is necessary and sufficient for phorbol ester-induced differentiation of HL60 promyelocytes. *J Biol Chem* **269**:4327–4331.

Maddy SQ, Chisholm GD, Busuttil A, Habib FK (1989) Epidermal growth factor receptors in human prostate cancer: correlation with histological differentiation of the tumour. *Br J Cancer* **60**:41–44.

Matz M, Usman N, Shagin D, Bogdanova E, Likyanov S (1997) Ordered differential display: a simple method for systematic comparison of gene expression profiles. *Nucleic Acids Res* **25**: 2541–2542.

Mellstrom B, Naranjo JR (2001) Mechanisms of Ca^{2+}-dependent transcription. *Curr Opin Neurobiol* **11**: 312–319.

Mohammed RM (1995) Bryostatin 1 induced apoptosis and augments inhibitory effects of vincristine in human diffuse large cell lymphoma. *Leuk Res* **19**:667–673.

Moscatello DK, Montgomery RB, Sundareshan P, *et al.* (1996) Transformational and altered signal transduction by a naturally occurring mutant EGF receptor. *Oncogene* **13**:85–96.

Muller A, Homey B, Soto H, *et al.* (2001) Involvement of chemokine receptors in breast cancer metastasis. *Nature* **410**:50–56.

Murray NR, Baumgardner GP, Burns DJ, Fields AP (1993) Protein kinase C isotypes in human erythroleukemia (k562) cell proliferation and differentiation. Evidence that beta II protein kinase C is required for proliferation. *J Biol Chem* **268**:15847–15853.

Mycielska M, Fraser SP, Szatkowski M, Djamgoz MBA (2001). Endocytic membrane activity in rat prostate cancer cell lines: Potentiation by functional voltage-gated sodium channels. *J Physiol* **531P**:81–82P.

Mycielska M, Szatkowski M, Djamgoz MBA (2003). Contribution of functional voltage-gated Na$^+$ channel expression to cell behaviours involved in the metastatic cascade in rat prostate cancer: I. Secretory membrane activity. *J Cell Physiol* **195**:461–469.

Nakayama T, Watanabe M, Yamanaka M, *et al.* (2001) The role of epigenetic modifications in retinoic acid receptor beta2 gene expression in human prostate cancers. *Lab Invest* **81**:1049–1057.

Niki I, Yokokura H, Sudo T, Kato M, Hidaka H (1996) Ca^{2+} signalling and intracellular Ca^{2+} binding proteins. *J Biochem* **120**:685–698.

North RA (1996) Families of ion channels with two hydrophobic segments. *Curr Opin Cell Biol* **8**:474–483.

Olapade-Olaopa EO, Moscatello DK, MacKay EH, *et al.* (2000) Evidence for the differential expression of a variant EGF receptor protein in human prostate cancer. *Br J Cancer* **82**:186–194.

Olumi AF, Grossfeld GD, Hayward SW, *et al.* (1999) Carcinoma-associated fibroblasts direct tumor progression of initiated human prostatic epithelium. *Cancer Res* **59**:5002–5011

Owen PJ, Johnson GD, Lord JM (1996) Protein kinase C-delta associates with vimentin intermediate filaments in differentiated HL-60 cells. *Exp Cell Res* **225**:366–373.

Pincelli C, Marconi A (2000) Autocrine nerve growth factor in human keratinocytes. *J Dermatol Sci* **22**:71–79.

Planz B, Wang Q, Kirley SD, Marberger M, McDougal WS (2001) Regulation of keratinocyte growth factor receptor and androgen receptor in epithelial cells of the human prostate. *J Urol* **166**:678–683.

Powell CT, Brittis NJ, Stec D, *et al.* (1996a) Persistent membrane translocation of protein kinase C alpha during 12-O-tetradecanoylphorbol-13-acetate-induced apoptosis of LNProstate cancer human prostate cancer cells. *Cell Growth Diff* **7**: 419–428.

Powell CT, Fair WR, Heston WD (1994) Differential expression of protein kinase C isoenzymes messenger RNAs in Dunning R-3327 rat prostatic tumors. *Cell Growth Diff* **5**:143–149.

Powell CT, Gschwend JE, Fair WR, *et al.* (1996b) Overexpression of protein kinase C-zeta (PKC-zeta) inhibits invasive and metastatic abilities of Dunning R-3327 MAT-LyLu rat prostate cancer cells. *Cancer Res* **56**:4137–4141.

Prashar Y, Weissman SM (1996) Analysis of differential gene expression by display of 3′ end restriction fragments of cDNAs. *Proc Natl Acad Sci USA* 93:659–663.

Prenzel N, Zwick E, Daub H, *et al.* (1999) EGF receptor transactivation by G-protein-coupled receptors requires metalloproteinase cleavage of proHB-EGF. *Nature* 402:884–888.

Riese DJ, Kim ED, Elenius K, *et al.* (1996) The epidermal growth factor receptor couples transforming growth factor-alpha, heparin-binding epidermal growth factor-like factor, and amphiregulin to Neu, ErbB-3, and ErbB-4. *J Biol Chem* 271:20047–20052.

Robertson CN, Roberson KM, Herzberg AJ, *et al.* (1994) Differential immunoreactivity of transforming growth factor alpha in benign, dysplastic and malignant prostatic tissues. *Surg Oncol* 3:237–242.

Robertson KD (2001) DNA methylation, methyltransferases and cancer. *Oncogene* 20:3139–3155.

Ropiquet F, Girl D, Lamb DJ, Ittmann M (1999) FGF7 and FGF2 are increased in benign prostatic hyperplasia and are associated with increased proliferation. *J Urol* 162:595–599.

Rowley DR (1998) What might a stromal response mean to prostate cancer progression? *Cancer Metastasis Rev* 17:411–419.

Rubenstein JL, Brice AE, Ciaranello RD, *et al.* (1990) Subtractive hybridization system using single-stranded phagemids with directional inserts. *Nucleic Acids Res* 18:4833–4842.

Rusnak JM, Lazo JS (1996) Downregulation of protein kinase C suppresses induction of apoptosis in human prostatic carcinoma cells. *Exp Cell Res* 224:189–199.

Sako Y, Minoghchi S, Yanagida T (2000) Single-molecule imaging of EGFR signalling on the surface of living cells. *Nat Cell Biol* 2:168–172.

Sanders JL, Chattopadhyay N, Kifor O, Yamaguchi T, Butters RR (2000) Extracellular calcium-sensing receptor expression and its potential role in regulating parathyroid hormone-related peptide secretion in human breast cancer cell lines. *Endocrinol* 141:4357–4364.

Schena M, Shalon D, Davis RW, Brown PO (1995) Quantitative monitoring of gene expression patterns with a complementary-DNA microarray. *Science* 270:467–470.

Sharpe JC, Abel PD, Gilbertson JA, Brawn P, Foster CS (1994) Modulated expression of HLA Class I and Class II determinants in hyperplastic and malignant human prostatic epithelium. *J Urol* 74:609–616.

Sherrill JM, Kyte J (1996) Activation of epidermal growth factor receptor by epidermal growth factor. *Biochemistry* 35:5705–5718.

Smith P, Rhodes NP, Shortland AP, *et al.* (1998) Sodium channel protein expression enhances the invasiveness of rat and human prostate cancer cells. *FEBS Lett* 423:19–24.

Sosnowski J, Stetter-Neel C, Cole D, Durham JP, Mawhinney MG (1997) Protein kinase C mediated anti-proliferative glucocorticoid-sphinganine synergism in cultured Pollard III prostate tumor cells. *J Urol* 158:269–274.

Spaargaren M, Defize LH, Boonstra J, de Laat SW (1991) Antibody-induced dimerization activates the epidermal growth factor receptor tyrosine kinase. *J Biol Chem* 266:1733–1739.

Sporn MB, Todaro GJ (1980) Autocrine secretion and malignant transformation of cells. *N Engl J Med* 303:878–880.

Stewart D, Djamgoz MBA (2001a). Modulation of voltage-gated Na^+ channel expression by its own activity in rat and human prostate cancer cells. *Soc Neurosci Abstr.* 27:46–52.

Stewart D, Foster CS, Smith P, Foster RG, Djamgoz MBA (1999). Expression of voltage-gated Na^+ channels in human prostate cancer. *Soc Neurosci Abstr* 25:208.

Stewart D, Mobasheri A, Djamgoz MBA (2001b). Tetrodotoxin down-regulates Na^+/K^+−ATPase α1 subunit expression in rat prostate cancer cell lines. *J Physiol* 531P:133–134P.

Szatkowski S, Mycielska M, Knowles R, Kho A-L, Djamgoz MBA (2000). Electrophysiological recordings from rat prostate gland in vitro: Identified single-cell and trans-epithelial potentials. *BJU Int* 86:1–8.

Tanabe T, Takeshima H, Mikami A, *et al.* (1987) Primary structure of the receptor for calcium channel blockers from skeletal muscle. *Nature* 328:313–318.

Taylor CW, Traynor D (1995) Calcium and inositol trisphosphate receptors. *J Membr Biol* 145:109–118.

Taylor CW, Genazzani AA, Morris SA (1999) Expression of inositol trisphosphate receptors. *Cell Calcium* 26:237–251.

Toledo-Aral JJ, Brehm P, Halegoua S, Mandel G (1995) A single pulse of nerve growth factor triggers long-term neuronal excitability through sodium channel gene induction. *Neuron* 14:607–611.

Toning N, Jorgensen PE, Sorensen BS, Nexo E (2000) Increased expression of heparin binding EGF (HB-EGF), amphiregulin, TGF alpha and epiregulin in androgen independent prostate cancer cell lines. *Anticancer Res* 20:91–95.

Turkeri LN, Sakr WA, Wykes SM, *et al.* (1994) Comparative analysis of epidermal growth factor receptor gene expression and protein product in benign, premalignant, and malignant prostate tissue. *Prostate* 25:199–205.

Wang G, Rudland PS, White MR, Barraclough R (2000) Interaction in vivo and in vitro of the metastasis-inducing S100 protein, S100A4 (p9Ka) with SIOOA1. *J Biol Chem* 275:11141–11146.

Wasilenko WJ, Palad AJ, Somers KD, *et al.* (1996) Effects of the calcium influx inhibitor carboxyamidotriazole on the proliferation and invasiveness of human prostate tumor cell lines. *Int J Cancer* 68:259–264.

Weinberg RA (1981) Use of transfection to analyze genetic information and malignant transformation. *Biochim Biophys Acta* 651:25–35.

Welsh J, Chada K, Dalal SS, *et al.* (1992) Arbitrary primed PCR fingerprinting of RNA. *Nucleic Acids Res* 20:4965–4790.

Wertz IE, Dixit VM (2000) Characterization of calcium release-activated apoptosis of LNCaP prostate cancer cells. *J Biol Chem* 275:11470–11477.

Wieland I, Bolger G, Asouuline G, Wigler M (1990) A method for different cloning: Gene amplification following subtractive hybridization. *Proc Natl Acad Sci USA* 87:2720–2724.

Wijetunge S, Hughes AD (1995) pp6Oc-src increases voltage-operated calcium channel currents in vascular smooth muscle cells. *Biochem Biophys Res Commun* 217:1039–1044.

Wijetunge S, Lymn JS, Hughes AD (2000) Effects of protein tyrosine kinase inhibitors on voltage-operated calcium channel currents in vascular smooth muscle cells and pp6O(c-src) kinase activity. *Br J Pharmacol* 129:1347–1354.

Young CY, Murtha PE, Zhang J (1994) Tumor promoting phorbol ester-induced cell death and gene expression in a human prostate adenocarcinoma cell line. *Oncol Res* 6:203–210.

Zakon HH (1998). The effects of steroid hormones on electrical excitability of excitable cells. *Trends Neurosci* 21:202–207.

3 Genetic susceptibility to prostate cancer

Olivier Cussenot

Abstract

The incidence of prostate cancer (CaP) is related to ageing, and its increase in the last 10 years varies from country to country and according to ethnic groups, being greatest among US black men and the lowest among Asian men. Just two risk factors are really established for CaP: familial aggregation of CaP and ethnic origin.

No dietary or environment-related cause has yet been identified in CaP. However, some variations in endogenous factors, such as sex steroids or insulin-like growth factor 1 (IGF1) circulating levels, may contribute to explain differences in risk observed between different populations. In this way, genetic polymorphisms of genes encoding for steroid receptor or enzymes involved in steroid metabolic pathways have been associated with different level of CaP risk, and could explain variations among ethnic group or geographic area.

Different studies support the hypothesis that familial CaP may be truly hereditary and not due to a similar lifestyle. In this way, familial inheritance is a parameter which has to be considered to advise screening in high-risk families. Indeed, the relative risk of first-degree relatives of CaP patients can reach 2, 5 and 11 when, respectively, 1, 2 and 3 first-degree relatives are affected. Some familial forms appear to be associated with transmission of a rare putative (0.003 to 0.06 allele frequency) autosomal dominant gene with a high penetrance (88% at age 85). Using this transmission model, and linkage analysis, three predisposing loci on chromosome 1: HPC-1 (hereditary prostate cancer 1: 1q24–25), PCaP (predisposing for prostate cancer: 1q42–43) and CAPB (predisposing for prostate and brain tumor: 1p36) and one locus on chromosome 20 (HPC20: 20q13) have been described. Moreover, X-linked transmission has been suggested and related to another predisposing gene locus: HPCX (Xq27–28). It is possible that a large proportion of familial CaP is due not to segregation of a few major gene mutations transmitted according to a monogenic inheritance but rather to familial sharing of alleles at many loci, each contributing to a small increase in cancer risk.

Introduction

Prostate cancer is the second most common malignancy in men in the European Union, with 135 000 new cancers and 55 000 deaths each year[1] (http 2000). Worldwide, prostate cancer incidence is steadily rising by 3% per annum, and has been called by expert epidemiologists the 'oncological time bomb'. Large variations in the incidence and mortality of prostate cancer have been observed among countries and ethnic groups. Many epidemiological studies have been conducted to evaluate the effects of environmental factors on the risk of prostate cancer, in an attempt to explain the large ethnic variations risk. However, any environmental or lifestyle factors have not been associated consistently with prostate cancer risk. Despite the absence of strong exogenous risk factor, some variations in endogenous genetic factors may contribute to explaining variation in risk among ethnic groups or geographic areas.

Family history data have provided suggestive evidence for a genetic component in prostate cancer aetiology. Further support that prostate cancer may be truly hereditary and not due to a similar lifestyle was provided by the twin studies. The concordance rate among heterozygotic twins was 0.06 (comparable with familial cancer as breast cancer), whereas the concordance rate in monozygotic twins was 0.21, almost three times higher (Grönberg *et al.* 1994). The risk of acquiring prostate cancer has been found to be much higher when the prostate cancer was diagnosed in the father before the age of 70 years than when it was diagnosed after 70 years. The risk for the sons gradually decreased with increasing age at diagnosis for the father, which suggested that the development of reliable tests could greatly help clinicians in genetic counselling. It is usual to consider as hereditary prostate cancer the cases where families express at least three first-degree relatives with the disease, or two relatives diagnosed below the age of 55 (Hopkins criteria: Carter *et al.* 1993). This definition results from the segregation analysis performed by Carter *et al.* (1992), in which the family clustering was best explained by autosomal dominant inheritance of a rare gene with a high age-dependent penetrance. This transmission model has been confirmed by two other studies conducted on American and

northern European populations, but X-linked or recessive transmission has also been suggested (Monroe *et al.* 1995). The Hopkins criteria of hereditary prostate cancer are well defined for prostate cancer, resulting from autosomal dominant inheritance; however, they don't take into account X-linked transmission, so that inherited cases could be missed. Indeed, hereditary cases criteria must be extended to the families with 3 second-degree relatives affected (Cussenot & Valeri 2001).

Other evidence suggesting genetic complexity included the significantly elevated age-adjusted risk of prostate cancer among brothers of probands, compared with their fathers. On the other hand, the fact that the frequency of prostate cancer shows a very steep increase with age in elderly men, and the improvement of early detection of insignificant prostate cancer in old men combine to find familial clustering in elderly men with no evidence of inheritance factors involvement (high age-dependent phenocopy rate). In the French ProGène study Valeri *et al.* (1996) have identified 8% of the families with hereditary criteria for prostate cancer. Interestingly, the age at diagnosis of this subset appeared earlier (65.9 years old) than in a control population of sporadic cases (68.9 years old).

What about genetic markers in familial prostate cancer?

Prostate cancer as a rare heritable monofactorial disease

In order to identify predisposing gene(s), several genome-wide screens with linkage analysis were performed on familial prostate cancer cases. This has led to the mapping of at least five predisposing loci. The first localized was HPC1 (hereditary prostate cancer 1) on 1q24–25 (Smith *et al.* 1996). This locus was identified in a study including North American and Swedish families with at least three affected individuals. Assuming heterogeneity, a maximum multipoint LOD score of 5.43 was found, with an estimated 34% of the families being linked. Extension of this analysis to a larger number of families from the same origin showed that a subset of pedigrees with an earlier age at diagnosis and at least five prostate cases was mostly responsible for the evidence of linkage (Gronberg *et al.* 1997). In order to confirm this localization, several linkage analyzes were performed with controversial results. Some studies concluded the absence of linkage within the selected population, whereas others show weak confirmation. The strongest confirmation for this localization was obtained by the examination of Utah families (Neuhausen *et al.* 1999), with a maximum three-point LOD score of 2.43. Again, in this study, younger age at diagnosis pedigrees provided stronger evidence of linkage to HPC1. Recently, a large linkage analysis performed by the International Consortium for Prostate Cancer Genetics (ICPCG) on 772 families from various origins has indicated that the estimated proportion of families linked to this locus was closer to 6% rather than 30% (Xu 2000).

The second locus called PCaP (predisposing for cancer prostate) was identified on 1q42.2–43 by our group on a combined analysis of French and German families (Berthon *et al.* 1998). This result wasn't confirmed by other groups working on whole populations but positive LOD scores suggestive of linkage were obtained when families were stratified. Indeed, evidence of linkage was observed among a small subset of families with ≥ 5 affected individuals (Gibbs *et al.* 1999) or with pedigrees fitting the same criterion, with an average age at diagnosis <66 years and male-to-male transmission (Berry *et al.* 2000a). The same author recently published evidence for a prostate cancer susceptibility locus on chromosome 20: HPC20 (20q13) on a set of 162 North American families (Berry *et al.* 2000b).

Examination of 360 families collected in North America, Finland and Sweden led to the identification of a fourth locus, termed HPCX, on Xq27–28 (Xu *et al.* 1998). In the overall population, the proportion of linked pedigrees was close to 16% but reached 41% in the Finnish subgroup. Results supporting this localization were further obtained in another analysis of 153 American families (Lange *et al.* 1999). In this report, the most significant evidence of linkage to this locus was found in pedigrees without male-to-male transmission and with early-onset prostate cancer.

The last gene which has been localized on 1p36 seemed to be predisposing for brain and prostate cancer. Indeed, strong evidence of linkage to this locus, CAPB, was obtained with 12 families showing both hereditary prostate cancer and a history of brain tumor (Gibbs *et al.* 1999).

Considering the genetic heterogeneity and the controversial results observed within the different populations, we have selected 64 families of south-western European origin and performed a linkage analysis with markers from the four candidate regions PCaP, HPC1, CAPB or HPCX in order to estimate the frequency of each locus in this subset of pedigrees. No significant evidence of linkage to HPC1, CAPB or HPCX was found either in the whole population or when pedigrees were stratified according to criteria specific for each locus. By contrast, results in favour of linkage to PCaP locus were observed. Homogeneity analysis performed with multipoint LOD scores gave an estimated proportion of families with linkage to this locus of up to 50%. In particular, families with an earlier age at diagnosis ($\leq$ 65 years old) contributed significantly to the evidence of linkage, with a maximum multipoint NPL score of 2.03. Those results suggest that PCaP is the most frequent known locus predisposing for hereditary prostate cancer cases from south-western European families (Cancel-Tassin et al. 2001).

Different epidemiological studies have observed coaggregation of prostate cancer and breast cancer in families (Tulinius et al. 1992). Several lines of evidence support the hypothesis that reported familial clustering of breast and prostate cancers could be due to the same inherited susceptibility. Recently, we have studied breast cancer occurrence in first-degree relatives of prostate cancer patients. We have observed a higher risk of breast cancer (1) in familial prostate cancer relatives compared to sporadic cases, and (2) in early onset prostate cancer relatives compared to late onset, suggesting a link between breast cancer risk in female and hereditary prostate cancer in men in some families (Valeri et al. 2000). Moreover, prostate cancer, in hereditary breast cancer syndromes, seems to be elevated among men who carry mutations of the BRCA1 or BRCA2 genes, located on chromosomes 17q12 and 13q14, respectively. Gao et al. (1995) supported the theory of a link between breast and prostate cancer by finding a high frequency of loss of BRCA1 in men with prostate cancer, but this was not based on linkages analysis. Recently, Gudmundsson et al. (1995) reported that six of seven prostate cancers from mutated BRCA2 carriers had lost their counterpart wild-type allele. But no evidence of loss of heterozygosity was found at the BCRA2 locus for sporadic prostate cancers. These facts, and reports of familial clustering of breast and prostate cancers, could suggest that the tumor suppressive gene for breast cancer may also be related to prostate cancer risk in some cases. However, the fraction where the familial aggregation for prostate cancer is due to a mutation of BRCA1 or BRCA2 genes seems rare and needs further proof.

Moreover, it is obvious that hereditary prostate cancer is dependent on different modulating genes in favour of familial genotype heterogeneity. It is possible that a large proportion of familial aggregation is due not to segregation of mutation in a few major genes but rather to familial sharing of alleles at many loci, each in itself exerting a small effect (low penetrance) of risk.

Recent linkage and association studies on prostate cancer susceptibility have claimed to identify candidate susceptibility genes for familial prostate cancer. These genes named HPC2/ELAC2 (17p) (Tavtigian et al. 2001) and PG1 (8p22–23) (Xu et al. 2001), have shown overtransmission of specific polymorphisms to case subjects. But, controversy on mutation screening probands suggests that these candidate genes play a limited and non-exclusive role in genetic susceptibility to hereditary prostate cancer.

Prostate cancer as a common familial multifactorial disease

The fact that genetic heritability explained 70% of the variance of plasma levels of androstanediols in male twins suggests that familial clustering may be due, at least in part, to familial correlation with hormonal status. Association between hormone levels and prostate cancer risk has been studied but it is unknown if serum androgenic hormone or IGF1 levels can explain population differences in prostate cancer incidence or can identify individuals at higher risk. However, circumstantial evidence exists that hormones play a supportive role in the progression of prostate cancer. Conversion of testosterone to its metabolite and active androgen on prostatic target cells, dihydrotestosterone (DHT), is catalysed in prostate by the enzyme 5α-reductase (5α-R). DHT is the androgen active on prostatic target cells and implied during the differentiation and growth of functional adult prostate gland. The two genes SRD5A1 and SRDA2, encoding for 5α-R isoforms type I and type II have been cloned recently and they are located on chromosomes 5p15 and 2p23, respectively, for isoforms type I and type II. The roles of the two isoforms in the adult tissue are still subject to controversy and it is believed that isoform type II predominates in the prostate. The 5α-R type I predominates in the skin and liver and contributes substantially to serum DHT levels. DHT is rapidly reduced to androstanediols by the more active 3-oxidoreductase enzymes in androgen target cells. Serum levels of androstanediols, as indices of the 5α-R activity, were measured in blacks, whites and native Asian young men: the DHT metabolites were higher in blacks and whites compared with Asian natives (Ross *et al.* 1992). The possibility that different alleles of the 5α-R gene (SRD5A2) may be associated with different levels of 5α-R activity and, consequently, different levels of prostate cancer risk has motivated studies of ethnic variation in alleles of this gene. The first DNA polymorphism described for the 5α-R type 2 gene as a susceptibility determinant in prostate cancer is a TA dinucleotide repeat. Three alleles have been considered but the allele with 18 TA repeats is common in Afro-American men (Davis & Russel 1993).

Two low-frequency missense mutations, VL89 and AT49, have also been studied in prostate cancer susceptibility. On the one

hand, the VL89 mutation reduces steroid 5α-reductase activity. This substitution is particularly common among Asians and may explain the low risk for prostate cancer in this population (Ross *et al.* 1998). On the other hand, the AT49 missense substitution increased conversion of testosterone to dihydrotestosterone and has been considered as a significant contributor to the incidence of prostate cancer in about 8% of African-American and Hispanic men in the United States. Furthermore, A49T has been correlated with a worse prognosis marker, such as differentiation score, in prostate cancer.

Two other genes encoding for cytochrome P450c androgen metabolism enzymes (CYP17 and CYP3A4-V) have been associated with prostate cancer risk. CYP17 encodes the enzyme which catalyses steroid 17α-hydroxylase/17,20-desmolase activities at key points in testosterone and estrogen biosynthesis in both gonads and adrenals. The CYP17 A2 allele contains a $T \rightarrow C$ transition polymorphism in the 5′ promoter region that creates an additional SP1-type (CCACC box) promoter site. Polymorphism is correlated with the promoter activity in the CYP17 gene and could predict circulating testosterone levels in male and estrogen levels in women. The A2 allele has been associated with an increased risk of baldness, polycystic ovarian cancer and, recently, prostate cancer (Lunn *et al.* 1999, Latil *et al.* 2001). The CYP3A4 enzyme catabolizes the testosterone. Rebbeck *et al.* (1998) identified a variant (CYP3A4-V) that is associated with poor prognosis of prostate cancer.

Ethnic variations of the androgen receptor (AR) have also been investigated as a possible explanation for ethnic differences in prostate cancer risk. Prostate cancer incidence differs considerably among the various racial–ethnic groups: it is highest in African-Americans (116 per 1000 person-years), intermediate in non-Hispanic whites (71 per 100 000 person-years), and lowest among Asians (Japanese at 39 per 100 000 person-years). The AR is encoded by a gene on the chromosome X (Xq11–13). One of the critical functions of the product of the androgen receptor gene is to activate the expression of target genes. This transactivation activity resides in the N-terminal domain of the protein, which is encoded in exon 1 and contains polymorphic CAG and GGC repeats (microsatellites). A smaller size of the CAG repeat is associated with a higher level of receptor transactivation function, thereby possibly resulting in a higher risk of prostate cancer. Schoenberg *et al.* (1994) demonstrated contraction in this microsatellite from 24 to 18 CAG units in an adenocarcinoma of the prostate, and the affects of the shorter allele were implicated in the development of the tumor. Edwards *et al.* (1992) and Irvine *et al.* (1995) showed that the prevalence of short CAG alleles was highest in African-American males, with the highest risk for prostate cancer, intermediate in intermediate-risk non-Hispanic whites and lowest in Asians at very low risk for prostate cancer. Irvine *et al.* (1995) found that high-risk African-Americans also had the lowest frequency of the GGC allele. Consistent with the interracial variation in CAG and GGC distributions, there was an excess of white patients with short CAG repeats relative to white controls. Irvine *et al.* found a statistically significant negative association between the number of CAG and GGC repeats among the prostate cancer patients. Overall, the data were interpreted to suggest a possible association between the polymorphisms of the androgen receptor gene and the development of prostate cancer. In the French–German collection (Progène study), Correa-Cerro *et al.* (1999a) have analyzed these polymorphisms of 105 controls, 132 sporadic

cases and a sample of families comprising 85 affected and 46 not-affected family members. The allele distributions were very similar in all subgroups of the sporadic cases defined by age classes or by Gleason score. So, we concluded that these AR polymorphisms cannot be used as predictive parameters for prostate cancer in the French or German population.

The inverse relationship between the geographical variations of sun exposure and the incidence of prostate cancer could be explained by vitamin D production, by the action of sun on the skin. Low serum levels of vitamin D could be associated with a high risk of prostate cancer. In the same way, a polymorphism between the different alleles of the vitamin D receptor gene (VDR gene localized on chromosome 2q12) could explain different levels of risk for prostate cancer, without link with the ethnic status. We studied three polymorphisms in the VDR gene (poly-A microsatellite, *Taq*I and *Fok*I RFLPs) in 105 controls and 132 sporadic PCA cases from France and Germany (Correa-Cerro *et al.* 1999b). The polymorphisms near the 3′ end of the gene were in linkage disequilibrium with an almost complete coincidence of the short poly-A alleles and t (cut) of the *Taq*I polymorphism. An association was found by logistic regression for the poly-A between prostate cancer and the heterozygous genotype (S/L; S <17, L ≥17, OR 0.44, 95% confidence interval, CI = 0.198–0.966, $p = 0.041$). OR was lower in patients ≤ 70 years old and patients with a Gleason score ≥ 6. The Tt genotype of the *Taq*I RFLP also showed an association with prostate cancer that was stronger for younger patients (≤ 70 years old). In the *Fok*I RFLP, the FF genotype had a lower risk (OR = 0.57, CI = 0.33–1.00, $p = 0.049$). In contrast to the polymorphisms in the androgen receptor gene, our present findings with the VDR gene agree well with those from North America, indicating a weak but general role of the VDR in prostate cancer susceptibility.

Conclusion

Prostate cancer risk associated with genetic status can result from two mechanisms. First, genetic predisposition associated with very high risk can explain hereditary prostate cancer in the case of an inherited mutation involving one of the five known predisposing loci. It is also possible that a proportion of familial aggregation is due not to segregation of mutation in a few major genes but rather to familial sharing of alleles at many loci, each in itself exerting a small effect of risk. The second genetic mechanism associated with prostate cancer risk can result from genetic susceptibility, via individual or ethnic polymorphisms that involve, especially, androgen metabolism: those polymorphisms could explain the variation of incidence according to geographic or ethnic status, and can increase prostate cancer risk, but not enough to trigger familial cases of prostate cancer.

Knowledge of prostate cancer genetics is essential in order to manage hereditary prostate cancer, including screening in high-risk families and searching for genetic–phenotype correlation; it is also necessary for identifing at-risk individuals, according to polymorphisms, who could benefit from prevention via pharmacogenomics tools.

References

Berry R, Schaid DJ, Smith JR, et al. (2000a) Linkage analyses at the chromosome 1 loci 1q24–25 (HPC1), 1q42.2–43 (PCAP), and 1p36 (CAPB) in families with hereditary prostate cancer. Am J Hum Genet 66:539–546.

Berry R, Schroeder JJ, French AJ, et al. (2000b) Evidence for a prostate cancer-susceptibility locus on chromosome 20. Am J Hum Genet 67:82–91.

Berthon P, Valeri A, Cohen Akenine A, et al. (1998) Predisposing gene for early onset prostate cancer localised on chromosome 1 q 42.2–43. Am J Hum Genet 62:416–424.

Cancel-Tassin G, Latil A, Valeri A, et al. (2001) PCAP is the major known prostate cancer predisposing locus in families from south and west Europe. Eur J Hum Genet 9(2):135–142.

Carter BS, Beaty TH, Steinberg GD, Childs B, Walsh PC (1992) Mendelian inheritance of familial prostate cancer. Proc Natl Acad Sci USA 89:3367–3371.

Carter BS, Bova GS, Beaty TH, et al. (1993) Hereditary prostate cancer: epidemiologic and clinical features. J Urol 150:797–802.

Correa-Cerro L, Berthon P, Häussler J, et al. (1999b) Vitamin D receptor polymorphisms as markers in prostate cancer. Hum Genet 105:281–287.

Correa-Cerro L, Wöhr G, Häussler J, et al. (1999a) (CAG)nCAA and GGN repeats in the human androgen receptor gene are not associated with prostate cancer in a French–German population. Eur J Hum Genet 7:357–362.

Cussenot O, Valeri A (2001) Heterogeneity in genetic susceptibility to prostate cancer. Eur J Intern Med 12(1):11–16.

Davis DL, Russel DW (1993) Unusual length polymorphism in human steroid 5α reductase type 2 gene (SRD5A2). Human Mol Ent 2: 820.

Edwards A, Hammond HA, Jin L, Caskey CT, Chakraborty R (1992) Genetic variation at five trimeric and tetrameric tandem repeat loci in four human population groups. Genomics 12:241–253.

Gao X, Zacharek A, Salkowski A, et al. (1995) Loss of heterozygosity of BRCA1 and other loci on chromosome 17q in human prostate cancer. Cancer Res 55:1002–1005.

Gibbs M, Stanford JL, McIndoe RA, et al. (1999) Evidence for a rare prostate cancer-susceptibility locus at chromosome 1p36. Am J Hum Genet 64: 776–787.

Gibbs M, Chakrabarti L, Stanford JL, et al. (1999) Analysis of chromosome 1 q 42.2–43 in 152 families with high risk of prostate cancer Am J Hum Genet 64:1087–1095.

Grönberg H, Damber L, Damber JE (1994). Studies of genetic factors in prostate cancer in twin population. *J Urol* **152**:1484–1489.

Gronberg H, Xu J, Smith JR, *et al*. (1997) Early age at diagnosis in families providing evidence of linkage to the Hereditary Prostate Cancer 1 *(HPC1)* locus on chromosome 1. *Cancer Res* **57**:4707–4709.

Gudmundsson J, Johannesdottir G, Bergthorsson JT, *et al*. (1995) Different tumor types from BRCA2 carriers show wild-type chromosome deletions on 13q12–q13. *Cancer Res* **55**:4830–4832.

http://www-dep.iarc.fr, 2000.

Irvine RA, Yu MC, Ross RK, Coetzee GA (1995) The CAG and GGC microsatellites of the androgen receptor gene are linkage disequilibrium in men with prostate cancer. *Cancer Res* **55**:1937–1940.

Lange EM, Chen H, Brierley K, *et al*. (1999) Linkage analysis of 153 prostate cancer families over a 30-cM region containing the putative susceptibility locus HPCX. *Clin Cancer Res* **5**:4013–4020.

Latil AG, Azzouzi R, Cancel GS, *et al*. Prostate carcinoma risk and allelic variants of genes involved in androgen biosynthesis and metabolism pathways. *Cancer* **92**(5):1130–1137.

Lunn RM, Bell DA, Mohler JL, Taylor JA (1999) Prostate cancer risk and polymorphism in 17 hydroxylase (CYP17) and steroid reductase (SRD5A2). *Carcinogenesis* **20**:1727–1731.

Monroe KR, Yu MC, Kolonel LN, *et al*. (1995) Evidence of an X-linked or recessive genetic component to prostate cancer risk. *Nature Med* **1**:827–829.

Neuhausen SL, Farnham JM, Kort E, *et al*. (1999) Prostate cancer susceptibility locus HPC1 in Utah high-risk pedigrees. *Hum Mol Genet* **8**:2437–2442.

Rebbeck TR, Jaffe JM, Walker AH, Wein AJ, Malkowicz SB. (1998) Modification of clinical presentation of prostate tumors by a novel genetic variant in CY3A4. *J Natl Cancer Inst* **90**:1225–1229.

Ross RK, Berstein L, Lobo RA, *et al*. (1992) 5 alpha reductase activity and risk of prostate cancer among Japanese and white and black males. *Lancet* **339**:887–889.

Ross RK, Pike MC, Coetzee GA, *et al*. (1998) Androgen metabolism and prostate cancer: establishing a model of genetic susceptibility. *Cancer Res* **58**:4497–4504.

Schoenberg MP, Hakimi JM, Wang S, *et al*. (1994) Microsatellite mutation (CAG (24-to-18)) in the androgen receptor gene in human prostate cancer. *Biochem Biophys Res Commun* **198**:74–80.

Smith JR, Freije D, Carpten JD, *et al*. (1996) Major susceptibility locus for prostate cancer on chromosome 1 suggested by a genome-wide search. *Science* **274**:1371–1374.

Tavtigian SV, Simard J, Teng DH, *et al*. (2001) A candidate prostate cancer susceptibility gene at chromosome 17p. *Nat Genet* **27**(2):172–180.

Tulinius H, Egilsson V, Otafsdottir H, Sigvaldason H (1992) Risk of prostate, ovarian and endometrial cancer among relatives of women with breast cancer. *BMJ* **305**:855–857.

Valeri A, Berthon Ph, Fournier G, *et al*. (1996) Etude PROGENE, projet français d'analyse génétique du cancer de la prostate familial: recrutement et analyse. *Progr Urol* **6**:226–235.

Valeri A, Fournier G, Morin V, *et al*. (2000) Early onset and familial predisposition to prostate cancer significantly enhance the probability of breast cancer in first degree relatives. *Int J Cancer* **86**:883–887.

Xu J and the International Consortium for Prostate Cancer Genetics (2000) Combined analysis of hereditary prostate cancer linkage to 1q 24–25: results from 772 hereditary prostate cancer families from the International Consortium for Prostate Cancer Genetics. *Am J Hum Genet* **66**:945–957.

Xu J, Meyers D, Freije D, *et al*. (1998) Evidence for a prostate cancer susceptibility locus on the X chromosome. *Nature Genetics* **20**:175–179.

Xu J, Zheng SL, Hawkins GA, *et al*. (2001) Linkage and association studies of prostate cancer susceptibility: evidence for linkage at 8p22–23. *Am J Hum Genet* **69**(2):341–350.

4 Molecular biology of progression of prostate cancer

Tapio Visakorpi

Introduction

Prostate cancer is the most common malignancy among men in many Western countries, and the incidence of the disease has sharply increased in recent decades (Kosary *et al.* 1995, Finnish Cancer Registry 2000). Localized prostate cancer is curable by radical prostatectomy or radiation therapy. However, many patients are diagnosed at the time when the disease has already spread beyond the prostate gland. In addition, about one-third of the patients that are assumed to have localized disease, and thus should be curable by prostatectomy or radiation therapy, later experience relapse (Gittes 1991, DeKernion *et al.* 1998). The growth of prostate cancer is highly dependent on androgens. Thus, androgen withdrawal, achieved by chemical or surgical castration, has become the treatment of choice for advanced prostate cancer. Initially, almost all patients respond to androgen ablation (Palmberg *et al.* 1999). Later, however, an androgen-independent or hormone-refractory tumor clone emerges, leading to clinical progression of the disease. The progression of prostate cancer during hormonal therapy is a major clinical problem, since there are no effective therapies available for such hormone-refractory disease (Gittes 1991). One major obstacle in developing treatment for hormone-refractory prostate cancer has been the lack of understanding of the mechanisms of the disease's progression. In the following chapters some of the aspects of the molecular basis of the progression of prostate cancer are discussed.

Chromosomal alterations

During the last decades, genetic aberrations underlying the development and progression of prostate cancer have been studied using several techniques, such as traditional cytogenetics, loss of heterozygosity analysis (LOH), fluorescence in-situ hybridization (FISH) and, especially, comparative genomic hybridization (CGH) (Kallioniemi & Visakorpi 1996). We have utilized CGH for screening prostate tumors for such genetic alterations. CGH is a fairly new molecular cytogenetic method that allows the detection of DNA sequence copy number changes throughout the genome in a single hybridization (Kallioniemi *et al.* 1992). It is helpful in both defining chromosomal regions that may harbour amplified oncogenes or deleted tumor suppressor genes and investigating the clonal evolution of tumor progression.

In order to study the clonal evolution of prostate cancer during the hormonal therapy, we analyzed primary untreated and corresponding hormone/refractory recurrent tumor pairs from 6 patients (Nupponen *et al.* 1998). Three of the cases showed a close genetic relationship, as evidenced by the high number of shared genetic alterations in the primary and the recurrent tumors, whereas in the rest of the cases such a relationship was not that evident. The result emphasizes that androgen ablation therapy can act as a selection force that may select a clone genetically very different from the primary tumor. The fact that recurrent tumors may share only few genetic alterations with the primary tumors suggests also that the analyzes of exclusively primary tumors give only a restricted view of the prostate cancer.

By screening larger number of untreated primary and hormonally treated recurrent prostate carcinomas, we have also found that the recurrent tumors contain about four times more genetic alterations than the untreated primary tumors. The most notable difference between these tumor types is that the gains and amplifications, which are almost completely missing in the hormone-dependent prostate carcinomas, are common in the hormone-refractory tumors. The results suggest that the early development of prostate cancer is attributable to the inactivation of tumor suppressor genes, whereas the late progression of the disease is also associated with activation of oncogenes (Visakorpi *et al.* 1995a, Nupponen *et al.* 1998). By CGH, the most common genetic alterations in the locally-recurrent hormone-refractory prostate carcinomas are losses of 1p, 6q, 8p, 10q, 13q, 16q, 19, and 22, as well as gains of 7q, 8q, 18q, and Xq.

Genes involved in the progression of prostate cancer

The chromosomal alterations found by CGH and other methods pinpoint the regions where the genes that are involved in the development and progression of malignancy are located. Based on this information, it is possible to identify the target genes of the chromosomal alterations. We have, so far, concentrated on two chromosomal regions, 8q and Xq, which are the most common regions of gains in hormone-refractory prostate cancer.

Putative target genes for the 8q gain

Gain of the whole long arm of chromosome 8 is the most common aberration in hormone-refractory prostate cancer observed in the CGH analyzes (Nupponen *et al.* 1998) and it is associated with an aggressive phenotype of the disease (Alers *et al.* 2000). Almost 90% of hormone-refractory and distant metastases, whereas only 5% of untreated prostate carcinomas, show gain of 8q (Visakorpi *et al.* 1995a, Nupponen *et al.* 1998, Cher *et al.* 1996). Within the q arm, two independently amplified subregions, 8q21 and 8q23–q24, have been identified by CGH, suggesting the presence of several target genes (Nupponen *et al.* 1998, Cher *et al.* 1996). One putative target gene for amplification is the well known oncogene MYC located at 8q24.1 (Dalla-Favera *et al.* 1982). Amplification of MYC has been found in about 8% of the primary and 11–30% of the advanced (hormone-refractory or metastatic lesions) prostate cancers (Nupponen *et al.* 1998, Jenkins *et al.* 1997, Bubendorf *et al.* 1999). The amplification seems to be associated with poor prognosis among patients with locally advanced prostate cancer (Sato *et al.* 1999). However, since there are at least two minimal commonly amplified regions at 8q, and since MYC amplification does not always correlate with overexpression of the gene, it is possible that there are other target genes for the gain at 8q (Nupponen *et al.* 1998, Bieche *et al.* 1999). Using a suppression subtractive hybridization technique, we have now been able to identify one such putative target gene, EIF3S3, located at 8q23 (Nupponen *et al.* 1999). Amplification and overexpression of EIF3S3 was found in about 30% of recurrent hormone-refractory prostate carcinomas, using FISH. Although the EIF3S3 was most often co-amplified with MYC, tumors in which EIF3S3 was highly amplified without MYC amplification were also found (Nupponen *et al.* 2000). In addition, the EIF3S3 is consistently overexpressed in tumors containing the gene amplification. The findings clearly suggest that EIF3S3 may be one of the putative target genes for the 8q gain.

The EIF3S3 (alias eIF3–p40) gene encodes for a p40 subunit of the largest eukaryotic translation initiation factor protein complex, eIF3, which has a central role in the initiation of translation. The eIF3 complex binds to 40S ribosomal subunits in the absence of other initiation factors and preserves the dissociated state of 40S and 60S ribosomal subunits. It also stabilizes eIF2·GTP·Met-tRNA, binding to 40S subunits and mRNA binding to ribosomes (Hershey *et al.* 1996). However, very little is known about the p40 subunit itself. Based on the sequence homology, it seems to be related to mouse protein Mov-34 (Asano *et al.*, 1997). The gene product of the human homologue of Mov-34 is a component of the 26S proteasome. However, based on current knowledge, it is not possible to draw conclusions on how EIF3S3 could be involved in the tumorigenesis.

Therefore, functional studies, in addition to studies aiming at defining the clinical significance, are required.

A third possible target gene as regards gain at 8q is prostate stem cell antigen (PSCA), which was recently cloned and localized to 8q24.2 (Reiter *et al.* 1998). Overexpression of PSCA has particularly been observed in poorly differentiated prostate tumors and bone metastases. The PSCA gene is often co-amplified with MYC. However, cases with MYC amplification without PSCA amplification have also been reported (Reiter *et al.* 2000).

Androgen receptor (AR) gene

As mentioned earlier, the gain of Xq is one of the most common chromosomal aberrations in the hormone-refractory prostate carcinomas. By CGH, we were able to narrow down the minimal commonly amplified region to Xq11–q13, in which androgen receptor (AR) gene is located. Subsequently, we showed by FISH that AR is highly amplified in 30% of hormone-refractory prostate carcinomas (Visakorpi *et al.* 1995b, Koivisto *et al.* 1997). No untreated prostate carcinomas have shown such amplification, suggesting that it occurs as a result of selection after androgen withdrawal (Visakorpi *et al.* 1995b, Koivisto *et al.* 1998, Bubendorf *et al.* 1999, Miyoshi *et al.* 2000). The amplification leads to the overexpression of the gene (Linja *et al.* 2001). In addition, it seems that practically all hormone-refractory prostate carcinomas (whether containing the amplification of the gene or not) express more AR than androgen-dependent prostate carcinomas, although the tumors with the gene amplification express the AR even more than tumors without the amplification (Linja *et al.* 2001, Latil *et al.* 2001). The data suggest that the AR signalling pathway is important even in the so-called androgen-refractory prostate cancer.

The precise mechanism by which amplification and overexpression of AR is involved in the emergence of hormone-refractory prostate cancer is not known. In a preliminary study, we have shown that tumors containing AR gene amplification respond better to so-called maximal androgen blockade, i.e. abolishing the effects of adrenal androgen remaining in the serum after castration (Palmberg *et al.* 2000). The finding indicates that the amplified and overexpressed AR is truly functional. We have suggested that amplification of the AR gene could hypersensitize the cells to low ligand concentrations. It is also possible that over-expressed AR is activated by ligands other than androgens. Activation of the AR has been described, in the absence of androgens, with specific growth factors such as IGF-1, KGF and EGF (Culig *et al.* 1994). In addition, it has been suggested that HER-2/neu (ERBB2) tyrosine kinase pathway could interact with AR, especially when androgen levels are reduced (Craft *et al.* 1999).

Certain point mutations are known to alter the transactivational properties of the AR molecule: for example, activating the receptor by other steroids than androgens or even by antiandrogens. Thus, the mutations of AR in prostate cancer have been extensively studied during the past 10 years. Still, the frequency of the mutations is under dispute. Most studies, including ours, suggest that mutations are rare (Wallen *et al.* 1999, reviewed in Koivisto *et al.* 1998). However, recent papers by Taplin and co-workers studying patients treated with an antiandrogen, flutamide, showed mutations in about one-third of the patients (Taplin *et al.* 1995, 1999). These mutations cluster to codon 877, modulating the receptor molecule in such a manner that it can be paradoxically activated by flutamide. Thus, it seems that flutamide is able to select a cell clone that contains a codon 877 mutation in the same way that castration selects the AR gene amplification.

Several co-regulators affecting the transactivational properties of AR have recently been cloned (reviewed in Elo & Visakorpi 2001). Some of the co-regulators, such as ARA70, may alter the function of AR in such a manner that the receptor molecule can be activated by antiandrogens or other steroid hormones than androgens. Thus, alterations in the co-regulators could be involved in the progression of prostate cancer (Miyamoto *et al.* 1998). However, the studies, so far, have mainly been done *in vitro*. And, almost nothing is known about, for example, the expression of these genes in prostate cancer *in vivo*.

Conclusions

Molecular genetic studies have now indicated several genes that may be involved in the progression of prostate cancer. In particular, the AR signalling pathway seems to have a central role in hormonal treatment failure. The chromosomal analyzes have also clearly indicated that gain of 8q is associated with an aggressive phenotype of the disease. One of the most important goals in future studies is to identify the possible several target genes of this amplification. It is hoped that by recognizing and understanding molecular mechanisms, new treatment strategies for prostate cancer could be developed. For example, it is evident that current hormonal therapies are not good enough to block the AR signalling pathways: new strategies directed against the AR could be developed.

References

Alers JC, Rochat J, Krijtenburg PJ, *et al.* (2000) Identification of genetic markers for prostatic cancer progression. *Lab Invest* **80**:931–942.

Asano K, Vornlocher HP, Richter-Cook NJ, *et al.* (1997) Structure of cDNAs encoding human eukaryotic initiation factor 3 subunits. Possible roles in RNA binding and macromolecular assembly. *J Biol Chem* **272**:27042–27052.

Bieche I, Laurendeau I, Tozlu S, *et al.* (1999) Quantitation of MYC gene expression in sporadic breast tumors with a real-time reverse transcription-PCR assay. *Cancer Res* **59**:2759–65.

Bubendorf L, Kononen J, Koivisto P, *et al.* (1999) Survey of gene amplifications during prostate cancer progression by high-throughout fluorescence in situ hybridization on tissue microarrays. *Cancer Res* **59**:803–806.

Cher ML, Bova GS, Moore DH, *et al.* (1996) Genetic alterations in untreated metastases and androgen independent prostate cancer detected by comparative genomic hybridization and allelotyping. *Cancer Res* **56**:3091–3102.

Craft N, Shostak Y, Carey M, Sawyers CL (1999) A mechanism for hormone-independent prostate cancer through modulation of androgen receptor signaling by the HER-2/neu tyrosine kinase. *Nature Med* **5**:280–285.

Culig Z, Hobisch A, Cronauer MV, *et al.* (1994) Androgen receptor activation in prostatic tumor cell lines by insulin-like growth factor-I, keratinocyte growth factor, and epidermal growth factor. *Cancer Res* **54**:5474–5478.

Dalla-Favera R, Bregni M, Erikson J, *et al.* (1982) Human c-myc onc gene is located on the region of chromosome 8 that is translocated in Burkitt lymphoma cells. *Proc Natl Acad Sci USA* **79**:7824–7827.

DeKernion J, Belldegrun A, Naitoh J (1998) Surgical treatment of localized prostate cancer: indications, technique and results. In: Belldegrun A, Kirby RS, Oliver T, eds, *New Perspectives in Prostate Cancer* (Isis Medical Media Ltd: Oxford) 185–203.

Elo J, Visakorpi T (2001) Molecular genetics of prostate cancer. *Ann Med* **33**:130–141.

Finnish Cancer Registry (2000) Cancer incidence in Finland 1996 and 1997. Cancer Society of Finland, Pub. No. 61, Helsinki.

Gittes RF (1991) Carcinoma of the prostate. *N Engl J Med* **324**:236–245.

Hershey JW, Asano K, Naranda T, *et al.* (1996) Conservation and diversity in the structure of translation initiation factor EIF3 from humans and yeast. *Biochimie* **78**:903–907.

Jenkins RB, Qian J, Lieber MM, Bostwick DG (1997) Detection of c-myc oncogene amplification and chromosomal anomalies in metastatic prostatic carcinoma by fluorescence in situ hybridization. *Cancer Res* **57**:524–531.

Kallioniemi O-P, Visakorpi T (1996) Genetic basis and clonal evolution of human prostate cancer. *Adv Cancer Res* **68**:225–255.

Kallioniemi A, Kallioniemi OP, Sudar D, *et al.* (1992) Comparative genomic hybridization for molecular cytogenetic analysis of solid tumors. *Science* **258**:818–821.

Koivisto P, Kolmer M, Visakorpi T, Kallioniemi OP (1998) Androgen receptor gene and hormonal therapy failure of prostate cancer. *Am J Pathol* **152**:1–9.

Koivisto P, Kononen J, Palmberg C, *et al.* (1997) Androgen receptor gene amplification: a possible molecular mechanism for failure of androgen deprivation therapy in prostate cancer. *Cancer Res* **57**:314–319.

Kosary CL, Ries LAG, Miller BA, *et al.* (1995) SEER Cancer Statistics Review, 1973–1992: tables and graphs. National Cancer Institute. NIH Pub. No. 96–2789, Bethesda, MD.

Latil A, Bieche I, Vidaud D, *et al.* (2001) Evaluation of androgen, estrogen (ERα and ERβ), and progesterone receptor expression in human prostate cancer by real-time quantitative reverse transcription-polymerase chain reaction assays. *Cancer Res* **61**:1919–1926.

Linja MJ, Savinainen KJ, Saramäki OR, *et al.* (2001) Amplification and overexpression of androgen receptor gene in hormone-refractory prostate cancer. *Cancer Res* **61**:3550–3555.

Miyamoto H, Yeh S, Wilding G, Chang C (1998) Promotion of agonist activity of antiandrogens by the androgen receptor coactivator, ARA70, in human prostate cancer DU145 cells. *Proc Natl Acad Sci USA* **95**:7379–7384.

Miyoshi Y, Uemura H, Fujinami K, *et al.* (2000) Fluorescence in situ hybridization evaluation of c-myc and androgen receptor gene amplification and chromosomal anomalies in prostate cancer in Japanese patients. *Prostate* **43**:225–232.

Nupponen NN, Isola J, Visakorpi T (2000) Mapping the amplification of EIF3S3 in breast and prostate cancer. *Genes Chrom Cancer* **28**:203–210.

Nupponen NN, Kakkola L, Koivisto P, Visakorpi T (1998) Genetic alterations in hormone-refractory recurrent prostate carcinomas. *Am J Pathol* **153**:141–148.

Nupponen NN, Porkka K, Kakkola L, *et al.* (1999) Amplification and overexpression of p40 subunit of eukaryotic translation initiation factor 3 in breast and prostate cancer. *Am J Pathol* **154**:1777–1783.

Palmberg C, Koivisto P, Kakkola L, *et al.* (2000) Androgen receptor gene amplification at the time of primary progression predicts response to combined androgen blockade as a second-line therapy in advanced prostate cancer. *J Urol* **164**:1992–1995.

Palmberg C, Koivisto P, Visakorpi T, Tammela TLJ (1999) PSA decline is an independent prognostic marker in hormonally treated prostate cancer. *Eur Urol* **36**:191–196.

Reiter RE, Gu Z, Watabe T, *et al.* (1998) Prostate stem cell antigen: a cell surface marker overexpressed in prostate cancer. *Proc Natl Acad Sci USA* **95**:1735–1740.

Reiter RE, Sato I, Thomas G, *et al.* (2000) Coamplification of prostate stem cell antigen (PSCA) and MYC in locally advanced prostate cancer. *Genes Chrom Cancer* **27**:95–103.

Sato K, Qian J, Slezak JM, *et al.* (1999), Clinical significance of alterations of chromosome 8 in high-grade, advanced, nonmetastatic prostate carcinoma. *J Natl Cancer Inst* **91**:1574–1580.

Taplin ME, Bubley GJ, Ko YJ, *et al.* (1999). Selection for androgen receptor mutations in prostate cancers treated with androgen antagonist. *Cancer Res* **59**:2511–2515.

Taplin ME, Bubley GJ, Shuster TD, *et al.* (1995). Mutation of the androgen-receptor gene in metastatic androgen-independent prostate cancer. *N Engl J Med* **332**:1393–1398.

Visakorpi T, Kallioniemi AH, Syvänen AC, *et al.* (1995a) Genetic changes in primary and recurrent prostate cancer by comparative genomic hybridization. *Cancer Res* **55**:342–347.

Visakorpi T, Hyytinen E, Koivisto P, *et al.* (1995b) In vivo amplification of the androgen receptor gene and progression of human prostate cancer. *Nature Genetics* **9**:401–406.

Wallen MJ, Linja M, Kaartinen K, Schleutker J, Visakorpi T (1999) Androgen receptor gene mutations in hormone-refractory prostate cancer. *J Pathol* **189**:559–563.

5 Human genetic variation at hormone-metabolic loci and prostate cancer risk

Nick M Makridakis, Ronald K Ross and Juergen KV Reichardt

Abstract

Prostate cancer is a serious and common malignancy in the United States and other industrialized countries: it is currently the most commonly diagnosed serious cancer and the second leading cause of cancer deaths in American men. Substantial epidemiologic evidence supports a role for race/ethnicity and androgen levels in prostate cancer. Furthermore, androgens have been shown to induce prostate adenocarcinomas in experimental rat models.

We review here epidemiologic data on SNPs (single nucleotide polymorphisms) in a series of androgen-metabolic loci:

1. the type II (or prostatic) steroid 5α-reductase (SRD5A2) gene
2. the type II 3β-hydroxysteroid dehydrogenase (HSD3B2) gene
3. other loci and potential candidate genes.

We conclude that, while early associations for certain polymorphisms are promising, further investigations of these and other candidate loci along with a systematic identification and functional characterization of SNPs are required.

Introduction

In the US some 198 100 men will be diagnosed with prostate cancer in 2001 alone and 31 500 men will die of the disease during the same year (Greenlee *et al.* 2001). In fact, prostate cancer is the most commonly diagnosed serious malignancy among men in the US and the second leading cause of male cancer deaths in this country (Greenlee *et al.* 2001).

Prostate cancer is rare before the age of 30, but the rate of increase thereafter is such that by the time a man is 90 years old, he has almost a 100% chance of having the disease (e.g. Peehl 1999). There is a large variation in prostate cancer incidence rates between racial/ethnic groups in the United States: highest in African-Americans, intermediate in Caucasians and Latinos and lowest in Asian-Americans (Bernstein & Ross 1991). These and other epidemiologic data provide support for a significant genetic component to prostate cancer risk, although environmental risk factors must also play an important role. In addition, epidemiologic and biochemical evidence suggests that variations on androgen levels may play a role in the risk for prostate cancer (Ross *et al.* 1992).

Two recent publications reported millions of SNPs (single nucleotide polymorphisms) in the human genome (Sachinandam *et al.* 2001, Venter *et al.* 2001). The systematic identification and careful functional characterization of

SNPs will aid human genetic association studies, including the dissection of prostate cancer, greatly.

Androgens and prostate cancer

Androgens play an important role in normal and abnormal prostate development. Studies of androgens and prostate cancer go back 60 years and were rewarded with a Nobel Prize (Huggins & Hodges 1941, Bosland 2000). Both testosterone (T) and dihydrotestosterone (DHT) have been shown to induce prostate adenocarcinomas in experimental rat models (Noble 1977). Normal prostate growth and development are both induced by DHT. In men, T is produced in large amounts by the testes (Cheng *et al.* 1993). It is then irreversibly metabolized to DHT, mainly in the prostate gland. DHT (or, much less efficiently, T) is bound by the androgen receptor (AR) (Figure 5.1). This complex then translocates to the cell nucleus where it activates transcription of several genes with androgen-responsive elements (AREs) in their promoters (Cheng *et al.* 1993). This process ultimately results in increased DNA synthesis (Figure 5.1). DHT is known to promote DNA synthesis and cell replication in the prostate (Cheng *et al.* 1993). Thus, increased prostatic DHT levels may increase the chance for prostate cancer.

Steroid 5α-reductase type II (SRD5A2) gene

Steroid 5α-reductase (testosterone 5α-reductase; EC 1.3.99.5) is a membrane-bound

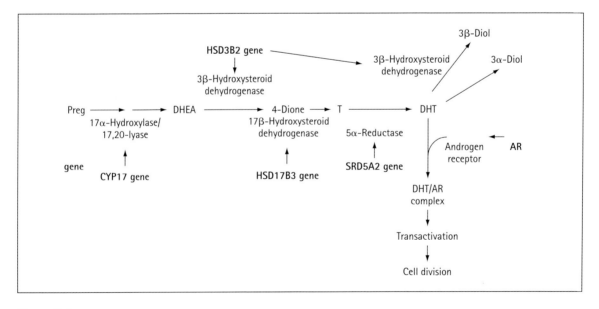

Figure 5.1
Human androgen metabolism. Steroid abbreviations are Preg = pregnenolone; DHEA = dehydro-epiandrosterone; 4-Dione = 4-androstenedione; T = testosterone; DHT = dihydrotestosterone; 3α-Diol = 3α-androstanediol; 3β-Diol = 3β-androstanediol.

enzyme that catalyzes the irreversible conversion of testosterone to dihydrotestosterone (Figure 5.1), with NADPH (nicotinamide adenine dinucleotide phosphate, reduced form) as a cofactor (Cheng *et al.* 1993). Two isozymes have been characterized so far in humans: the type I enzyme with an alkaline pH optimum, encoded by the SRD5A1 gene, and the type II enzyme with an acidic pH optimum *in vitro*, encoded by the SRD5A2 gene (Thigpen *et al.* 1993). Thigpen *et al.* (1993) showed that the type I isozyme is expressed primarily in newborn scalp, skin and liver, while the type II isozyme protein is expressed primarily in genital skin and the prostate gland.

Cloning and characterization of the SRD5A2 gene has demonstrated that it is located on the short arm of human chromosome 2 (band 2p23) and that it is comprised of five exons and four introns (Thigpen *et al.* 1992). A rare disorder of male sexual differentiation, male pseudohermaphroditism due to 5α-reductase deficiency (originally called pseudovaginal perineoscrotal hypospadias; Wilson *et al.* 1993), is caused by inactivating germline mutations in the SRD5A2 gene (reviewed by Russell & Wilson 1994). 46 X, Y affected males exhibit genital ambiguity and external female characteristics until puberty, at which point there is some development of male secondary sex characteristics, but the prostate remains highly underdeveloped (Wilson *et al.* 1993). Thus, normal prostate development requires the normal function of the SRD5A2 gene.

Makridakis *et al.* (1999) reported data on a missense mutation, also known as non-synonymous SNP: A49T (alanine at codon 49 replaced by threonine), that is associated with a 7.2-fold increased risk of advanced prostate cancer in African-American men ($p = 0.001$) and a 3.6-fold increased risk in Latino men ($p = 0.04$). Significantly, this mutation also increases steroid 5α-reductase activity five-fold *in vitro* (when measured as apparent V_{max}; Makridakis *et al.* 1999), providing a biochemical rationale for the increased risk. Jaffe *et al.* (2000) subsequently showed a significant association between the presence of the A49T mutation and a greater frequency of extracapsular prostate cancer as well as a higher pathological tumor–lymph node–metastasis (pTNM) stage and poor disease prognosis, in mostly Caucasian patients.

Interestingly, the SRD5A2 locus also encodes significant pharmacogenetic variation for different competitive steroid 5α-reductase inhibitors, such as finasteride (Makridakis *et al.* 1999, Makridakis *et al.* 2000). For example, finasteride has a 12-fold lower affinity (measured as apparent K_i) in the A49T mutant enzyme than for the wild-type protein (Makridakis *et al.* 1999). This and other pharmacogenetic variation at the SRD5A2 locus should be taken into account when prescribing steroid 5α-reductase inhibitors for the chemoprevention or treatment of prostatic and other diseases (Makridakis *et al.* 2000). In summary, there is a 200-fold natural variation in V_{max} and a 60-fold natural variation in K_i at the SRD5A2 locus (Makridakis *et al.* 2000). This significant biochemical and pharmacogenetic variation has important implications for prostate cancer risk in particular and human genetics in general.

3α-Hydroxysteroid dehydrogenase type II (HSD3B2) gene

As discussed above, DHT is the most active androgen in the prostate gland (Cheng *et al.* 1993). It is synthesized from T by the enzyme steroid 5α-reductase and it is inactivated through a reductive reaction catalyzed by either 3α- or 3β-hydroxysteroid dehydrogenase (Figure 5.1; Cheng *et al.* 1993). Both reductions use NAD(P)H (nicotinamide adenine dinucleotide (phosphate), reduced form) as a cofactor (Cheng *et al.* 1993). Thus, the 3β-hydroxysteroid dehydrogenase enzyme (EC 1.1.1.210) is one of the two enzymes that initiate the irreversible inactivation of DHT in the prostate. In addition, 3β-hydroxysteroid dehydrogenase is responsible for the production of androstenedione in the adrenals, which in subsequent steps is converted to DHT in the prostate (Figure 5.1). Thus, 3β-hydroxysteroid dehydrogenase may affect both the synthesis and degradation of DHT. Finally, it has been reported that the activity of the two 3-hydroxysteroid dehydrogenase enzymes is significantly lower in abnormal prostatic tissue (Bartsch *et al.* 1990). Thus, DHT might accumulate in the prostate because of slower degradation (Figure 5.1).

3β-Hydroxysteroid dehydrogenase in humans can act on a number of steroid substrates, including DHT (Labrie *et al.* 1992). This enzyme activity is encoded by two closely linked yet distinct loci: the HSD3B1 and HSD3B2 genes, which are both located in chromosome band 1p13 (Berube *et al.* 1989). The type I gene (HSD3B1) encodes the isoform present in the placenta and peripheral tissues such as skin and mammary gland, while expression of the type II enzyme is restricted to adrenals and gonads (Labrie *et al.* 1992, Rheaume *et al.* 1992).

Cloning and characterization of the human HSD3B2 gene has revealed that it spans about 7.8 kb of genomic DNA in four exons (Lachance *et al.* 1991). Mutations in this gene cause male pseudohermaphroditism with congenital adrenal hyperplasia (e.g. Simard *et al.* 1993), but no mutations have yet been reported in prostate cancer patients.

A complex dinucleotide repeat polymorphism has been reported in the third intron of the HSD3B2 gene (Verreault *et al.* 1994). These authors discovered nine alleles of a $(TG)_n$ $(TA)_n$ $(CA)_n$ STR (short tandem repeat). Devgan *et al.* (1997) exploited this finding and subsequently reported substantial allelic differences, which include at least 25 different alleles, at the HSD3B2 locus among African-Americans, Asians and Caucasians. Some of these alleles appear at higher frequencies in prostate cancer cases than in controls, in distinct racial/ethnic groups (Devgan *et al.* 1997). This racial/ethnic diversity at the HSD3B2 locus suggests that it may play a role in the racial/ethnic variation in prostate cancer risk. Additional screening of the HSD3B2 gene should be carried out for the systematic identification and characterization of SNPs and mutations that may predispose to prostate cancer.

Other loci

Both T and DHT exert their androgenic effects through the androgen receptor (AR) protein (Figure 5.1), a transcription factor that transactivates genes with androgen receptor elements (AREs) in their promoters (Cheng *et al.* 1993). The AR gene is located on the long arm of the X-chromosome, and its large exon 1 is responsible for the transactivation activity of its mature gene product (e.g. Barrack *et al.* 1996). Increased activity or levels of the AR protein are expected to increase prostate cancer risk.

The AR gene has been the focus of intense molecular epidemiologic investigations. It appears that a polymorphic $(CAG)_n$ trinucleotide repeat in the exon 1 of the AR gene which encodes a polyglutamine stretch plays a role in predisposition to prostate cancer. In fact, shorter alleles of the $(CAG)_n$ repeat seem to be associated with a modest (specifically 1.5- to 2.1-fold) increase in prostate cancer risk (e.g. Giovannucci *et al.* 1997, Ingles *et al.* 1997, Xue *et al.* 2000). Other studies, however, reported no significant associations (e.g. Correa-Cerro *et al.* 1999, Edwards *et al.* 1999, Bratt *et al.* 1999), or weak and statistically insignificant association (Stanford *et al.* 1997), between the presence of shorter $(CAG)_n$ repeat alleles and prostate cancer. The polymorphic polyglutamine stretch also appears to have biochemical consequences *in vitro* (Tut *et al.* 1997). AR receptors with expanded $(CAG)_n$ repeats cloned from patients with Kennedy disease (an adult-onset X-linked disease associated with low virilization, decreased sperm production, testicular atrophy and reduced fertility; Tut *et al.* 1997), exhibit 50% lower transactivation activity but normal androgen-binding activity (Tut *et al.* 1997). Thus, it is likely that shorter $(CAG)_n$ repeats are causing increased prostate cancer risk through increased AR transactivation (Figure 5.1).

Another androgen metabolic locus that may play a role in prostate cancer predisposition is the HSD17B3 gene, which encodes 17β-hydroxysteroid dehydrogenase (HSD) type III, the testicular 17-ketoreductase (Geissler *et al.* 1994). This enzyme utilizes NADP(H) as a cofactor and favors the reduction of androstenedione to testosterone, in the testis (Geissler *et al.* 1994). Thus, mutations in this gene may increase the production of T in the testes, which can directly or indirectly (through DHT) activate the AR, potentially increasing prostate cancer risk (Figure 5.1). The HSD17B3 gene is located in chromosomal band 9q22 and contains 11 exons (Geissler *et al.* 1994). No mutations of this gene have yet been reported in prostate cancer, but several inactivating HSD17B3 mutations have been reported to cause another form of male pseudohermaphroditism, called 17β-hydroxysteroid dehydrogenase deficiency (e.g. Geissler *et al.* 1994).

Estrogens are also suspected to contribute to the etiology of prostate cancer and BPH (e.g. Tsugaya *et al.* 1996, Bonkhoff *et al.* 1999, Bosland, 2000). The aromatase cytochrome p450 enzyme which is encoded by the CYP19 gene is mainly localized in the ovary and the placenta, and it converts androgens to estrogens (Harada *et al.* 1993). Aromatase mRNA and protein have both been detected in BPH and prostate cancer tissue, but not at significantly different levels between cancerous and non-cancerous tissue (Tsugaya *et al.* 1996, Hiramatsu *et al.* 1997). Several CYP19 polymorphisms have been investigated in breast cancer (e.g. Probst-Hensch *et al.* 1999, Kristensen *et al.* 2000), but none in prostate cancer.

Conclusions

Despite the ample evidence linking androgens and prostate cancer, convincing molecular epidemiologic evidence for the involvement of androgen metabolic loci in prostate cancer exists for only one single-point mutation so far: the A49T non-synonymous SNP in the SRD5A2 gene. Two independent studies confirm a significant association between the presence of the A49T mutation and the presence of advanced prostate cancer in three racial/ethnic groups. Mechanistic/biochemical evidence also exists that provides a plausible etiologic mechanism for this increased prostate cancer risk: enhanced DHT production by the mutant allele (Figure 5.1). Other polymorphisms, though, yielded mixed results. The $(CAG)_n$ repeat in the AR gene, for example, has been shown by several studies both to be associated with – and not to be associated with – prostate cancer in Caucasians, even though mechanistic/biochemical data supportive of an etiologic association exists.

An important goal of the Human Genome Project is the systematic identification of SNPs (Sachinandam *et al.* 2001, Venter *et al.* 2001). Molecular investigations of prostate cancer show that:

- it is important to identify all SNPs, including rare ones such as the A49T mutation
- a complete functional analysis of SNPs allows for the identification of functionally significant 'candidate alleles' for mechanistically based association studies (cf. the A49T SNP)
- there is astounding biochemical and pharmacogenetic natural variation in humans that may lead to many phenotypes (see V_{max} and K_i variation at the SRD5A2 locus).

Future investigations of other loci should incorporate these important 'lessons'.

Acknowledgements

This work was supported by grants from the NCI (CA68581 and CA83112), the California CRP (99-0053V-10150), the DoD (PC992018 and PC001280) and the TJ Martell Foundation to JKVR and RKR.

References

Barrack ER (1996) Androgen receptor mutations in prostate cancer. *Mt Sinai J Med* **63**:403–412.

Bartsch W, Klein H, Schiemann U, Bauer HW, Voigt KD (1990) Enzymes of androgen formation and degradation in the human prostate. *Ann NY Acad Sci* **595**:53–66.

Berube D, Luu-The V, Lachance Y, Gagne R, Labrie F (1989) Assignment of the human 3B-hydroxysteroid dehydrogenase gene to the p13 band of chromosome 1. *Cytogen Cell Genet* **52**:199–200.

Bernstein L, Ross RK (1991) *Cancer in Los Angeles County, A Portrait of Incidence and Mortality* (USC Press: Los Angeles, CA).

Bonkhoff H, Fixemer T, Hunsicker I, Remberger K (1999) Estrogen receptor expression in prostate cancer and premalignant prostatic lesions. *Am J Pathol* **155**:641–647.

Bosland MC (2000) The role of steroid hormones in prostate carcinogenesis. *J Natl Cancer Inst Monographs* **27**:39–66

Bratt O, Borg A, Kristoffersson U, *et al.* (1999) CAG repeat length in the androgen receptor gene is related to age at diagnosis of prostate cancer and response to endocrine therapy, but not to prostate cancer risk. *Br J Cancer* **81**:672–676.

Cheng E, Lee C, Grayhack J (1993) Endocrinology of the prostate. In: Lepor, H and Lawson RK, eds, *Prostate Diseases* (WB Saunders: Philadelphia) 57–71.

Correa-Cerro L, Wohr G, Haussler J, *et al.* (1999) (CAG)n CAA and GGN repeats in the human androgen receptor gene are not associated with prostate cancer in a French–German population. *Eur J Hum Genet* **7**:357–362

Devgan SA, Henderson BE, Yu MC, *et al.* (1997) Genetic variation of 3beta-hydroxysteroid dehydrogenase type II in three racial/ethnic groups: implications for prostate cancer risk. *The Prostate* **33**:9–12.

Edwards SM, Badzioch MD, Minter R, *et al.* (1999) Androgen receptor polymorphisms: association with prostate cancer risk, relapse and overall survival. *Int J Cancer* **84**:458–465.

Geissler WM, Davis DL, Wu L, *et al.* (1994) Male pseudohermaphroditism caused by mutations of testicular 17 beta-hydroxysteroid dehydrogenase 3. *Nature Genet* **7**:34–39.

Giovannucci E, Stampfer MJ, Krithivas K, *et al.* (1997) The CAG repeat within the androgen receptor gene and its relationship to prostate cancer. *Proc Natl Acad Sci* **94**:3320–3323.

Greenlee RT, Hill-Harmon MB, Murray T, Thun M (2001) Cancer statistics, 2001, CA. *Cancer J Clin* **51**:15–36.

Harada N, Utsumi T, Takagi Y (1993) Tissue-specific expression of the human aromatase cytochrome P-450 gene by alternative use of multiple exons 1 and promoters, and switching of tissue-specific exons 1 in carcinogenesis. *Biochemistry* **90**:11312–11316.

Hiramatsu M, Maehara I, Ozaki M, Harada N, Orikasa S, Sasano H (1997) Aromatase in hyperplasia and carcinoma of the human prostate, *Prostate* **31**:118–124.

Huggins C, Hodges CV (1941) Studies on prostate cancer. *Cancer Res* **1**:293–297.

Ingles SA, Garcia DG, Wang W, *et al.* (2000) Vitamin D receptor genotype and breast cancer in Latinas (United States). *Cancer Causes Control* **11**:25–30.

Jaffe JM, Malkowicz SB, Walker AH, *et al.* (2000) Association of SRD5A2 genotype and pathologic characteristics of tumors. *Cancer Res* **60**:1626–1630.

Kristensen VN, Harada N, Yoshimura N, *et al.* (2000) Genetic variants of CYP19 (aromatase) and breast cancer risk. *Oncogene* **19**:1329–1333.

Labrie F, Simard J, Luu-The V, Belanger B, Pelletier G (1992) Structure, function and tissue-specific expression of 3beta-hydroxysteroid dehydrogenase/5ene-4ene isomerase enzymes in classical and peripheral intracrine steroidogenic tissue. *J Steroid Biochem Molec Biol* **43**:805–826.

Lachance Y, Luu-The V, Verreault H, *et al.* (1991) Structure of the human type II 3beta-hydroxysteroid dehydrogenase/delta^5-delta^4 isomerase (3beta-HSD) gene: adrenal and gonadal specificity. *DNA and Cell Biol* **10**:701–711.

Makridakis N, Ross RK, Pike MC, *et al.* (1999) A missense substitution in the *SRD5A2* gene is associated with prostate cancer in African-American and Hispanic men in Los Angeles. *Lancet* **354**:975–978.

Makridakis NM, di Salle E, Reichardt JKV (2000) Biochemical and pharmacogenetic dissection of human steroid 5α-reductase type II. *Pharmacogenetics* **10**:407–413.

Noble RL (1977). The development of prostate adenocarcinoma in Nb rats following prolonged sex hormone administration. *Cancer Res* **37**:1929–1933.

Peehl DM (1999) Vitamin D and prostate cancer risk. *Eur Urol* **35**:392–394.

Probst-Hensch NM, Ingles SA, Diep AT, *et al.* (1999) Aromatase and breast cancer susceptibility. *Endocr Relat Cancer* **6**:165–173.

Rheaume E, Simard J, Morel Y, *et al.* (1992) Congenital adrenal hyperplasia due to point mutations in the type II 3beta-hydroxysteroid dehydrogenase gene. *Nature Gen* **1**:239–245.

Ross RK, Bernstein L, Lobo RA, *et al.* (1992) 5-α Reductase activity and risk of prostate cancer among Japanese and US white and black males. *Lancet* **339**:887–889.

Ross RK, Pike MC, Coetzee GA, Reichardt JKV, *et al.* (1998) Androgen metabolism and prostate cancer: establishing a model of genetic susceptibility. *Cancer Res* **58**:4497–4504.

Russell DW, Wilson JD (1994) Steroid 5α-reductase: two genes /two enzymes. *Annu Rev Biochem* **63**:25–61.

Sachidanandam R, Weissman D, Schmidt SC, *et al.* (2001) A map of human genome sequence variation containing 1.42 million single nucleotide polymorphisms. The International SNP Map Working Group. *Nature* **409**:928–933.

Simard J, Rheaume E, Sanchez R, *et al.* (1993) Molecular basis of congenital adrenal hyperplasia due to 3β-hydroxysteroid dehydrogenase deficiency. *Molec Endocrinol* **7**:716–728.

Stanford JL, Just JJ, Gibbs M, *et al.* (1997) Polymorphic repeats in the androgen receptor gene: molecular markers of prostate cancer risk. *Cancer Res* **57**:1194–1198.

Thigpen AE, Davis DL, Milatovich A, *et al.* (1992) Molecular genetics of steroid 5α-reductase 2 deficiency. *J Clin Invest* **90**:799–809.

Thigpen AE, Silver RI, Guileyardo JM, *et al.* (1993) Tissue distribution and ontogeny of steroid 5alpha-reductase isozyme expression. *J Clin Invest* **92**:903–910.

Tsugaya M, Harada N, Tozawa K, *et al.* (1996) Aromatase mRNA levels in benign prostatic hyperplasia and prostate cancer. *Int J Urol* **3**:292–296.

Tut TG, Ghadessy FJ, Trifiro MA, *et al.* (1997) Long polyglutamine tracts in the androgen receptor are associated with reduced trans-activation, impaired sperm production, and male infertility. *J Clin Endocrinol Metab* **82**:3777–3782.

Venter JC, Adams MD, Myers EW, *et al.* (2001) The sequence of the human genome. *Science* **291**:1304–1351.

Verreault H, Dufort I, Simard J, Labrie F, Luu-The V (1994) Dinucleotide repeat polymorphisms in the HSD3B2 gene. *Hum Molec Genet* **3**:384.

Wilson JD, Griffin JE, Russell DW (1993) Steroid 5α-reductase 2 deficiency. *Endocrine Rev* **14**:577–593.

Xue W, Irvine RA, Yu MC, *et al.* (2000) Susceptibility to prostate cancer: interaction between genotypes at the androgen receptor and prostate-specific antigen loci. *Cancer Res* **60**:839–841.

6 Ligand-dependent and independent activation of the androgen receptor and implications for therapy

Helmut Klocker, Zoran Culig, Iris Eder, Claudia Nessler-Manardi, Iveta Iotova, Alfred Hobisch and Georg Bartsch

Introduction

There is currently no curative treatment available for non-organ confined prostate cancer. Only when a tumor is detected at an early, organ-confined stage – for example, through prostate specific antigen (PSA) based screenings (Horninger *et al.* 2000) – can curative surgery be performed. The main choice of palliative treatment of non-organ confined prostate cancer is androgen ablation, which allows controlling tumor growth at least for some time (Auclerc *et al.* 2000). Deprivation of tumor cells from androgen supply by surgical or pharmacological castration (alone or in combination with antiandrogen treatment) results in inhibition of proliferation and induction of programmed cell death. However, almost all tumors develop resistance to endocrine therapy, and develop into an androgen-insensitive stage (Crawford *et al.* 1999).

The target of hormone ablation therapy and the central regulator of androgen effects is the androgen receptor (AR). Recent findings gave new insight into the molecular structure and function of the AR and improved our understanding about prostate cancer progression. It became clear that the AR is expressed in all tumor stages and can be activated ligand-dependently by androgens as well as ligand-independently by other hormones and various growth factors, respectively. Moreover, it was shown that the interaction of the AR with other proteins of the intracellular signal transduction cascade may promote prostate tumor growth. Further understanding of the role and function of the AR in prostate diseases and therapy failures will give us the basis to develop new treatment strategies.

The androgen receptor

The AR is a member of the superfamily of nuclear transcription factors, which includes the steroid hormone receptors retinoid and thyroid hormone receptors, receptors for vitamin D_3 and a number of so-called orphan receptors (Whitfield *et al.* 1999, Hager 2000). All members of this family share a unique molecular structure comprising a C-terminal ligand-binding domain, a DNA-binding domain that is built up of two zinc finger motifs, a hinge region, and an N-terminal transactivation domain (Figure 6.1) (Tilley *et al.* 1989, Fuller 1991). Through ligand binding or ligand-independent activation the AR is transformed into a transcription factor that interacts with so-called hormone-responsive elements in the DNA. This binding of the receptor to DNA in turn induces transcription of so-called androgen-regulated genes, such as for example prostate specific antigen (PSA) (Tsai & O'Malley 1994, Riegman *et al.* 1991, Rennie *et al.* 1993). With androgen ablation or antiandrogen treatment one blocks AR transcriptional activity – at least for some time. Then tumor cells develop resistance and androgen signalling is reactivated despite continuation of therapy. Immunohistochemical studies revealed that the AR is expressed in primary prostate tumors (van der Kwast *et al.* 1991, de Winter *et al.* 1990) as well as in metastatic lesions (Figure 6.2) (Hobisch *et al.* 1995a, 1995b). Moreover, Visakorpi and coworkers found amplifications of the AR gene and increased AR expression in tumors that recurred after androgen ablation therapy. This indicates that increased AR levels may facilitate tumor cell growth in a low-androgen environment and play an important role during progression of the disease (Palmberg *et al.* 1997, Koivisto *et al.* 1998, Nupponen *et al.* 1998). Because of these findings it became evident that androgen-independent prostate tumor cell growth is not caused by a loss of AR expression, as was assumed some years ago.

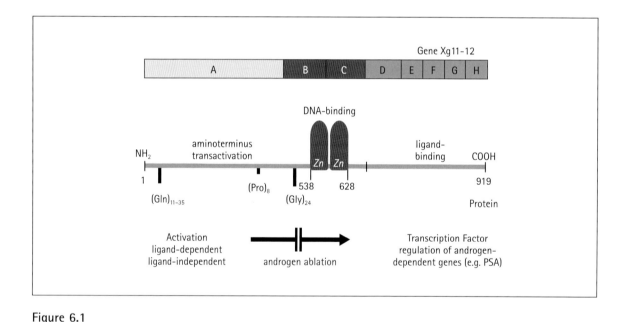

Figure 6.1

The androgen receptor gene and protein. The androgen receptor is a member of the superfamily of nuclear receptors; the gene is located on the long arm of the X chromosome at position Xq11–12. The AR comprises an N-terminal domain (amino acids 1–537), a DNA-binding domain (DBD) with two zinc finger motifs (amino acids 538–611), a hinge region (amino acids 612–661), and a ligand-binding domain at the C-terminus (amino acids 662–919). Two regions with activation function have been identified, AF-1 and AF-2. AF-1 is located in the N-terminal domain, whereas AF-2 was found in the ligand-binding domain. In the N-terminal domain there are also amino acid repeat regions such as the highly polymorphic glutamine repeat. Activation of the androgen receptor transforms it to an active transcription factor regulating the expression of androgen-sensitive genes such as prostate specific antigen (PSA). Androgen ablation therapy aims to block the transformation into a transcription factor.

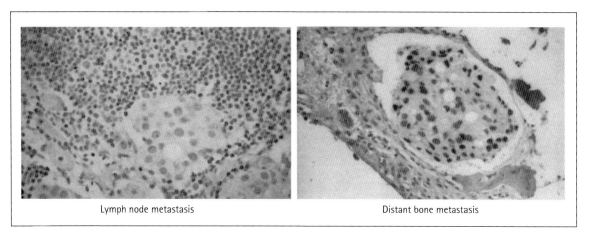

Lymph node metastasis   Distant bone metastasis

Figure 6.2
Androgen receptor expression in tumour metastasis. Immunohistochemical analysis revealed expression of androgen receptor in all stages of prostate cancer. Strong nuclear staining was found in primary tumours, lymph node and bone metastases. The picture shows a prostate cancer lymph node and a bone metastasis specimen, respectively, stained with a polyclonal anti–AR antibody.

LNCaP tumor progression model

Development of therapy resistance can be demonstrated in a cell culture model with the androgen-sensitive tumor cell line LNCaP. We kept these cells in an androgen-depleted medium for more than half a year and established a new subline, LNCaP-abl, which shows many characteristics resembling the situation in patients after escape from endocrine therapy (Culig *et al.* 1999). LNCaP-abl cells display a hypersensitive biphasic proliferative response to androgen. In comparison to parental LNCaP cells, maximal proliferation of LNCaP-abl cells was achieved at 10 times lower concentrations of androgen. At later passages, after more than a year in steroid-depleted culture medium, androgens exerted an inhibitory effect on growth of LNCaP-abl cells.

AR protein expression in LNCaP-abl cells increased approximately 4-fold. The basal AR transcriptional activity, assessed by trans-activation assay using the reporter plasmid ARE_2TATA-CAT, was 30-fold higher in LNCaP-abl than in LNCaP cells: 10 pmol of methyltrienolone (R1881) and 10 μmol of the antiandrogen hydroxyflutamide stimulated reporter gene activity in LNCaP-abl 3.2 and 4.1 times better than in parental LNCaP cells (Table 6.1). Noteworthy bicalutamide, that acts as a pure antagonist in parental LNCaP cells showed agonistic effects on AR trans-activation activity in LNCaP-abl cells and was not able to block the effects of androgen in these cells (Table 6.1). The changes in AR activity were associated neither with a new alteration of the AR cDNA sequence nor with amplification of the AR gene.

Growth of LNCaP-abl tumors in nude mice was stimulated by bicalutamide and repressed by testosterone (Figure 6.3). These results show for the first time that the non-steroidal antiandrogen bicalutamide acquires agonistic properties during long-term androgen ablation and these cells are a model to

Table 6.1 Hypersensitive androgen receptor on long–term androgen ablated cells.*

Stimulation	AR activity in LNCaP-abl (fold of parental LNCaP)	
No, 5% serum	30	
No, without serum	10	
10 pmol R1881	3.2	
1 nmol R1881	1.3	
10 μmol hydroxyflutamide	4.1	
Inhibition of AR activity	LNCaP	LNCaP-abl
1 μmol bicalutamide	90%	0%

*LNCaP and the long-term androgen ablated LNCaP-abl cells were transfected with the androgen-inducible reporter plasmid ARE_2TATA-CAT and treated with androgens and/or antiandrogens. Thereafter reporter gene activity was measured in the cell extracts. AR activity in LNCaP-abl cells was correlated to the activity of the parental LNCaP cells. Inhibition was calculated in percent.

study the causes of the antiandrogen with-drawal syndrome *in vitro* and *in vivo*. This phenomenon is observed in about one-third of patients treated with antiandrogens. When antiandrogens are withdrawn in these patients after escape from therapy, a decrease of PSA serum levels and an improvement of symptoms is observed, suggesting that the antiandrogens functioned as androgen receptor stimulators in these patients (Moul *et al.* 1995, Fuhrmann *et al.* 1998).

hormone binds to the LBD of the receptor, an activation cascade is induced, including release of heat-shock proteins, hyperphosphorylation, dimerization and conformational changes of the receptor (Prins 2000, McEwan 2000). This converts the AR into a transcription factor that is transported to the nucleus and regulates transcription of androgen-regulated genes (Riegman *et al.* 1992, Rennie *et al.* 1993, Murtha *et al.* 1993, Xu *et al.* 2000, Ulrix *et al.* 1999, Prescott & Tindall 1998).

Alteration of AR activation in prostate cancer

In the absence of hormone, the AR forms a complex with heat-shock proteins and is thus inactive (Smith & Toft 1993). As soon as a

Androgen receptor mutations

One mechanism that is involved in escape from therapy is mutation of the androgen receptor. Some 50 mutations were detected in prostate cancer specimens (for a comprehensive list visit

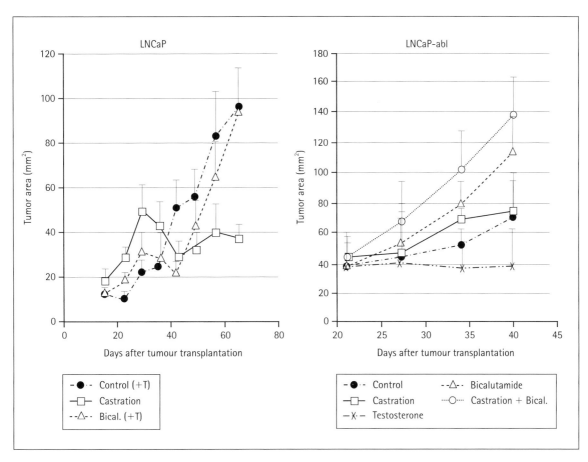

Figure 6.3

Androgen receptor activity in long-term androgen-ablated LNCaP cells. Tumours from parental (LNCaP) and long-term androgen-ablated (LNCaP-abl) cells were established in nude mice. Twenty days after transplantation the animals were treated as indicated and tumour growth was followed by determination of the tumour area. The long-term androgen-ablated cells show reversal of antagonist to agonist and vice versa. The parental LNCaP cells are stimulated by testosterone and moderately inhibited by the antiandrogen bicalutamide. LNCaP-abl cells are stimulated by bicalutamide and inhibited by testosterone.

the AR-mutations database: *http://ww2.mcgill.ca/androgendb/*). The fast majority are point mutations resulting in single amino acid exchanges; only a few mutations were detected that introduce a premature stop codon or affect non-coding regions of the AR gene. With two exceptions, androgen receptor mutations in prostate cancer are somatic mutations in the tumors of patients with an otherwise normal AR sequence. Most studies on prostate cancer revealed that AR mutations are rare in primary tumors from patients with localized prostate cancer and obviously do not account for prostate carcinogenesis. However, the frequency of AR mutations is mostly higher in distant metastases as compared with primary tumors (Marcelli *et al.* 2000, Suzuki *et al.* 1993, Taplin *et al.* 1995, Culig *et al.* 1998,

Klocker *et al.* 1996), indicating that AR mutations may play a crucial role in prostate cancer progression.

Some of the mutant receptors were characterized with regard to their functional properties. Their predominate feature is loss of androgen specificity and promiscuous activation by different steroids and antiandrogens (Tan *et al.* 1996, Culig *et al.* 1996b, Zhao *et al.* 2000). This may improve the survival conditions of a tumor during androgen ablation therapy. Among the ligands that activate one or several mutant androgen receptors in prostate tumor cells are estradiol, progesterone, glucocorticoids, adrenal androgens, androgen metabolites and the antiandrogens cyproterone acetate, hydroxyflutamide and nilutinamide. In the treatment of patients it has to be considered that androgen receptor mutations may convert the effect of antiandrogens into activating instead of blocking AR activity (Fenton *et al.* 1997, Wang *et al.* 2000).

Androgen receptor overexpression

Besides recruitment of non-classical AR ligands for activation, the increase of receptor concentration in the tumor cells seems to be another mode for circumventing the effects of androgen withdrawal. AR gene amplification is observed in about one-third of tumors after they escaped therapy. In these but also in tumors with only a single AR gene increased AR mRNA levels were measured by FISH techniques (Nupponen *et al.* 1998, Palmberg *et al.* 1997, Koivisto *et al.* 1998).

Ligand-independent androgen receptor activation

An important finding of androgen receptor research of recent years was the detection of androgen-independent AR activation through crosstalk with other signalling pathways: Ligand-independent AR activation by growth factors such as IGF-I and EGF or the cytokine IL6, neuropeptides and activators of protein kinase A (Culig *et al.* 1994, 1995, Culig *et al.* 1996a). Most important for the physiological situation and the situation in patients receiving endocrine prostate cancer treatment is the fact that ligand-independent AR activation acts synergistically together with very low concentrations of androgens. Androgen ablation nowadays is usually achieved by LHRH treatment, which inhibits testosterone biosynthesis. Most striking, this substance can also act directly in prostate tumor cells by activating the AR, which may counteract the inhibitory effects on androgen levels (Culig *et al.* 1997). LHRH induces adenylate cyclase in the tumor cells and since cAMP analogues show the same effect on AR activity, this indicates that LHRH effects on AR are mediated through the protein kinase A pathway.

The crosstalk with growth factor pathways needs an active mitogen-activated protein kinase (MAPK). Inhibition of MAPK activity with the specific inhibitor PD 98059 abrogates the effects of IGF-I or EGF on AR activity (Figure 6.4). In the same way, growth factor activation is strongly reduced when serine residue 515 in the AR is mutated to alanine, indicating that this is a site of interaction with MAPK. This site in the AR has the consensus recognition sequence for MAPK and is probably directly phosphorylated by activated

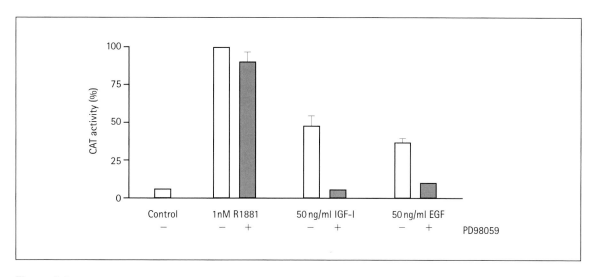

Figure 6.4

MAP kinase inhibition abrogates ligand-independent androgen receptor activation. An androgen-inducible reporter gene and an AR expression vector were cotransfected into Du-145 cells and cells were stimulated with the synthetic androgen R1881 or growth factors IGF-1 or EGF in the absence or presence of the MAP kinase inhibitor PD98059. Reporter gene activity was measured after 2 days and correlated to the activity induced by 1 nmol of R1881. Reporter gene induction by the growth factors was almost completely inhibited by the MAP kinase inhibitor, whereas androgen-induced activity was unchanged.

MAPK. Wen *et al.* (2000) recently also established an activation of the androgen receptor by protein kinase B (pKB, Akt-1), which phosphorylates the AR at sites 213 and 791, thus enhancing its transactivation activity.

Taken together, these findings revealed that the AR has more functions than those of the classical steroid receptor model. It is part of the cellular signalling network, interacting with several other regulatory pathways of the cell, which modulate its activity (Figure 6.5).

Androgen receptor coactivators

Steroid receptor cofactors are indispensable in steroid hormone action. They function as costimulators, corepressors or bridging molecules. A misbalanced cofactor expression may contribute to tumor progression. We analyzed cofactor expression in a panel of prostate cancer cell culture models and in prostate stromal cells using RT-PCR. This study revealed expression of a broad cofactor spectrum in the cells tested (Nessler-Menardi *et al.* 2000). All general nuclear receptor coactivators, such as the SRC family (SRC-1, TIF2, AIB1), were expressed in all cells. The same is true for the bridging molecule CBP, which is considered a mediator of 'cross-coupling' between different signal pathways. Of the ARA (androgen receptor activator) proteins, ARA54 and 70 are expressed in all cells, whereas ARA55 is not contained in LNCaP and DU-145 cells. We also checked two proteins which act as repressors – SMRT and Cyclin D1; both of them were expressed in all

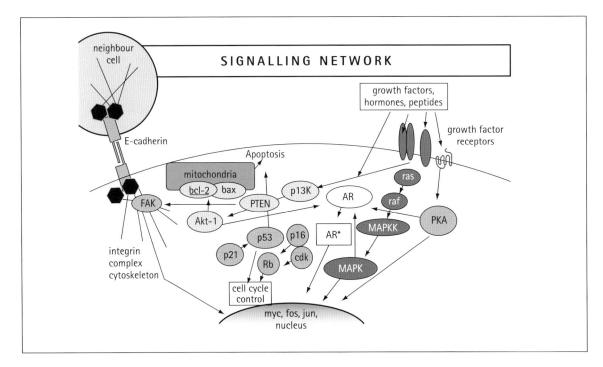

Figure 6.5

The cellular signalling network. The different cellular signalling pathways such as the MAP kinase, the protein kinase-A or the phosphatidylinositol-3 kinase–protein kinase B (pKB, Akt-1) pathway crosstalk among each other, forming the cellular regulatory signalling network. The androgen receptor is part of this network, and interacts with other signalling pathways, which modulate its activity.

cell lines. BAG-1L was reported to enhance AR and vitamin D receptor activity (Guzey *et al.* 2000, Froesch *et al.* 1998). It is also expressed in all cell lines analyzed.

The expression of coregulatory proteins in prostate cancer tissue has to be analyzed in detail; however, it is obvious that inappropriate expression and function of coactivators or corepressors can have great implications on AR activity. In cell culture systems, overexpression of coactivators resulted in enhancement of transactivation activity and antagonist-to-

agonist reversal of antiandrogens (Miyamoto *et al.* 1998, Culig *et al.* 2001).

The hyperreactive androgen receptor prostate cancer model

Founded on the novel findings on androgen receptor signalling in prostate cancer, we

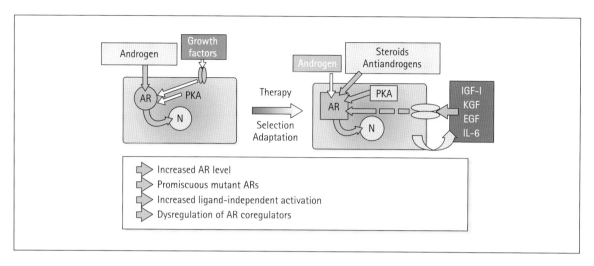

Figure 6.6

The hyperreactive androgen receptor model of therapy resistance. The selective pressure of androgen ablation therapy forces surviving prostate cancer cells to adapt to an androgen-deprived environment by development of a hyperreactive androgen receptor signalling. This enables prostate cancer cells to survive and proliferate in the absence of androgens, and results in failure of hormonal withdrawal therapies. Several mechanisms seem to be involved in this process. Cells from therapy-resistant tumours may contain promiscuous ARs generated by mutation of the wild-type AR. These receptors can be activated by various steroid hormones and antiandrogens. Alternatively, the AR may be activated ligand-independently through a panel of different growth factors or cytokines such as IGF-I, KGF, EGF and IL-6 and the protein kinase A pathway. Other reasons for AR hyperreactivity may be increased AR levels and/or AR gene amplifications found in about one-third of therapy-resistant tumours, or a dysregulation of the expression of coregulatory proteins: the latter modulate AR activity as a transcription factor and their expression was shown to enhance the agonist activity of antiandrogens.

propose the hyperreactive androgen receptor model as a working model for tumor progression (Figure 6.6). In this model androgen receptor activity in normal prostate cells and untreated prostate tumor cells is mainly regulated by androgenic hormones; other activation pathways play a minor role. With androgen ablation therapy, tumor cells are forced either to die through programmed cell death or to adapt to the conditions of androgen deprivation. Adaptation is achieved by generation of promiscuous mutant receptors, increase of androgen receptor expression levels, enhancement of ligand-independent activation or dysregulation of androgen receptor coregulatory proteins.

Elimination of AR protein as an alternative to inhibition of AR function

The results summarized above demonstrate that currently used modes of endocrine therapy for prostate cancer, which aim to inhibit AR function, are not sufficient to block androgen receptor action in the long run. A promising alternative to inhibition of AR function would be to eliminate the androgen receptor protein. We evaluated this possibility using antisense technology. AR antisense

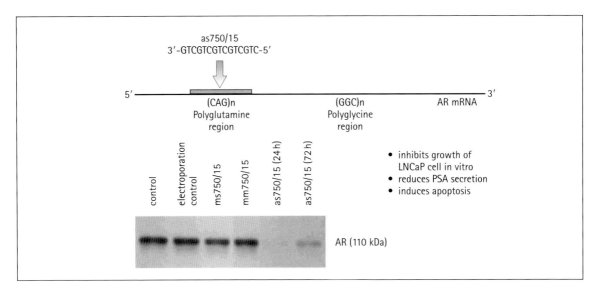

Figure 6.7
Inhibition of androgen receptor expression by antisense oligonucleotides. Introduction of androgen receptor antisense oligonucleotides targeting the polyglutamine-encoding CAG-triplet repeat region in the AR mRNA (as750/15) into LNCaP cells by electroporation caused downregulation of AR protein levels to below 10% within 24 hours. Electroporation alone or electroporation of a missense (ms750/15) or mismatch (mm750/15) control oligonucleotide had no effect on AR protein levels. Inhibition of AR protein synthesis led to inhibition of growth, reduction of PSA secretion and increase of the rate of apoptosis.

oligonucleotides, which allow efficient inhibition of AR expression, were identified. One of them targets the CAG-repeat in the mRNA region encoding the N-terminal domain (Figure 6.7). Treatment of LNCaP cells with this antisense oligonucleotide resulted in a significant inhibition of basal and androgen-induced proliferation, a reduced PSA secretion and decreased EGF receptor levels, respectively. In addition, antisense treatment increased the rate of apoptosis (Eder *et al.* 2000). As expected, the AR antisense treatment was equally effective in the parental cell line and in the LNCaP-abl subline that has increased AR levels.

The promising results in cell culture studies encouraged us to test the efficacy of our antisense oligonucleotides in an in-vivo system, in LNCaP tumors bearing nude mice. The results also supported the efficacy of AR antisense treatment. Tumor growth was inhibited significantly, without adverse side effects, thus providing a first proof-of-principle of elimination of AR protein as a promising treatment for prostate cancer.

References

Auclerc G, Antoine EC, Cajfinger F, *et al.* (2000) Management of advanced prostate cancer. *Oncologist* 5:36–44.

Crawford ED, Rosenblum M, Ziada AM, Lange PH (1999) Hormone refractory prostate cancer. *Urology* 54:1–7.

Culig L, Lambrinidis L, Hobisch A, Klocker H, Bartsch G (2001) The transcriptional integrator CBP preferentially enhances agonistic effect of hydroxyflutamide in prostate cancer cells [Abstract]. *Proc AACR* 42:546.

Culig Z, Hobisch A, Cronauer MV, et al. (1994) Androgen receptor activation in prostatic tumor cell lines by insulin-like growth factor-I, keratinocyte growth factor, and epidermal growth factor. Cancer Res 54:5474–5478.

Culig Z, Hobisch A, Cronauer MV, et al. (1995) Androgen receptor activation in prostatic tumor cell lines by insulin-like growth factor-I, keratinocyte growth factor and epidermal growth factor. Eur Urol 2:45–47.

Culig Z, Hobisch A, Cronauer MV, et al. (1996a). Regulation of prostatic growth and function by peptide growth factors. Prostate 28:392–405.

Culig Z, Hobisch A, Hittmair A, et al. (1997) Synergistic activation of androgen receptor by androgen and luteinizing hormone-releasing hormone in prostatic carcinoma cells. Prostate 32:106–114.

Culig Z, Hobisch A, Hittmair A, et al. (1998) Expression, structure, and function of androgen receptor in advanced prostatic carcinoma. Prostate 35:63–70.

Culig Z, Hoffmann J, Erdel M, et al. (1999) Switch from antagonist to agonist of the androgen receptor bicalutamide is associated with prostate tumour progression in a new model system. Br J Cancer 81:242–251.

Culig Z, Stober J, Gast A, et al. (1996b) Activation of two mutant androgen receptors from human prostatic carcinoma by adrenal androgens and metabolic derivatives of testosterone. Cancer Detect Prev 20:68–75.

de Winter JA, Trapman J, Brinkmann AO, et al. (1990) Androgen receptor heterogeneity in human prostatic carcinomas visualized by immunohistochemistry. J Pathol 160:329–332.

Eder I, Culig Z, Ramoner R, et al. (2000) Inhibition of LNCaP prostate cancer cells by means of androgen receptor antisense oligonucleotides. Cancer Gene Ther 7:997–1007.

Fenton MA, Shuster TD, Fertig AM, et al. (1997) Functional characterization of mutant androgen receptors from androgen-independent prostate cancer. Clin Cancer Res 3:1383–1388.

Froesch BA, Takayama S, Reed JC (1998) BAG–1L protein enhances androgen receptor function. J Biol Chem 273:11660–11666.

Fuhrmann U, Parczyk K, Klotzbucher M, Klocker H, Cato AC (1998) Recent developments in molecular action of antihormones. J Mol Med 76:512–524.

Fuller PJ (1991) The steroid nuclear receptor superfamily: mechanisms of diversity. FASEB J 5:2243–2249.

Guzey M, Takayama S, Reed JC (2000) BAG1L enhances trans-activation function of the vitamin D receptor. J Biol Chem 275:40749–40756.

Hager GL (2000) Understanding nuclear receptor function: from DNA to chromatin to the interphase nucleus. Prog Nucleic Acid Res Mol Biol 66: 279–305.

Hobisch A, Culig Z, Radmayr C, et al. (1995a) Androgen receptor status of lymph node metastases from prostatic carcinoma. Prostate 29:129–136.

Hobisch A, Culig Z, Radmayr C, et al. (1995b) Distant metastases from prostatic carcinoma express androgen receptor protein. Cancer Res 55:3068–3072.

Horninger W, Reissigl A, Rogatsch H, et al. (2000) Prostate cancer screening in the Tyrol, Austria. Experience and results. Eur J Cancer 36:1322–1335.

Klocker H, Culig Z, Hobisch A, et al. (1996) Androgen receptor alterations in prostatic carcinoma. In Schnorr D, Loening SA, Dinges S, Budach V, eds. Locally Advanced Prostate Cancer T3/C, Berlin: Blackwell Wissenschafts-Verlag, pp. 57–67.

Koivisto P, Kolmer M, Visakorpi T, Kallioniemi OP (1998) Androgen receptor gene and hormonal therapy failure of prostate cancer. Am J Pathol 152:1–9.

Marcelli M, Ittmann M, Mariani S, et al. (2000) Androgen receptor mutations in prostate cancer. Cancer Res 60:944–949.

McEwan IJ (2000) Gene regulation through chromatin remodelling by members of the nuclear receptor superfamily. Biochem Soc Trans 28:369–373.

Miyamoto H, Yeh S, Wilding G, Chang C (1998) Promotion of agonist activity of antiandrogens by the androgen receptor coactivator, ARA70, in human prostate cancer DU145 cells. Proc Natl Acad Sci U S A 95:7379–7384.

Moul JW, Srivastava S, McLeod DG (1995) Molecular implications of the antiandrogen withdrawal syndrome. Semin Urol 13:157–163.

Murtha P, Tindall DJ, Young CY (1993) Androgen induction of a human prostate-specific kallikrein, hKLK2: characterization of an androgen response element in the 5′ promoter region of the gene. Biochemistry 32:6459–6464.

Nessler-Menardi C, Jotova I, Culig Z, et al. (2000) Expression of androgen receptor coregulatory proteins in prostate cancer and stromal-cell culture models. Prostate 45:124–131.

Nupponen NN, Kakkola L, Koivisto P, Visakorpi T (1998) Genetic alterations in hormone-refractory recurrent prostate carcinomas. Am J Pathol 153:141–148.

Palmberg C, Koivisto P, Hyytinen E, et al. (1997) Androgen receptor gene amplification in a recurrent prostate cancer after monotherapy with the non-steroidal potent antiandrogen Casodex (bicalutamide) with a subsequent favorable response to maximal androgen blockade. *Eur Urol* 31:216–219.

Prescott JL, Tindall DJ (1998) Clathrin gene expression is androgen regulated in the prostate. *Endocrinology* 139:2111–2119.

Prins GS (2000) Molecular biology of the androgen receptor. *Mayo Clin Proc* 75 Suppl, S32–35.

Rennie PS, Bruchovsky N, Leco KJ, *et al.* (1993) Characterization of two cis-acting DNA elements involved in the androgen regulation of the probasin gene. *Mol Endocrinol* 7:23–36.

Riegman PH, Vlietstra RJ, Suurmeijer L, Cleutjens CB, Trapman J (1992) Characterization of the human kallikrein locus. *Genomics* 14:6–11.

Riegman PH, Vlietstra RJ, van der Korput JA, Brinkmann AO, Trapman J (1991) The promoter of the prostate-specific antigen gene contains a functional androgen responsive element. *Mol Endocrinol* 5:1921–1930.

Smith DF, Toft DO (1993) Steroid receptors and their associated proteins. *Mol Endocrinol* 7:4–11.

Suzuki H, Sato N, Watabe Y, *et al.* (1993) Androgen receptor gene mutations in human prostate cancer. *J Steroid Biochem Mol Biol* 46:759–765.

Tan J, Sharief J, Hamil KG, *et al.* (1996) Altered ligand specificity of a mutant androgen receptor (AR) in the androgen dependent human prostate cancer cenograft, CWR–22: Comparison with the LNCaP mutant AR. *J Urol* 155:340A [Abstract].

Taplin ME, Bubley GJ, Shuster TD, *et al.* (1995) Mutation of the androgen-receptor gene in metastatic androgen-independent prostate cancer. *N Engl J Med* 332:1393–1398.

Tilley WD, Marcelli M, Wilson JD, McPhaul MJ (1989) Characterization and expression of a cDNA encoding the human androgen receptor. *Proc Natl Acad Sci U S A* 86:327–331.

Tsai MJ, O'Malley BW (1994) Molecular mechanisms of action of steroid/thyroid receptor superfamily members. *Ann Rev Biochem* 63:451–486.

Ulrix W, Swinnen JV, Heyns W, Verhoeven G (1999) The differentiation-related gene 1, Drg1, is markedly upregulated by androgens in LNCaP prostatic adeno-carcinoma cells. *FEBS Lett* 455:23–26.

van der Kwast T, Schalken J, Ruizeveld de Winter J, *et al.* (1991) Androgen receptors in endocrine therapy-resistant human prostate cancer. *Int J Cancer* 48:189.

Wang C, Young WJ, Chang C (2000) Isolation and characterization of the androgen receptor mutants with divergent transcriptional activity in response to hydroxyflutamide. *Endocrine* 12:69–76.

Wen Y, Hu MC, Makino K, *et al.* (2000) HER–2/neu promotes androgen-independent survival and growth of prostate cancer cells through the Akt pathway. *Cancer Res* 60:6841–6845.

Whitfield GK, Jurutka PW, Haussler CA, Haussler MR (1999) Steroid hormone receptors: evolution, ligands, and molecular basis of biologic function. *J Cell Biochem* Suppl 32:110–122.

Xu LL, Srikantan V, Sesterhenn IA, *et al.* (2000) Expression profile of an androgen regulated prostate specific homeobox gene NKX3.1 in primary prostate cancer. *J Urol* 163:972–979.

Zhao XY, Malloy PJ, Krishnan AV, *et al.* (2000) Glucocorticoids can promote androgen-independent growth of prostate cancer cells through a mutated androgen receptor. *Nat Med* 6:703–706.

7 Estrogen receptor beta in the prostate

Zhang Weihua, Sari Mäkelä, Stefan Nilsson, Margaret Warner and Jan-Åke Gustafsson

Summary

In mice whose estrogen receptor β (ERβ) gene has been inactivated (BERKO mice) epithelial cells in the ventral prostate are not at G0 but are always in the cell cycle. As BERKO mice age, there is a progressive hyperplasia and at 2 years of age PIN lesions are present. One possible mechanism for this prostate phenotype is that ERβ is a pro-apoptotic gene and that its inactivation results in accumulation of cells normally destined for death. If this is the role for ERβ in the prostate, BERKO mice will be very useful for the *in-vivo* study of estrogen effects on the cell cycle and for characterization of the cellular changes which occur as epithelium progresses from hyperplasia to dysplasia and carcinoma. If ERβ does have a regulatory function in the prostate, ligands for this receptor might be useful in controlling proliferative diseases of the prostate. The major estrogen in mouse ventral prostate extracts is not estradiol, but 5α-androstane-3β, 17β-diol (3βAdiol). If 3βAdiol is the ligand for ERβ in the prostate, inhibition of 5α-reductase would be expected to have adverse effects on the prostate. This may explain the apparent increase in prostate cancer in men treated with the 5α-reductase inhibitor finasteride.

17β-estradiol (E2) effects on the prostate

E2 exposure has effects in both the developing and adult male urogenital tract, but it is not clear to what extent these effects are due to direct E2 actions mediated via ERs in reproductive tissues or to indirect effects. Indirect effects are caused by actions of E2 on the hypothalamic–pituitary–gonadal axis, and result in insufficient androgen production.

Exposure to a differentiation hormone at an inappropriate stage during tissue development can change the balance between proliferating and differentiated cells and lead to proliferative abnormalities in the mature tissue. Inappropriate exposure to estrogen, in fact, does have adverse effects on the prostate. Exposure of male rats to estrogens during the neonatal period retards prostate branching morphogenesis, blocks epithelial differentiation and predisposes the adult prostate to hyperplasia and dysplasia (Chang *et al.* 1999). Transient nuclear localization of the cyclin-dependent kinase inhibitor p21 is normally observed in epithelial cells between days 6 and 15 and is associated with entry of cells into a terminal differentiation pathway. Neonatal estrogenization prevented this transient expression of p21.

One source of confusion in the estrogen field is the role of phytoestrogens in prostatic disease. Epidemiological studies indicate that consumption of phytoestrogens offers protection against prostate cancer and is a contributing factor to the lower incidence of cancers in the Asian population (Messina 1999, Davis *et al.* 1998).

Genistein, one of the major phytoestrogens in soy, causes a G2/M cell cycle arrest and thus inhibits growth of prostate cancer cells in culture (Aronson *et al.* 1999, Choi *et al.* 2000). Along with growth suppression, there is upregulation of the p21 growth-inhibitory protein, and induction of apoptosis. In apparent contradiction, the antiestrogen tamoxifen also induces p21 and causes G1/S phase cell cycle arrest in prostate cancer cells (PC3, PC3-M and DU145) (Rohlf *et al.* 1998).

The existence of two estrogen receptors offers one possibility to understand these apparent contradictions in the actions of estrogens and antiestrogens. The fact is that ERα and ERβ have different affinities for phytoestrogens (Keiper *et al.* 1997, 1998) and have different, sometimes opposing, biological functions (Paech *et al.* 1997). Genistein is a better ligand for ERβ than for ERα. In addition to their well-characterized transcriptional activation of genes containing estrogen response elements (EREs) (Beato 1989), both receptors stimulate gene expression by indirect binding of the receptor to DNA through physical interaction with the Sp1 transcription factor (Battistuzzo de Medeiros *et al.* 1997, Porter *et al.* 1999, Qin *et al.* 1999). Both ERα and ERβ activate retinoic acid receptor α1 (RARα1) gene expression, by the formation of an ER:Sp1 complex on GC-rich Sp1 sites in the RARα1 promoter (Sun *et al.* 1998) but in this case the two estrogen receptors have opposing effects. ERβ activates RARα1 promoter reporter constructs in the presence of estrogen

antagonists such as 4-OH-tamoxifen, raloxifene and ICI 164,384, but not in the presence of E2, which instead blocks the effect of the antagonists (Zou *et al.* 1999). Since activation of RARα is of advantage in cancer, through its induction of cell adhesion molecules (Zhu *et al.* 1999), antiestrogens interacting with ERβ should be beneficial. There are probably many, as yet uncharacterized, alternative pathways through which estrogen receptors could affect gene transcription and the role of ERα and ERβ in such pathways will have to be examined.

In breast cancer cells, estrogen-induced cell proliferation is caused by stimulating progression through the G(1) phase of the cell cycle and this is mediated through induction of cyclin D1. The region in the cyclin D1 promoter that confers regulation by estrogens in these cells is not a classical ERE but has the sequence of a potential cAMP response element (CRE-D1) (Sabbah *et al.* 1999). How estrogen receptors mediate their action in this system and what are the differences between the two estrogen receptors on this gene remain to be determined.

ERβ in the prostate

With specific ERβ antibodies, immunohistochemical studies show that the nuclei of most cells of normal adult human, rat and mouse prostatic epithelium harbor ERβ (Figure 7.1).

Several splice variants of ERβ have been described. Some have extended N-termini and others have truncations and/or insertions at the C-terminus and in the LBD. ERβ 530 (Ogawa *et al.* 1998a) differs (Kuiper *et al.* 1996) from the original rat ERβins, an isoform with an in-frame insertion of 18 amino acids in the LBD (Chu & Fuller 1997, Petersen *et al.*

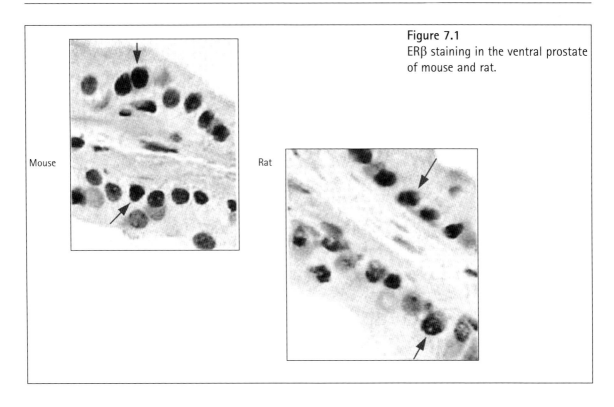

Figure 7.1
ERβ staining in the ventral prostate of mouse and rat.

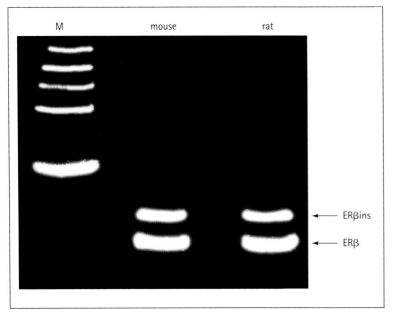

Figure 7.2
RT-PCR detection of ERβ isoforms in the rodent ventral prostate.

1998, Hanstein *et al.* 1999). In contrast to the N-terminally extended ERβ isoforms, the affinity of ERβ-503 for E2 and other known ER ligands is lower than for ERβ-485, or ERβ-530. ERβ-503 acts as a dominant negative regulator by suppressing E2-dependent ERα- and ERβ-mediated activation of gene transcription, but does not bind E2 (Maruyama *et al.* 1998).

ERβ isoforms with variations at the extreme C-terminus have been found (Ogawa *et al.* 1998b, Moore *et al.* 1998). In ERβcx the last 61

C-terminal amino acids (exon 8) have been replaced by 26 unique amino acid residues. ERβcx lacks amino acid residues important for ligand binding and those that constitute the core of the AF2 domain. ERβcx does not bind E2 and has no capacity to activate transcription of an E2-sensitive reporter gene (Ogawa *et al.* 1998). Functionally, the heterodimerization of ERβcx with ERα and ERβ has a dominant negative effect on ligand-dependent ER reporter-gene transactivation (Inoue *et al.* 2000).

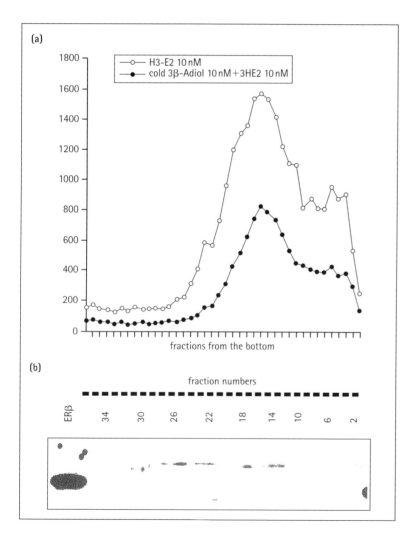

Figure 7.3
Sucrose gradient sedimentation combined with Western blotting detections of ERβ with 17β-estradiol and 3βAdiol as ligands in the rat ventral prostate cystosol. (a) Sucrose gradient sedimentation assay. (b) Western blot detection of ERβ from the fractions of A.

Five ERβ isoforms (ERβ1–5) have been found in rats (Moore *et al*. 1998). ERβ1 corresponds to ERβ-530 and the ERβ2 variant is ERβcx. However, ERβ3–5 are novel splice variants with exchanges of the last exon of ERβ-530 for previously unknown exons.

By N-terminal amino acid sequencing of high salt extracts of mouse prostates, 549 and 530 molecular weight isoforms of ERβ were identified and by RT-PCR the non-estrogen binding ERβ isoforms ERβcx (in human) and ERβins (in rodents) were found to be expressed at levels similar to ERβ1 (Figure 7.2).

5α-androstane-3β, 17β-diol (3βAdiol), an estrogenic metabolite of 5α-dihydrotestos-terone, binds to both ERα and ERβ with quite similar dissociation constants of approximately $1–2 \times 10^{-8}$ mol (Kuiper *et al*. 1997). Its affinity for the androgen receptor is negligible (Turcotte *et al*. 1998). Both 17β-estradiol and 3βAdiol are good ligands for ERβ (Figure 7.3). When ventral prostates of rats raised on a soy-free diet were extracted with ethyl acetate, there was estrogenic activity in the extract. This was assessed in a cell assay in which cells harbored an ERE-luc reporter (Barkhem *et al*. 1998). Surprisingly, when the extract was fractionated by HPLC, the major estrogenic component of the prostate co-eluted with 3βAdiol. There was very little E2 in the extract.

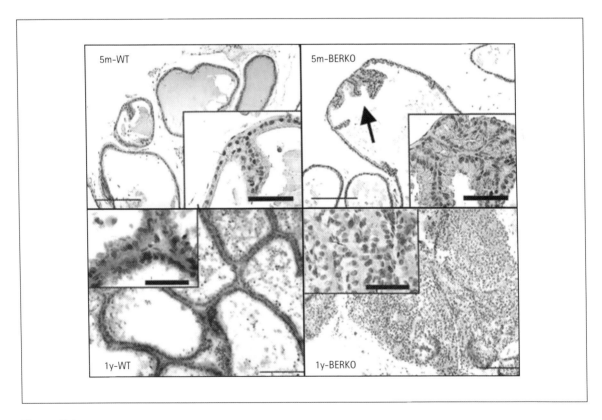

Figure 7.4
Prostate morphology of wild-type and BERKO mice. Arrows: cribriform hyperplasia at 5 months old and PIN lesion at 1 year old.

Prostate phenotype in ERβ knock out (BERKO) mice

Perhaps not surprisingly, in view of the abundance of ERβ in the prostate epithelium, mice lacking ERβ have abnormal prostates. BERKO mice develop prostatic hyperplasia by 3 months of age and, as they get older, this hyperplasia becomes more pronounced. All of the epithelial cells in the prostate of BERKO mice at 5 months of age express the proliferation marker Ki67 protein, indicating that they are not in G0 but have all entered the cell cycle, a highly abnormal situation. Interestingly, at 5 months of age, most of these cells are not proliferating, so they must be arrested at some stage in the cell cycle (Figure 7.4).

Although the role of ERβ in control of prostatic growth is not understood, one interesting gene appears to be under the control of ERβ. This is the androgen receptor (AR). AR is highly expressed in BERKO mouse prostates. In addition, 3βAdiol downregulates AR in the prostates of +/+ but not −/− mice. Regulation of AR by 3βAdiol suggests that one possible mechanism through which ERβ could regulate prostatic growth is by altering the sensitivity of the prostate to androgens.

Conclusions

ERβ is the dominant estrogen receptor in prostatic epithelium and loss of ERβ results in proliferation of prostatic epithelium. We anticipate that ERβ ligands will have a role in controlling proliferative diseases of the prostate.

References

Aronson WJ, Tymchuk CN, Elashoff RM, *et al.* (1999) Decreased growth of human prostate LNCaP tumors in SCID mice fed a low-fat, soy protein diet with isoflavones. *Nutr Cancer* **35**:130–136.

Barkhem T, Carlsson B, Nilsson Y, *et al.* (1998) Differential response of estrogen receptor alpha and estrogen receptor beta to partial estrogen agonists/antagonists. *Mol Pharmacol* **54**:105–112.

Batistuzzo de Medeiros SR, Krey G, Hihi AK, Wahli W (1997) Functional interaction between the estrogen receptor and the transcription activator Sp1 regulates the estrogen-dependent transcriptional activity of the vitellogenin A1 promoter. *J Biol Chem* **272**:18250–18260.

Beato M (1989) Gene regulation by steroid hormones. *Cell* **56**:335–344.

Chang WY, Birch L, Woodham C, Gold LI, Prins GS (1999) Neonatal estrogen exposure alters the transforming growth factor-beta signaling system in the developing rat prostate and blocks the transient p21(cip1/waf1) expression associated with epithelial differentiation. *Endocrinology* **140**:2801–2813.

Choi YH, Lee WH, Park KY, Zhang L (2000) p53-independent induction of p21 (WAF1/CIP1), reduction of cyclin B1 and G2/M arrest by the isoflavone, genistein, in human prostate carcinoma cells. *Jpn J Cancer Res* **91**:164–173.

Chu S, Fuller PJ (1997) Identification of a splice variant of the rat estrogen receptor beta gene. *Mol Cell Endocrinol* **132**:195–199.

Davis JN, Singh B, Bhuiyan M, Sarkar FH (1998) Genistein-induced upregulation of p21WAF1, downregulation of cyclin B, and induction of apoptosis in prostate cancer cells. *Nutr Cancer* **32**:123–131.

Hanstein B, Liu H, Yancisin M, Brown M (1999) Functional analysis of a novel estrogen receptor-β isoform. *Mol Endocrinol* **13**:129–137.

Inoue S, Ogawa S, Horie K, *et al.* (2000) An estrogen receptor beta isoform that lacks exon 5 has dominant negative activity on both ERalpha and ERbeta. *Biochem Res Comm* **279**:814–819.

Kuiper GG, Carlsson B, Grandien K, *et al.* (1997) Comparison of the ligand binding specificity and transcript tissue distribution of estrogen receptors alpha and beta. *Endocrinology* **138**:863–887.

Kuiper GG, Enmark E, Pelto-Huikko M, Nilsson S, Gustafsson J-Å (1996) Cloning of a novel receptor expressed in rat prostate and ovary. *Proc Natl Acad Sci USA* 93:5925–5930.

Kuiper GG, Lemmen JG, Carlsson B, *et al.* (1998) Interaction of estrogenic chemicals and phyto-estrogens with estrogen receptor beta. *Endocrinology* 139:4252–4263.

Maruyama K, Endoh H, Sasaki-Iwaoka H, *et al.* (1998) A novel isoform of rat estrogen receptor beta with 18 amino acid insertion in the ligand binding domain as a putative dominant negative regular of estrogen action. *Biochem Biophys Res Comm* 246:142–147.

Messina MJ (1999) Legumes and soybeans: overview of their nutritional profiles and health effects. *Am J Clin Nutr* 70:439S–450S.

Moore JT, McKee DD, Slentz-Kesler K, *et al.* (1998) Cloning and characterization of human estrogen receptor beta isoforms. *Biochem Biophys Res Comm* 247:75–78.

Ogawa S, Inoue S, Watanabe T, *et al.* (1998a) The complete primary structure of human estrogen receptor β(hEβ) and its heterodimerization with ERα in vivo and in vitro. *Biochem Biophys Res Comm* 243: 122–126.

Ogawa S, Inoue S, Watanabe T, *et al.* (1998b) Molecular cloning and characterization of human estrogen receptor βcx: a potential inhibitor of estrogen action in human. *Nucleic Acids Res* 26:3505–3512.

Paech K, Webb P, Kuiper GG, *et al.* (1997) Differential ligand activation of estrogen receptors ERalpha and ERbeta at AP1 sites. *Science* 277:1508–1510.

Petersen DN, Tkalcevic GT, Koza-Taylor PH, Turi TG, Brown TA (1998) Identification of estrogen receptor beta2, a functional variant of estrogen receptor beta expressed in normal rat tissues. *Endocrinology* 139:1082–1092.

Porter W, Saville B, Hoivik D, Safe S (1999) Functional synergy between the transcription factor Sp1 and the estrogen receptor. *Mol Endocrinol* 11:1569–1580.

Qin C, Singh P, Safe S (1999) Transcriptional activation of insulin-like growth factor-binding protein-4 by 17β-estradiol in MCF-7 cells: Role of estrogen receptor-SP1 complexes. *Endocrinology* 140:2501–2508.

Rohlf C, Blagosklonny MV, Kyle E, *et al.* (1998) Prostate cancer cell growth inhibition by tamoxifen is associated with inhibition of protein kinase C and induction of p21(waf1/cip1). *Prostate* 37:51–59.

Sabbah M, Courilleau D, Mester J, Redeuilh G (1999) Estrogen induction of the cyclin D1 promoter: involvement of a cAMP response-like element. *Proc Natl Acad Sci USA* 96:11217–11222.

Sun G, Porter W, Safe S (1998) Estrogen-induced retinoic acid receptor α1 gene expression: role of estrogen receptor-Sp1 complex. Mol Endocrinol 12:882–890.

Turcotte G, Chapdelaine A, Roberts KD, Chevalier S (1988) Androgen binding as evidenced by a whole cell assay system using cultured canine prostatic epithelial cells. *J Steroid Biochem* 29:69–76.

Zhu WY, Jones CS, Amin S, *et al.* (1999) Retinoic acid increases tyrosine phosphorylation of focal adhesion kinase and paxillin in MCF-7 human breast cancer cells. *Cancer Res* 59:85–90.

Zou A, Marschke KB, Arnold KE, *et al.* (1999) Estrogen receptor activates the human retinoic acid receptor-1 promoter in response to tamoxifen and other estrogen receptor antagonists, but not in response to estrogen. *Mol Endocrinol* 13:418–430.

8 Vitamin D deficiency increases risk of prostate cancer

*Pentti Tuohimaa, Merja H Ahonen, Merja Bläuer, Ilkka Laaksi,
Yan-Ru Lou, Paula Martikainen, Susanna Miettinen, Pasi Pennanen,
Sami Purmonen, Annika Vienonen, Timo Ylikomi and Heimo Syvälä*

Introduction

The etiology of cancer of the prostate remains unclear. Epidemiological studies have suggested that the cause of prostate cancer (PCa) is multifactorial, involving both genetic and environmental risk factors (age, race, geography, diet and hereditary factors) (Ruijter 1999). Some of these risk factors may be related to conditions that can alter vitamin D status. It has been estimated that approximately 10% of prostate cancer cases are hereditary, the majority of PCa (90%) being sporadic. A number of genes have been suggested to be associated with PCa risk, including androgen (AR) and vitamin D receptors (VDR), 5α-reductase, 1α-hydroxylase, 24-hydroxylase, cell cycle regulators and several growth factors (Cussenot *et al*. 1998, Ylikomi *et al*. 2001). Many of these genes are regulated by androgens and/or vitamin D. It has been estimated that approximately 6% of prostate cancer mortality is caused by vitamin D deficiency (Hanchette & Schwartz 1992, Schwartz & Hulka 1990). However, the estimate may be influenced by the geographic location. Our own estimation is significantly higher, with the possibility of 26% of PCa cases in Finland being related to vitamin D deficiency due to low UV radiation during the 7 months of the winter season (Ahonen *et al*. 2000a).

Surprisingly, alongside the cloning of the nuclear receptor for vitamin D it became obvious that this receptor, although in low concentration, could be found in most tissues and cells, including malignant cells not previously appreciated as targets of vitamin D action (Bouillon *et al*. 1995). The results suggested that the functions of vitamin D might be more prevalent than previously anticipated. Moreover, the role of vitamin D as a hormone and para- and autocrine factor became evident. It was shown that vitamin D is an important regulator of growth, differentiation and apoptosis in many tissues (Botling *et al*. 1996, Demay *et al*. 1992, Norman *et al*. 1980, Smith *et al*. 1986, Suda *et al*. 1992). In most normal and cancer cells, vitamin D acts as an antiproliferative factor, but there are exceptions where vitamin D at certain concentrations may stimulate cell proliferation. These effects are believed to be mediated mainly by the nuclear VDR, which is also expressed in cancer cells; therefore there has been increasing interest in the role of vitamin D in carcinogenesis (van Leeuwen & Pols, 1997), and the exact mechanisms whereby vitamin D exerts its antiproliferative action are under an intense investigation. This chapter is a general review of the role of vitamin D in prostate cancer, with a focus on local vitamin D metabolism and interaction with androgens as well as on the possibilities of preventing PCa with different vitamin D treatments.

Epidemiology of prostate carcinoma

Early epidemiological studies based on indirect evidence suggested a relationship between vitamin D (sunlight) and colon cancer (Garland & Garland 1980) as well as breast cancer (Garland et al. 1990). The protective action of vitamin D against carcinogenesis became evident on the basis of several epidemiological studies (Corder et al. 1993, Doll & Peto 1981, Hanchette & Schwartz 1992). This action of vitamin D is thought to be due to its antiproliferative effect, but differentiation and apoptosis might also be involved (Ylikomi et al. 2001). There seems to be widespread vitamin D deficiency in elderly people, which was suggested to be an important factor in the progression of cancer. Schwartz and Hulka (1990) put forward the hypothesis that vitamin D deficiency also increases the risk of PCa. The hypothesis was supported by the findings that the mortality rates from PCa in the United States are inversely proportional to incident ultraviolet radiation (Hanchette & Schwartz 1992) and that serum $1,25(OH)_2D_3$ is a predictor for the development of PCa (Corder et al. 1993). However, other reports have questioned these findings (Braun et al. 1995, Gann et al. 1996, Nomura et al. 1998). It also seems evident that prostate cancer by itself can have an adverse effect on vitamin D homeostasis and various treatments for prostate cancer may alter circulating $1,25(OH)_2D_3$ levels (Miller 1998).

In Finland, the age-adjusted incidence of prostate cancer is continuously increasing and, during the last decade, PCa has been the most common cancer among males (Teppo 2000). It is interesting that 25-OH-vitamin D_3 ($25(OH)D_3$) serum levels in the Finnish population have been decreasing since 1979 (Figure 8.1), which may contribute to the accelerating increase of the PCa incidence. Although the $25(OH)D_3$ levels cannot be directly compared because of the methodological differences – the assay for the year 1979 was competitive protein binding assay (Lamberg-Allardt et al. 1983), whereas the other values are determined with radioimmunoassay (Ahonen et al. 2000a) – a decreasing trend is obvious. There are several possible explanations (dietary, etc.) for the decrease of serum $25(OH)D_3$ among Finns, but one of the key factors could, nevertheless, be lower UV exposure, because people spend more and more time indoors. The main source (two-thirds) of vitamin D is previtamin D_3 produced in the skin upon exposure to sunlight (Holick et al. 1980a). It seems that UV exposure throughout the year is needed for the maintenance of an adequate vitamin D balance. Vitamin D deficiency is believed to develop slowly after the fat stores of the vitamin, where excess of cutaneously produced vitamin D is stored, have been consumed (Mawer et al. 1972). It has also been noted that UVB radiation is inadequate for the synthesis of previtamin D_3 in northern countries during winter (Webb et al. 1988). In addition, sunscreen use and clothing prevent the synthesis of previtamin D_3 (Alagol et al. 2000). During the past few decades there has been a significant population shift in Finland from rural to urban areas and, therefore, Finns are less exposed to sunlight. It is interesting to note that, in winter, serum $25(OH)D_3$ levels in the more rural Northern Finland (72 ± 28 nmol/l) are significantly higher than in Southern Finland (56 ± 28 nmol/l) (Lamberg-Allardt et al. 1983). It seems obvious that both the total exposure to sunlight and vitamin D stores as well as dietary supplementation of the vitamin determine the development of vitamin D deficiency. During the past two decades vitamin D deficiency has become more common in Finland and, therefore, it is reasonable to study the association between vitamin D deficiency and cancer in Finland.

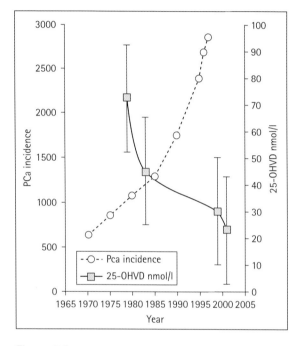

Figure 8.1
The age-adjusted prostate cancer (Pca) incidence rate per 100 000 person-years and serum 25-OH vitamin D_3 (25-OHVD) winter level (nmol/l) in Finland in 1965–1997. The rate of increase of cancer incidence was moderate until 1985, after which there has been an accelerating rate. Serum 25-OH vitamin D_3 winter levels show a decreasing slope since 1979, when most of the values were above the internationally recommended level (50 nmol/l). In Finland, the recommended 25-OH vitamin D_3 level is 40 nmol/l. In 1999 and 2001, most of the winter 25-OH vitamin D_3 levels are below the recommended one (assayed for this study by radioimmunoassay from 65 volunteers as described by Ahonen et al. (2000a)). Vitamin D values in 1979 are from the study of Lamberg-Allardt et al. (1983) and in 1983 from the study of Ahonen et al. (2000a).

We performed a prediagnostic nested case–control study on the 19 000 Finnish men who attended the first screening visit within the Helsinki Heart Study (Frick et al. 1984). We decided to assay only the major serum metabolite, 25(OH)D_3, which reflects vitamin D deficiency better than 1,25(OH)$_2$D$_3$ and which is an important precursor of 1,25(OH)$_2$D$_3$ in the prostate (Hsu et al. 2001, Schwartz et al. 1998). Our study (Ahonen et al. 2000a) brought out the following interesting aspects concerning prostate cancer:

1. vitamin D deficiency may be an important cause of cancer in countries having seasonally low UV irradiation
2. the prostate cancer risk attributable to vitamin D deficiency is higher among preandropausal (3.5-fold) than postandropausal men (1.2-fold)
3. vitamin D probably plays a role in the initiation, promotion and progression of cancer
4. the protective action of vitamin D seems to be dependent on androgens
5. high serum vitamin D levels delay the development of prostate cancer.

The results are summarized in Figure 8.2.

Our epidemiological results can be explained on the basis of experimental data. Proliferation of normal and malignant human prostate cells can be inhibited by vitamin D (Peehl et al. 1994, Skowronski et al. 1993, Tuohimaa et al. 2000). The vitamin D-induced antiproliferative action is mediated predominantly through a G1/S phase block of the cell cycle (for review see Ylikomi et al. 2001). The blocking of the G1/S phase by vitamin D is known to be associated with alteration of protein levels or kinase activity of CDK2, CDK4 and CDK6, ultimately leading to inhibition of phosphorylation of the retinoblastoma protein.

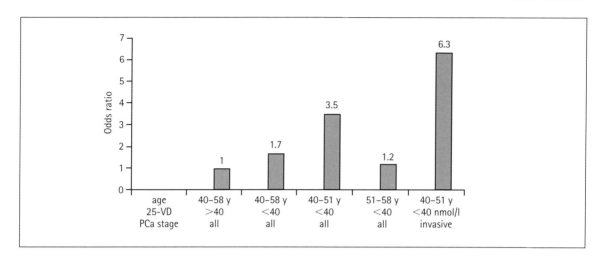

Figure 8.2
The risk of prostate cancer in Finland according to serum 25-OH vitamin D, age and stage (Ahonen *et al.* 2000a). In the whole material, odds ratio for prostate cancer is 1.7-fold ($p = 0.01$), when the serum 25(OH) vitamin D_3 level is below 40 nmol/l. When the men had a serum level below 40 nmol/l and were younger than 51 years old at entry, the risk of prostate cancer (invasive or non-invasive) was 3.5-fold ($p = 0.0006$) and the risk for invasive cancer 6.3-fold ($p = 0.02$). Low serum vitamin D comprises only a 1.2-fold risk (non-significant) for men over 51 years of age at entry.

In the LNCaP prostate cancer cell line, CDK2 kinase activity has been shown to decrease by vitamin D (Zhuang & Burnstein 1998).

The antiproliferative action of vitamin D is not only due to its direct effects on cell cycle but also includes differentiation of cancer cells, as described below, and an increased apoptosis (Ylikomi *et al.* 2001). LNCaP prostate cancer cells have been shown to undergo apoptosis after $1,25(OH)_2D_3$ treatment, although there are varying reports concerning the extent of the induced cell death (Blutt *et al.* 2000, Fife *et al.* 1997, Hsieh & Wu 1997). In the study by Blutt *et al.* (2000) $1,25(OH)_2D_3$ was shown to induce a 5-fold increase in the apoptosis of LNCaP cells accompanied by downregulation of Bcl-2 and Bcl-X_L anti-apoptotic proteins. The association of Bcl-2 downregulation with apoptosis was assessed with cells overexpressing Bcl-2 gene. In these cells, although failing to induce apoptosis, $1,25(OH)_2D_3$ was still able to cause

marked growth inhibition. This indicates that in LNCaP cells both cell cycle arrest and apoptosis are involved in the action of $1,25(OH)_2D_3$. Likewise, neither the capability of $1,25(OH)_2D_3$ to trigger apoptosis nor the downregulation of Bcl-2 in the apoptotic process is straightforward but displays cell specificity.

The antitumor effect of vitamin D can also be modified by induction or inhibition of the expression of growth factors (Ylikomi *et al.* 2001). Vitamin D regulates the expression of several growth factors and their receptors and possibly also the availability of the growth factors in tissues. The efficacy of $1,25(OH)_2D_3$ in the regulation of cell differentiation and growth might thus critically depend on its ability to regulate specific paracrine–autocrine signalling in tissues. Growth factors such as EGF, FGFs, TGF-β, and IGF, as well as some lymphokines, have been shown to be affected by vitamin D and its analogues (Ylikomi *et al.*

2001). TGF-β has been shown to reduce the proliferation of many cell types such as epithelial, leukaemic and bone cells. In breast cancer cells vitamin D inhibits cell proliferation in a dose-dependent manner and the growth inhibition is accompanied by an increase in the expression of TGF-β1. The growth inhibition can be blocked by neutralizing anti-TGF-β antibodies (Mercier *et al.* 1996). Vitamin D has also been shown to inhibit the signal transduction pathways of growth factors whose functions are associated with an increase in cell proliferation, such as EGF, IGF and interleukins. Paradoxically, FGF-7 expression is increased in LNCaP prostate cancer cells, although cell proliferation is inhibited (Lyakhovich *et al.* 2000).

We found a 6.3-fold increase of non-localized PCa in men with low $25(OH)D_3$ serum levels. It has been demonstrated experimentally that vitamin D inhibits the invasion of prostate cancer cells (Schwartz *et al.* 1997). Furthermore, metastasis of rat Dunning tumor has been largely inhibited by vitamin D and by its less calcaemic analogue EB1089 (Lokeshwar *et al.* 1999). Vitamin D may also exert its antitumor effects through antiangiogenic activity (Majewski *et al.* 1996).

The role of local metabolism of vitamin D

Under an adequate exposure to UVB, 7-dehydrocholesterol is photolysed in the skin to form previtamin D_3, which is transformed to vitamin D_3 and enters the circulation (Holick *et al.* 1980b). Vitamin D_3 is hydroxylated to 25-hydroxyvitamin D_3 ($25(OH)D_3$) in the liver and undergoes another hydroxylation mainly in the kidney, resulting in 1α,25-dihydroxyvitamin D_3

($1,25(OH)_2D_3$), the most active metabolite of vitamin D (Holick 1995). $25(OH)D_3$ has also been reported to display biological activity, but 500–1000-fold less than $1,25(OH)_2D_3$ (Reichel *et al.* 1989). Since the serum concentration of $25(OH)D_3$ is about 1000-fold over that of $1,25(OH)_2D_3$, $25(OH)D_3$ can be regarded as a biologically active metabolite. However, $25(OH)D_3$ might also be a substrate for the synthesis of biologically more active $1,25(OH)_2D_3$ within the prostate (Figure 8.3).

$1,25(OH)_2D_3$ is synthesized from $25(OH)D_3$ mainly in the kidney by mitochondrial cytochrome P450 enzyme $25(OH)D_3$-1α-hydroxylase (CYP27B), which is expressed along the human nephron (Zehnder *et al.* 1999). Because $1,25(OH)_2D_3$ acts humorally on distant target cells, vitamin D is regarded as a hormone. However, recent studies have demonstrated that there is significant extrarenal 1α-hydroxylase activity in several tissues such as lymphocytes (Reichel *et al.* 1987), alveolar macrophages (Adams & Gacad 1985), bone,

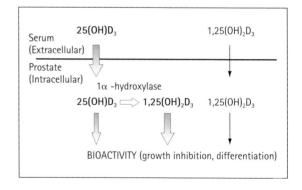

Figure 8.3
Hypothesis on the role of local activation of vitamin D in the prostate. Availability of the precursor ($25(OH)D_3$) might be more important for the biological response of the target cell than the concentration of serum-derived $1,25(OH)_2D_3$, if there is a sufficient amount of 1α-hydroxylase in the cell, resulting in a high intracellular concentration of $1,25(OH)_2D_3$.

liver, placenta, pancreas, colon, parathyroids, adrenal medulla, cerebellum (Hewison *et al.* 2000), skin (Horst & Reinhardt 1997), prostate carcinoma cell lines and normal prostatic cells (Schwartz *et al.* 1998). Therefore, vitamin D functions as an auto- and paracrine factor. Parathyroid hormone (PTH), extracellular calcium, calcitonin, acidosis, sex steroids, prolactin, growth hormone, glucocorticoids, thyroid hormone and pregnancy are also potential regulators of $1,25(OH)_2D_3$ synthesis (Henry 1997). It is interesting that LNCaP cells contain no measurable 1α-hydroxylase (Schwartz *et al.* 1998). These cells cannot respond to $25(OH)D_3$ unless they are transfected with 1α-hydroxylase cDNA plasmid (Hsu *et al.* 2001, Whitlach *et al.* 2001). This suggests that the more 1α-hydroxylase activity in the cell the more antiproliferative activity $25(OH)D_3$ possesses.

The 24-hydroxylation, which inactivates both $25(OH)D_3$ and $1,25(OH)_2D_3$, takes place mainly in the kidney; however, local inactivation in the prostate also seems to occur. The 25-hydroxyvitamin D 24-hydroxylase enzyme (CYP24) controls the first step in the inactivation process of $25(OH)D_3$ and $1,25(OH)_2D_3$. The 24-hydroxylase is widely distributed throughout the body and is strongly induced by $1,25(OH)_2D_3$. There are several prostate cancer cell lines among target cells shown to increase 24-hydroxylase activity after treatment with $1,25(OH)_2D_3$ (Miller *et al.* 1995). However, Skowronski *et al.* (1993) were unable to show enhanced CYP24 expression after $1,25(OH)_2D_3$ administration. It might be due to a short time course only up to 6 h, since we found significantly enhanced gene expression at 48 h after vitamin D (Figure 8.4). Breakdown of $1,25(OH)_2D_3$ by 24-hydroxylase

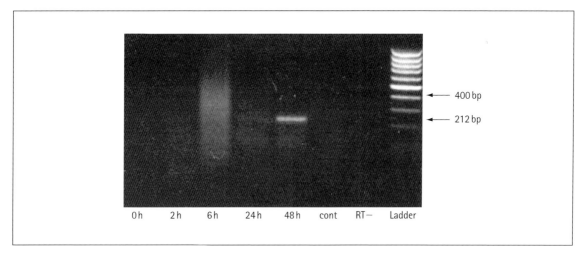

Figure 8.4
Induction of 24-hydroxylase by $1,25(OH)_2D_3$ in LNCaP cells. LNCaP cells were treated with 10 nM $1,25(OH)_2D_3$ for the times indicated: cont = control LNCaP cells treated with vehicle (0.1% ethanol); RT– = sample without reverse transcriptase. Oligonucleotide primers were synthesized by Amersham Pharmacia Biotech based on the sequence for CYP24 (Genbank access No L13286). The forward primer was 5′-TGATCCTGGAAGGGAAGAC-3′ (833–852) and the reverse primer was 5′-CACGAGGCAGATACTTTCAAAC-3′ (1023–1044). RobusT RT-PCR kit (Finnzymes) was used to perform one-tube RT-PCR. A weak induction can be observed at 24 h and a clear band of 212 bp at 48 h after treatment.

in target cells is likely to modify the growth inhibition effect of $1,25(OH)_2D_3$ and the use of cytochrome P450 enzyme inhibitors renders cells more sensitive to the antiproliferative action of $1,25(OH)_2D_3$ (Ly *et al.* 1999, Zhao *et al.* 1996). For instance, the ability of $1,25(OH)_2D_3$ to inhibit the growth of DU145 cells is substantially increased by liarozole, which blocks 24-hydroxylase activity in these cells (Ly *et al.* 1999). A recent report has indicated that CYP24 may have an oncogenic role in breast cancer (Albertson *et al.* 2000). It appeared that expression of CYP24, when normalized with that of VDR, correlates with the copy number of the CYP24 locus in breast tumors, suggesting that overexpression of CYP24 is due to amplification of the corresponding gene and may thus interfere with control of growth by vitamin D. A similar role for CYP24 in prostatic carcinogenesis has not yet been shown.

Vitamin D receptor

It has been clearly demonstrated that the antiproliferative effects of $1,25(OH)_2D_3$ are mediated through genomic pathways and therefore require the expression of nuclear VDR. Cells which fail to express VDR are not growth-inhibited by $1,25(OH)_2D_3$. For example, the prostatic carcinoma cell line JCA-1 neither expresses VDR nor is its growth affected by $1,25(OH)_2D_3$. When stably transfected with VDR cDNA, however, the cells are growth-inhibited by $1,25(OH)_2D_3$ in a dose-dependent manner (Hedlund *et al.* 1996a). Similarly, cells expressing VDR in high levels lose their ability to respond to $1,25(OH)_2D_3$ when transfected with VDR antisense mRNA, as shown with another prostatic carcinoma cell line, ALVA-31 (Hedlund *et al.* 1996b).

Zhuang *et al.* (1997) compared VDR content and growth response to $1,25(OH)_2D_3$ in four prostatic cancer cell lines: LNCaP, DU145, PC-3 and ALVA-31. PC-3 and DU145 cells contain low levels of VDR and are poorly growth-inhibited by $1,25(OH)_2D_3$, whereas LNCaP cells have high levels of VDR and are highly sensitive to $1,25(OH)_2D_3$ (approximately 55% inhibition). However, ALVA-31 cells contain the highest levels of VDR of the four cell lines, but display only 20% growth inhibition by $1,25(OH)_2D_3$, without any decrease in the general transcriptional activity. This suggests that the putative membrane receptor for vitamin D might play some role in the mitotic inhibition by vitamin D (Dormanen *et al.* 1994). It is thus obvious that nuclear VDR is needed for $1,25(OH)_2D_3$ growth suppression, but the sensitivity to growth inhibition does not necessarily correlate with VDR content and transcriptional activity. The relationship between VDR and mitotic response might be the gene regulation of proteins involved in mitotic control such as cell cycle proteins and growth factors (for review see Ylikomi *et al.* 2001). Some of the effects of vitamin D on MAP kinases in LNCaP cells are rapid (within 5 min) and, therefore, may not involve genomic action (Tuohimaa *et al.* 2000).

Vitamin D receptor polymorphism in cancer cells may influence cancer progression. When comparing newly diagnosed breast cancers with relapsed, metastasized disease, Ruggiero *et al.* (1998) found vitamin D receptor gene polymorphism to be associated with the metastatic disease. Polymorphism of VDR gene may influence tumor progression and response to tamoxifen treatment in early-onset breast cancer (Lundin *et al.* 1999). Although VDR polymorphism has been associated with prostate cancer in some studies (Ingles *et al.* 1997, Taylor *et al.* 1996), no association, however, was found between vitamin D receptor genotype and lethal prostate cancer in another study (Kibel *et al.* 1998).

Cross-talk with androgen signalling system

Our epidemiological study (Ahonen *et al.* 2000a) suggests that the cancer-protective action of vitamin D is androgen-dependent. Preandropausal men having vitamin D deficiency have a significantly higher risk for prostate cancer than postandropausal men. Thus, it seems that vitamin D protects against androgen-induced prostate cancer. Androgens play an important role in the development, growth and progression of PCa (McConnell 1991). A correlation between serum testosterone level and increased risk of PCa has been shown (Carter *et al.* 1990). It is not known how this cross-talk between androgen and vitamin D signalling is mediated. Crosstalk between vitamin D and androgens has been studied in prostate and ovarian cancer cells. Vitamin D ($1,25(OH)_2D_3$) has been shown to have an antiproliferative effect on different prostate cancer cell lines; however, the mechanism of action seems to be dependent on the cell line (Peehl *et al.* 1994, Schwartz *et al.* 1994, Skowronski *et al.* 1993, Esquenet *et al.* 1996, Miller *et al.* 1992). Although an increasing body of data indicates a role for vitamin D in prostate cancer, little is known as to the role of this hormone in the non-cancerous prostate. Examination of the effect of $1,25(OH)_2D_3$ on the growth of non-cancerous rat prostates indicates that in the absence of testosterone, $1,25(OH)_2D_3$ may exert a growth-promoting effect on the prostatic stroma *in vivo*. In concert with testosterone, it may play an impor-

tant role in the growth and differentiation of the normal rat prostate (Konety *et al.* 1996). In LNCaP cells which have high-affinity receptors for androgen, the mechanism is AR-dependent (Zhao *et al.* 1999). Treatment with $1,25(OH)_2D_3$ indirectly induced the expression of AR and the antiproliferative effect was blocked by the pure AR antagonist, Casodex. In MDA PCa 2a and 2b cells, which have low-affinity receptors for androgen, $1,25(OH)_2D_3$ increased the mRNA level of AR; however, the antiproliferative effect is not blocked by AR antagonists, suggesting an AR-independent mechanism (Zhao *et al.* 2000). Cross-talk between $1,25(OH)_2D_3$ and androgens has also been studied in ovarian cancer cell line OVCAR-3, which is both VDR- and AR-positive and in which both $1,25(OH)_2D_3$ and DHT upregulated VDR and AR expression (Ahonen *et al.* 2000b). Treatment with $1,25(OH)_2D_3$ inhibited growth and even reduced DHT-induced cell proliferation. In conclusion, androgens can enhance vitamin D effect by inducing VDR. Whether this could explain the androgen dependency of vitamin D action on cell proliferation is not clear.

Possibilities of differentiation therapy and cancer prevention with vitamin D

On the basis of our epidemiological study (Ahonen *et al.* 2000a), it would seem reasonable to examine the possibility of preventing PCa with vitamin D, since 26% of the prostate cancer cases in Finland appear to be due to vitamin D deficiency during the winter season. Vitamin D supplementation could be given at the population level, because it might also prevent breast cancer (Gulliford *et al.* 1998). There are two forms of vitamin D: animal-derived vitamin D$_3$ and plant-derived vitamin D$_2$. Both are metabolized in a similar fashion to produce a hormonally active form. Both can be used in the supplementation of animal and human diets (Horst & Reinhardt, 1997).

As seen in Figure 8.5, vitamin D supplementation (ergocalciferol or fish liver oil) improves the serum 25(OH)D$_3$ levels significantly. However, there is always a risk of overdose in oral administration of vitamin D, since the intestinal absorption of vitamin D cannot be controlled. Therefore, we studied the effect of different skin exposures of UVB on serum 25(OH)D$_3$. Sixty-five volunteers from our Medical School participated in the study. They were exposed for 1 year to full-spectrum light emitting weak UVB irradiation in the

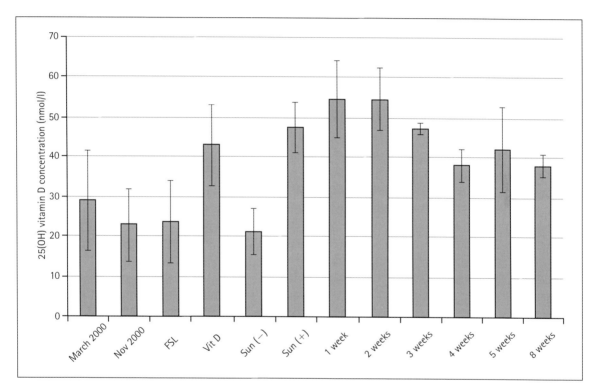

Figure 8.5
Serum 25-OH vitamin D$_3$ levels (nmol/l) of normal volunteers during winters 2000 and 2001. Serum 25(OH)D$_3$ was assayed using radioimmunoassay (Incstar Co) from 65 volunteers working at the Tampere Medical School (with permission of the local Ethical Committee). March 2000 = serum 25(OH)D$_3$ level of 65 volunteers in March 2000; Nov 2000 = serum 25(OH)D$_3$ level of 42 volunteers in November 2000; FSL = serum 25(OH)D$_3$ level of 30 volunteers after 1 year exposure to full-spectrum light (True Lite) for working hours (about 8 h per day) (Tuohimaa *et al.* 2000); Vit D = serum 25(OH)D$_3$ level of 30 volunteers taking ergocalciferol pills or fish liver oil daily according to manufacturer's suggestion; Sun(−) = serum 25(OH)D$_3$ level of 8 volunteers before visiting southern countries for sun tour of 2 weeks; Sun(+) = serum 25(OH)D$_3$ level of 8 volunteers immediately after return from visit to southern countries for sun tour of 2 weeks; 1, 2, 3, 4, 5, 8 weeks = serum 25(OH)D$_3$ level of 8 volunteers 1, 2 , 3, 4, 5 and 8 weeks after return from visit to southern countries for sun tour of 2 weeks.

laboratory and office (for methodological details see Tuohimaa *et al.* 2000); the controls were under normal fluorescent lamps. No difference was found between the groups (Figure 8.5). On the other hand, a 2-week tourist visit to southern countries improved serum 25(OH)D$_3$ to the normal level and the level remained normal for weeks (Figure 8.5). The long-lasting effect might be due to fat storage and slow release of vitamin D from fat storage. The inefficiency of full-spectrum light in improving serum vitamin D levels might be due to the low energy of the lamps and the small skin surface exposed in our study, since in another study significant improvement of vitamin D status was observed after full-spectrum light exposure (Gloth *et al.* 1999). It is also possible to give a single annual intramuscular injection of ergocalciferol and cause continuous normalization of vitamin D for 1 year (Heikinheimo *et al.* 1991). This would be an optimal cancer prevention for men aged 40–51 years old.

Prostate cancer treatment with differentiating agents has been proposed (Walczak *et al.* 2001). The use of vitamin D is limited by its hypercalcaemic property, a problem to which the new less calcaemic derivatives of vitamin D might provide a solution (Blutt & Weigel 1999). 1,25(OH)$_2$D$_3$ evinces differentiating and growth-controlling activity in a wide range of tissues and cell types. These include keratinocytes (Hosomi *et al.* 1983), lung cells (Marin *et al.* 1993), adipocytes (Sato & Hiragun 1988), activated lymphocytes (Tsoukas *et al.* 1984), breast (Frappart *et al.* 1989), prostate (Esquenet *et al.* 1996, Miller *et al.* 1992, Skowronski *et al.* 1993) and colon carcinoma cell lines (Brehier & Thomasset 1988; Zhao & Feldman 1993) and several leukaemia cell lines (Abe *et al.* 1981, Tanaka *et al.* 1982).

It has been demonstrated that 1,25(OH)$_2$D$_3$ regulates the growth and differentiation of both female and male reproductive organs (Kinuta *et al.* 2000, Konety *et al.* 1996, Yoshizawa *et al.* 1997). VDR knock-out studies show that, after weaning, female mice lacking a functional vitamin D receptor exhibit uterine hypoplasia and folliculogenesis is impaired (Kinuta *et al.* 2000, Yoshizawa *et al.* 1997). In male mice, decreased sperm counts and sperm motility with histological abnormality of the testis can be observed (Kinuta *et al.* 2000). In prostate cancer cell lines 1,25(OH)$_2$D$_3$ promotes differentiation. Studies with a normal epithelial cell line derived from rat dorsal–lateral prostate show that autocrine production of TGF-beta may play a significant role in 1,25(OH)$_2$D$_3$-induced prostate differentiation (Danielpour 1996).

The great majority of causal relationships suggested by epidemiology have not been validitated by intervention trials and, therefore, caution in interpreting epidemiological findings is warranted (Young & Lee 1999). Largely, the lack of vitamin D intervention studies in humans is due to the known toxicity of the active form of vitamin D, calcitriol, resulting in induction of hypercalcaemia. However, Smith *et al.* (1999) demonstrated that substantial doses of calcitriol can be administered subcutaneously every other day with tolerable toxicity. The newly developed less calcaemic analogues provide even better tools for the treatment trials (Blutt & Weigel 1999). A phase I study of the effects of vitamin D analogue EB 1089 in advanced breast and colon cancer showed this analogue to be less calcaemic than 1,25-dihydroxyvitamin D$_3$, and showed stabilization of the disease in 6/36 patients, but with no complete responses (Gulliford *et al.* 1998). There have also been only limited trials to study the effects of 1,25(OH)$_2$D$_3$ or its analogues on prostate cancer in vivo (Feldman *et al.* 2000), including a small phase II trial of calcitriol in hormone refractory metastatic carcinoma (Osborn *et al.* 1995) and a small trial with non-metastasized prostate cancer in patients who were having a rising PSA as the only measure of recurrent disease (Gross *et al.* 1998). In spite of the scanty results of these trials, in his review Miller (1998) concludes that the time is ripe to consider the use of vitamin D as a clinical tool in the treatment of prostate cancer, whether it would be in the form of chemoprevention trials or treatment trials, up to hormone refractory advanced disease.

Conclusions

Vitamin D has a potent growth inhibitory function in prostate cancer, with a multitude of mechanisms. It can regulate cell cycle regulatory proteins, expression of growth factors and their receptors, nuclear receptor expression and local metabolism of nuclear receptor ligands (Ylikomi *et al.* 2001). The growth inhibition aspect is associated with the differentiation-promoting effects of prostate cancer cells. In certain cell types vitamin D can also induce apoptosis or sensitize cells for apoptosis. Thus, vitamin D has a wide range of potential therapeutic uses in treating cellular defects characterized by increased cell proliferation and decreased differentiation, as in prostate cancer, among many other cancer types. Epidemiological studies have demonstrated that vitamin D exerts a protective effect against carcinogenesis, suggesting that it might not only be involved in regulating the growth of cancer cells but could also have a role in regulating cancer initiation, promotion and progression (Ahonen *et al.* 2000a).

Cross-talk between vitamin D and androgen signalling systems suggests the possibility of using combinatory therapy whereby the serum androgen level is decreased and the serum vitamin D level increased. In Figure 8.6, we illustrate the important steps in the cross-talk between androgen and vitamin D signalling. The local metabolism of both steroids might be of crucial importance for prostate cancer development and treatment, as discussed above. The usefulness of vitamin D is limited by reason of the severe harmful effects arising from its hypercalcaemic property. Much effort has therefore been directed to identifying new vitamin D analogues with potent cell regulatory effects but with less calcaemic effect. In prostate cancer prevention, it is important to adjust vitamin D balance in the case of

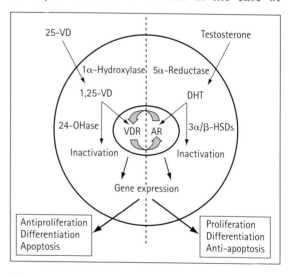

Figure 8.6
A model of the interaction between androgens and vitamin D in the regulation of the growth of the prostate. The local metabolism (= activation and inactivation) of both steroids is important. The steroids can mutually regulate the expression of their receptors. Therefore the antiproliferative action of vitamin D may depend on androgen action and the differentiation markers of vitamin D action are similar to those of androgen: $3\alpha/\beta HSDs = 3\alpha/3\beta$-hydroxysteroid dehydrogenases; 24-OHase = 1,25-dihydroxyvitamin D_3 24-hydroxylase; VDR = vitamin D receptor; AR = androgen receptor.

seasonal vitamin D deficiency and deficient nutritional intake by dietary vitamin D supplementation and by higher UV exposure.

Acknowledgements

Work in this laboratory was financially supported by grants from Medical Research Fund of Tampere University Hospital and the Finnish Cancer Foundation. We thank Arja Ahola, Taina Eskola and Janette Hinkka for their skillful assistance in blood sampling.

References

Abe E, Miyaura C, Sakagami H, et al. (1981) Differentiation of mouse myeloid leukemia cells induced by 1 alpha, 25-dihydroxyvitamin D3. *Proc Natl Acad Sci USA,* 78:4990–4994.

Adams JS, Gacad MA (1985) Characterization of 1 alpha-hydroxylation of vitamin D3 sterols by cultured alveolar macrophages from patients with sarcoidosis. *J Exp Med* 161:755–765.

Ahonen MH, Tenkanen L, Teppo L, Hakama M, Tuohimaa P (2000a) Prostate cancer risk and prediagnostic serum 25-hydroxyvitamin D levels (Finland). *Cancer Causes and Control* 11:847–852.

Ahonen MH, Zhuang YH, Aine R, Ylikomi T, Tuohimaa P (2000b) Androgen receptor and vitamin D receptor in human ovarian cancer: growth stimulation and inhibition by ligands. *Int J Cancer* 86:40–46.

Alagol F, Shihadeh Y, Boztepe H, et al. (2000) Sunlight exposure and vitamin D deficiency in Turkish women. *J Endocrinol Invest* 23:173–177.

Albertson DG, Ylstra B, Segraves R, et al. (2000) Quantitative mapping of amplicon structure by array CGH identifies CYP24 as a candidate oncogene. *Nat Genet* 25:144–146.

Blutt SE, Weigel NL (1999) Vitamin D and prostate cancer. *Proc Soc Exp Biol Med* 221:89–98.

Blutt SE, McDonnell TJ, Polek TC, Weigel NL (2000) Calcitriol-induced apoptosis in LNCaP cells is blocked by overexpression of Bcl-2. *Endocrinology* 141:10–17.

Botling J, Oberg F, Torma H, et al. (1996) Vitamin D3- and retinoic acid-induced monocytic differentiation: interactions between the endogenous vitamin D3 receptor, retinoic acid receptors, and retinoid X receptors in U-937 cells. *Cell Growth Differ* 7:1239–1249.

Bouillon R, Okamura WH, Norman AW (1995) Structure–function relationships in the vitamin D endocrine system. *Endocr Rev* 16:200–257.

Braun MM, Helzlsouer KJ, Hollis BW, Comstock GW (1995) Prostate cancer and prediagnostic levels of serum vitamin D metabolites (Maryland, United States). *Cancer Causes and Control* 6:235–239.

Brehier A, Thomasset M (1988) Human colon cell line HT-29: characterisation of 1,25-dihydroxyvitamin D3 receptor and induction of differentiation by the hormone. *J Steroid Biochem* 29:265–270.

Carter BS, Carter HB, Isaacs JT (1990) Epidemiologic evidence regarding predisposing factors to prostate cancer. *Prostate* 16:187–197.

Corder EH, Guess HA, Hulka BS, et al. (1993) Vitamin D and prostate cancer: a prediagnostic study with stored sera. *Cancer Epidemiol Biomarkers Prev* 2:467–472.

Cussenot O, Valeri A, Berthon P, Fournier G, Mangin P (1998) Hereditary prostate cancer and other genetic predispositions to prostate cancer. *Urol Int* 60:30–44; discussion 35.

Danielpour D (1996) Induction of transforming growth factor-beta autocrine activity by all-trans-retinoic acid and 1 alpha, 25-dihydroxyvitamin D3 in NRP-152 rat prostatic epithelial cells. *J Cell Physiol* 166:231–239.

Demay MB, Kiernan MS, DeLuca HF, Kronenberg HM (1992) Sequences in the human parathyroid hormone gene that bind the 1,25-dihydroxyvitamin D3 receptor and mediate transcriptional repression in response to 1,25-dihydroxyvitamin D3. *Proc Natl Acad Sci USA,* 89:8097–8101.

Doll R, Peto R (1981) The causes of cancer: quantitative estimates of avoidable risks of cancer in the United States today. *J Natl Cancer Inst* 66:1191–1308.

Dormanen MC, Bishop JE, Hammond MW, et al. (1994) Nonnuclear effects of the steroid hormone 1 alpha, 25(OH)2-vitamin D3: analogs are able to functionally differentiate between nuclear and membrane receptors. *Biochem Biophys Res Comm* 201:394–401.

Esquenet M, Swinnen JV, Heyns W, Verhoeven G (1996) Control of LNCaP proliferation and differentiation: actions and interactions of androgens, 1alpha, 25-dihydroxycholecalciferol, all-trans retinoic acid, 9-cis retinoic acid, and phenylacetate. *Prostate* 28:182–194.

Feldman D, Zhao XY, Krishnan AV (2000) Vitamin D and prostate cancer. *Endocrinology* **141**:5–9.

Fife RS, Sledge GW Jr, Proctor C (1997) Effects of vitamin D3 on proliferation of cancer cells in vitro. *Cancer Lett* **120**:65–69.

Frappart L, Falette N, Lefebvre MF, *et al.* (1989) In vitro study of effects of 1,25 dihydroxyvitamin D3 on the morphology of human breast cancer cell line BT.20. *Differentiation* **40**:63–69.

Frick MH, Elo EO, Haapa K, *et al.* (1984) Helsinki Heart Study: primary-prevention trial with gemfibrozil in middle-aged men with dyslipidemia. Safety of treatment, changes in risk factors, and incidence of coronary heart disease. *N Engl J Med* **317**:1237–1245.

Gann PH, Ma J, Hennekens CH, *et al.* (1996) Circulating vitamin D metabolites in relation to subsequent development of prostate cancer. *Cancer Epidemiol Biomarkers Prev* **5**:121–126.

Garland CF, Garland FC (1980) Do sunlight and vitamin D reduce the likelihood of colon cancer? *Int J Epidemiol* **9**:227–231.

Garland FC, Garland CF, Gorham ED, Young JF (1990) Geographic variation in breast cancer mortality in the United States: a hypothesis involving exposure to solar radiation. *Prev Med* **19**:614–622.

Gloth FM 3rd, Alam W, Hollis B (1999) Vitamin D vs broad spectrum phototherapy in the treatment of seasonal affective disorder. *J Nutr Health Aging* **3**:5–7.

Gross C, Stamey T, Hancock S, Feldman D (1998) Treatment of early recurrent prostate cancer with 1,25-dihydroxyvitamin D3 (calcitriol) [published erratum appears in *J Urol* 1998 Sep;**160**(3 Pt 1):840]. *J Urol* **159**:2035–2039; discussion 2039–2040.

Gulliford T, English J, Colston KW, *et al.* (1998) A phase I study of the vitamin D analogue EB 1089 in patients with advanced breast and colorectal cancer. *Br J Cancer* **78**:6–13.

Hanchette CL, Schwartz GG (1992) Geographic patterns of prostate cancer mortality. Evidence for a protective effect of ultraviolet radiation. *Cancer* **70**:2861–2869.

Hedlund TE, Moffatt KA, Miller GJ (1996a) Stable expression of the nuclear vitamin D receptor in the human prostatic carcinoma cell line JCA-1: evidence that the antiproliferative effects of 1 alpha, 25-dihydroxyvitamin D3 are mediated exclusively through the genomic signaling pathway. *Endocrinology* **137**:1554–1561.

Hedlund TE, Moffatt KA, Miller GJ (1996b) Vitamin D receptor expression is required for growth modulation by 1 alpha, 25-dihydroxyvitamin D3 in the human prostatic carcinoma cell line ALVA-31. *J Steroid Biochem Mol Biol* **58**:277–288.

Heikinheimo RJ, Haavisto MV, Harju EJ, *et al.* (1991) Serum vitamin D level after an annual intramuscular injection of ergocalciferol. *Calcif Tissue Int* **49**:S87.

Henry HL (1997) The 25-hydroxyvitamin D 1a-hydroxylase. In: Feldman D, Glorieux FH, Pike JW, eds, *Vitamin D* (Academic Press: San Diego) 57–68.

Hewison M, Zehnder D, Bland R, Stewart PM (2000) 1 alpha-hydroxylase and the action of vitamin D. *J Mol Endocrinol* **25**:141–148.

Holick MF (1995) Defects in the synthesis and metabolism of vitamin D. *Exp Clin Endocrinol Diabetes* **103**:219–227.

Holick MF, MacLaughlin JA, Clark MB, *et al.* (1980a) Photosynthesis of previtamin D3 in human skin and the physiologic consequences. *Science* **210**:203–205.

Holick MF, Uskokovic M, Henley JW, *et al.* (1980b) The photoproduction of 1 alpha, 25-dihydroxyvitamin D3 in skin: an approach to the therapy of vitamin-D-resistant syndromes. *N Engl J Med* **303**:349–354.

Horst RL, Reinhardt TA (1997) Vitamin D metabolism. In: Feldman D, Glorieux FH, Pike JW, eds, *Vitamin D.* (Academic Press: San Diego) 13–31.

Hosomi J, Hosoi J, Abe E, Suda T, Kuroki T (1983) Regulation of terminal differentiation of cultured mouse epidermal cells by 1 alpha, 25-dihydroxyvitamin D3. *Endocrinology* **113**:1950–1957.

Hsieh T, Wu JM (1997) Induction of apoptosis and altered nuclear/cytoplasmic distribution of the androgen receptor and prostate-specific antigen by 1 alpha, 25-dihydroxyvitamin D3 in androgen-responsive LNCaP cells. *Biochem Biophys Res Comm* **235**:539–544.

Hsu JY, Feldman D, McNeal JE, Peehl DM (2001) Reduced 1 alpha-hydroxylase activity in human prostate cancer cells correlates with decreased susceptibility to 25-hydroxyvitamin D3-induced growth inhibition. *Cancer Res* **61**:2852–2856.

Ingles SA, Ross RK, Yu MC, *et al.* (1997) Association of prostate cancer risk with genetic polymorphisms in vitamin D receptor and androgen receptor. *J Natl Cancer Inst* **89**:166–170.

Kibel AS, Isaacs SD, Isaacs WB, Bova GS (1998) Vitamin D receptor polymorphisms and lethal prostate cancer. *J Urol* **160**:1405–1409.

Kinuta K, Tanaka H, Moriwake T, *et al.* (2000) Vitamin D is an important factor in estrogen biosynthesis

of both female and male gonads. *Endocrinology*
141:1317–1324.

Konety BR, Schwartz GG, Acierno JS, Jr, Becich MJ,
Getzenberg RH (1996) The role of vitamin D in nor-
mal prostate growth and differentiation. *Cell Growth
Differ* **7**:1563–1570.

Lamberg-Allardt C, Kirjarinta M, Dessypris AG (1983)
Serum 25-hydroxy-vitamin D, parathyroid hormone
and calcium levels in adult inhabitants above Arctic
circle in northern Finland. *Ann Clin Res* **15**:142–145.

Lokeshwar BL, Schwartz GG, Selzer MG, *et al*. (1999)
Inhibition of prostate cancer metastasis in vivo: a
comparison of 1,23-dihydroxyvitamin D (calcitriol) and
EB1089. *Cancer Epidemiol Biomarkers Prev* **8**:241–248.

Lundin AC, Soderkvist P, Eriksson B, Bergman-
Jungestrom M and Wingren S (1999) Association of
breast cancer progression with a vitamin D receptor
gene polymorphism. South-East Sweden Breast Cancer
Group. *Cancer Res* **59**:2332–2334.

Ly LH, Zhao XY, Holloway L, Feldman D (1999)
Liarozole acts synergistically with 1 alpha, 25-dihy-
droxyvitamin D3 to inhibit growth of DU 145 human
prostate cancer cells by blocking 24-hydroxylase
activity. *Endocrinology* **140**:2071–2076.

Lyakhovich A, Aksenov N, Pennanen P, *et al*. (2000)
Vitamin D induced up-regulation of keratinocyte
growth factor (FGF-7/KGF) in MCF-7 human breast
cancer cells. *Biochem Biophys Res Comm* **273**:675–680.

McConnell JD (1991) Physiologic basis of endocrine therapy for prostatic cancer. *Urol Clin North Am* **18**:1–13.

Majewski S, Skopinska M, Marczak M, *et al*. (1996)
Vitamin D3 is a potent inhibitor of tumor cell-induced
angiogenesis. *J Investig Dermatol Symp Proc* **1**:97–101.

Marin L, Dufour ME, Nguyen TM, Tordet C,
Garabedian M (1993) Maturational changes induced
by 1 alpha, 25-dihydroxyvitamin D3 in type II cells
from fetal rat lung explants. *Am J Physiol* **265**:L45–52.

Mawer EB, Backhouse J, Holman CA, Lumb GA,
Stanbury SW (1972) The distribution and storage of
vitamin D and its metabolites in human tissues. *Clin
Sci* **43**:413–431.

Mercier T, Chaumontet C, Gaillard-Sanchez I, Martel
P, Heberden C (1996) Calcitriol and lexicalcitol
(KH1060) inhibit the growth of human breast adenocarcinoma cells by enhancing transforming growth factor-beta production. *Biochem Pharmacol* **52**:505–510.

Miller GJ (1998) Vitamin D and prostate cancer: biologic
interactions and clinical potentials. *Cancer Metastasis
Rev* **17**:353–360.

Miller GJ, Stapleton GE, Ferrara JA, *et al*. (1992) The
human prostatic carcinoma cell line LNCaP expresses
biologically active, specific receptors for 1 alpha, 25-
dihydroxyvitamin D3. *Cancer Res* **52**:515–520.

Miller GJ, Stapleton GE, Hedlund TE, Moffat KA (1995)
Vitamin D receptor expression, 24-hydroxylase activity, and inhibition of growth by 1 alpha, 25-dihydroxy-
vitamin D3 in seven human prostatic carcinoma cell
lines. *Clin Cancer Res* **1**:997–1003.

Nomura AMY, Stemmermann GN, Lee J, *et al*. (1998)
Serum vitamin D metabolite levels and the subsequent
development of prostate cancer (Hawaii, United
States). *Cancer Causes and Control* **9**:425–432.

Norman AW, Frankel JB, Heldt AM, Grodsky GM (1980)
Vitamin D deficiency inhibits pancreatic secretion of
insulin. *Science* **209**:823–825.

Osborn JL, Schwartz GG, Smith DC, *et al*. (1995) Phase
II trial of oral 1,25-dihydroxyvitamin D (calcitriol) in
hormone refractory prostate cancer. *Urol Oncol*
1:195–198.

Peehl DM, Skowronski RJ, Leung GK, *et al*. (1994)
Antiproliferative effects of 1,25-dihydroxyvitamin D3
on primary cultures of human prostatic cells. *Cancer
Res* **54**:805–810.

Reichel H, Koeffler HP, Norman AW (1987) 25-
Hydroxyvitamin D3 metabolism by human T-
lymphotropic virus-transformed lymphocytes. *J Clin
Endocrinol Metab* **65**:519–526.

Reichel H, Koeffler HP, Norman AW (1989) The role of
the vitamin D endocrine system in health and disease.
N Engl J Med **320**:980–991.

Ruggiero M, Pacini S, Aterini S, *et al*. (1998) Vitamin D
receptor gene polymorphism is associated with
metastatic breast cancer. *Oncol Res* **10**:43–46.

Ruijter E, van de Kaa C, Miller G, *et al*. (1999) Molecular
genetics and epidemiology of prostate carcinoma.
Endocrine Rev **20**:22–45.

Sato M, Hiragun A (1988) Demonstration of 1 alpha, 25-
dihydroxyvitamin D3 receptor-like molecule in ST 13
and 3T3 L1 preadipocytes and its inhibitory effects
on preadipocyte differentiation. *J Cell Physiol* **135**:
545–550.

Schwartz GG, Hulka BS (1990) Is vitamin D deficiency
a risk factor for prostate cancer? (Hypothesis).
Anticancer Res **10**:1307–1311.

Schwartz GG, Oeler TA, Uskokovic MR, Bahnson RR
(1994) Human prostate cancer cells: inhibition of
proliferation by vitamin D analogs. *Anticancer Res*
14:1077–1081.

Schwartz GG, Wang M-H, Zhang RK, *et al*. (1997) 1α,
25-dihydroxyvitamin D (calcitriol) inhibits the

invasiveness of human prostate cancer cells. *Cancer Epidemiol Biomarkers Prev* 6:727–732.

Schwartz GG, Whitlatch LW, Chen TC, Lokeshwar BL, Holick MF (1998) Human prostate cells synthesize 1,25-dihydroxyvitamin D3 from 25-hydroxyvitamin D3. *Cancer Epidemiol Biomarkers Prev* 7:391–395.

Skowronski RJ, Peehl DM, Feldman D (1993) Vitamin D and prostate cancer: 1,25 dihydroxyvitamin D3 receptors and actions in human prostate cancer cell lines. *Endocrinology* 132:1952–1960.

Smith DC, Johnson CS, Freeman CC, et al. (1999) A Phase I trial of calcitriol (1,25-dihydroxycholecalciferol) in patients with advanced malignancy. *Clin Cancer Res* 5:1339–1345.

Smith EL, Walworth NC, Holick MF (1986) Effect of 1 alpha, 25-dihydroxyvitamin D3 on the morphologic and biochemical differentiation of cultured human epidermal keratinocytes grown in serum-free conditions. *J Invest Dermatol* 86:709–714.

Suda T, Takahashi N, Martin TJ (1992) Modulation of osteoclast differentiation [published erratum appears in *Endocr Rev* (1992) 13(2):191]. *Endocr Rev* 13:66–80.

Tanaka H, Abe E, Miyaura C, et al. (1982) 1 alpha, 25-dihydroxycholecalciferol and a human myeloid leukaemia cell line (HL-60). *Biochem J* 204:713–719.

Taylor JA, Hirvonen A, Watson M, et al. (1996) Association of prostate cancer with vitamin D receptor gene polymorphism. *Cancer Res* 56:4108–4110.

Teppo L (2000) Cancer incidence in Finland 1996 and 1997. *Cancer Soc Finland Publ* 61:10.

Tsoukas CD, Provvedini DM, Manolagas SC (1984) 1,25-dihydroxyvitamin D3: a novel immunoregulatory hormone. *Science* 224:1438–1440.

Tuohimaa P, Ahonen MH, Lyakhovitch A, et al. (2000) Vitamin D and prostate cancer. *J Steroid Biochem Mol Biol* 76:

van Leeuwen JPTM, Pols HAP (1997) Vitamin D: anti-cancer and differentiation. In: Feldman D, Glorieux FH, Pike JW, eds, *Vitamin D* (Academic Press: San Diego) 1089–1105.

Walczak J, Wood H, Wilding G, et al. (2001) Prostate cancer prevention strategies using antiproliferative or differentiating agents. *Urology* 57:81–85.

Webb AR, Kline L, Holick MF (1988) Influence of season and latitude on the cutaneous synthesis of vitamin D3: exposure to winter sunlight in Boston and Edmonton will not promote vitamin D3 synthesis in human skin. *J Clin Endocrinol Metab* 67:373–378.

Whitlach LW, Young MV, Wang L, et al. (2001) Vitamin D autocrine system and prostate cancer. *International Symposium 'Disorders of the Prostate' Abstract Book*, 43.

Ylikomi T, Laaksi I, Lou Y-L, et al. (2002) Antiproliferative action of vitamin D. *Vitam Horm* 64:357–406.

Yoshizawa T, Handa Y, Uematsu Y, et al. (1997) Mice lacking the vitamin D receptor exhibit impaired bone formation, uterine hypoplasia and growth retardation after weaning. *Nat Genet* 16:391–396.

Young KJ, Lee PN (1999) Intervention studies on cancer. *Eur J Cancer Prev* 8:91–103.

Zehnder D, Bland R, Walker EA, et al. (1999) Expression of 25-hydroxyvitamin D3-1 alpha-hydroxylase in the human kidney. *J Am Soc Nephrol* 10:2465–2473.

Zhao X, Feldman D (1993) Regulation of vitamin D receptor abundance and responsiveness during differentiation of HT-29 human colon cancer cells. *Endocrinology* 132:1808–1814.

Zhao J, Tan BK, Marcelis S, Verstuyf A, Bouillon R (1996) Enhancement of antiproliferative activity of 1 alpha, 25-dihydroxyvitamin D3 (analogs) by cytochrome P450 enzyme inhibitors is compound- and cell-type specific. *J Steroid Biochem Mol Biol* 57:197–202.

Zhao XY, Ly LH, Peehl DM, Feldman D (1999) Induction of androgen receptor by 1 alpha, 25-dihydroxyvitamin D3 and 9-cis retinoic acid in LNCaP human prostate cancer cells. *Endocrinology* 140:1205–1212.

Zhao XY, Peehl DM, Navone NM, Feldman D (2000) 1 alpha, 25-dihydroxyvitamin D3 inhibits prostate cancer cell growth by androgen-dependent and androgen-independent mechanisms. *Endocrinology* 141:2548–2556.

Zhuang SH, Burnstein KL (1998) Antiproliferative effect of 1 alpha, 25-dihydroxyvitamin D3 in human prostate cancer cell line LNCaP involves reduction of cyclin-dependent kinase 2 activity and persistent G1 accumulation. *Endocrinology* 139:1197–1207.

Zhuang SH, Schwartz GG, Cameron D, Burnstein KL (1997) Vitamin D receptor content and transcriptional activity do not fully predict antiproliferative effects of vitamin D in human prostate cancer cell lines. *Mol Cell Endocrinol* 126:83–90.

9 A novel gene therapeutic strategy co-targeting tumor epithelium and stroma

Leland WK Chung, Andrew Law, Hong Rhee, Shigeji Matsubara, Chia-Ling Hsieh, Masayuki Egawa, Moon-Soo Park, Kenneth Koeneman, Fan Yeung and Haiyen E Zhau

Introduction

Cancer cells and their genetic constituents may be altered during disease progression (Nowell 1976, Hanahan & Weinberg 2000, Compagni & Christoferi 2000). The type of genetic alteration and the resultant changes in gene expression can be attributed either to inherited or acquired factors, or to both. The hierarchical genetic alteration of cancer cells precedes alterations in gene expression. Mechanisms include the overexpression of tumor-causing genes and metastasis-associated genes (Baker *et al.* 1990), loss of the expression of tumor suppressors through promoter silencing by hypermethylation (Baylin *et al.* 1998), gene deletion/mutation/re-arrangement (Ni *et al.* 2000), or modulation of specific intracellular signaling pathways (Chen *et al.* 2000) with the participation of key transcription factors that may affect the overall transcriptional/translational efficiency of specific target genes (Rhee *et al.* 2001). This chapter addresses three related points concerning tumor–stroma interaction:

1. Human prostate cancer epithelial cells interact with stromal cells in a reciprocal manner. We documented that permanent genetic and phenotypic alterations of human prostate cancer and prostate and bone stromal cells can be achieved through co-culture of tumor epithelial cells with either prostate or bone stromal cells under three-dimensional (3-D) rotating wall vessel conditions (Rhee *et al.* 2001, and unpublished results). The resulting genetically altered prostate cancer and stromal cells can trigger a further cascade of tumor–stromal interaction, resulting in enhanced tumorigenic, androgen-independent and metastatic progression of prostate tumor epithelial cells.

2. As prostate tumor cells acquire increasing tumorigenic and metastatic potential in bone, they also acquire the ability to synthesize and deposit noncollagenous bone matrix proteins such as osteopontin, osteocalcin (OC), bone sialoprotein and osteonectin. These 'bone-like' properties of prostate cancer cells are termed 'osteomimetic' and may enhance the ability of tumor cells to adhere, invade and survive in the skeleton (Koeneman *et al.* 1999).

3. Because of the osteomimetic properties of prostate tumor epithelial cells in bone, we propose a novel co-targeting strategy using tissue-specific and tumor-restrictive

promoters to co-target tumor epithelium and its supporting stroma to maximize cell kill and minimize further genetic and phenotypic alterations induced through tumor–stroma interaction (Koeneman *et al.* 1999, Matsubara *et al.* 2001, Gardner *et al.* 1998). We predict that this strategy will improve tumor cell kill, and minimize subsequent phenotypic and genotypic drifts of tumor cells and their resistance to hormone, radiation and chemotherapy.

Stroma–epithelium interaction in normal prostate development and prostate cancer progression

The intricate intercellular communication between stromal and epithelial cells involves cell–cell, cell-insoluble extracellular matrix proteins (ECMs) and cell-soluble factor mediated processes (Anastasiadis & Reynold 2000, Song *et al.* 2000). The 'cross-talk' between cells mediated by factors synthesized, secreted and/or deposited is highly complex and often interactive and redundant, involving intracellular signaling pathways and cell surface receptors that coordinate and interpret external stimuli. It remains a challenge to assess how cells mediate specific and dynamic inter- and intracellular signaling cascades. It is intriguing to observe that under some conditions such communication may be reversible (Song *et al.* 2000, Levine *et al.* 1995), while under other conditions, as described herein, the structure, function and behavior of cancer cells subsequent to cell–cell interaction can be altered permanently (Rhee *et al.* 2001, Chung & Zhau

2001). These early publications indicate that some important features of stromal–epithelial interaction deserve special attention.

First, intracellular transcription factors such as androgen receptor (AR) could play a role in mediating intracellular communication and mediating downstream signal cascades that involve 'cross-talk' between external soluble and insoluble factor stimuli and intracellular signaling network (Qiu *et al.* 1998, Wen *et al.* 2000). Recent research has made it increasingly clear that specific extracellular ligands can interact with cell surface receptors and mediate a set of intracellular signaling cascades involving protein tyrosine kinases, phosphatases, transcription factors, and cell structure-associated molecules that ultimately determine cell growth, cell cycle arrest, apoptosis and survival of cells (Wen *et al.* 2000, Culig *et al.* 1994). In addition, cell behaviors such as attachment, detachment, migration, invasion and metastasis could be altered through cell–cell communication (McCawley & Matrisian 2000, Fuseniz & Boukamp 1998, Chung & Davis 1996). Tissue and cell recombination studies have demonstrated that AR in fetal prostate stroma may be responsible for driving prostate development (Chung *et al.* 1981, Cunha *et al.* 1981). AR in the epithelium could assume the regulatory function and determine the ultimate growth and differentiation potential of adult normal and tumor epithelium (Kokotis & Liao 1999). Experimental evidence from co-cultured human BPH-derived stromal and epithelial cells indicates that the expression of AR, prostate-specific antigen (PSA) and 5-α-reductase in the epithelial cells relies on the inductive influence of neighboring stromal cells (Bayne *et al.* 1998, Grant *et al.* 1996). Similarly, in co-cultured rat prostatic epithelial and fibroblast cells, AR-mediated growth responses can be conferred by the presence of prostate fibroblasts (Chang &

Chung 1989). However, in transplantable PC-82 human prostate cancer xenografts maintained in Tfm/y athymic mice, AR in the epithelium rather than the stroma is required for androgen responsiveness of the prostate tumors *in vivo*. Once prostate cancer cells acquire the ability to grow autonomously as xenografts and are passaged in immune-compromised competent hosts (Gao & Isaacs 1998), AR in the epithelium rather than in the stroma may play a regulatory role.

Secondly genetic changes in the tumor epithelium are required but are insufficient in themselves to drive the metastatic cascade. Using a human prostate cancer epithelial cell line, LNCaP, as a model, we and others demonstrated that despite its extensive chromosomal changes, this cell line remained non-tumorigenic and non-metastatic in castrated hosts (Gleave *et al.* 1992, Wu *et al.* 1998). We observed that by growing LNCaP cells as chimeric tumors with either prostate or bone fibroblasts followed by *in-vitro* cell cultures revealed subtle and nonrandom genetic changes in LNCaP cells, which had acquired tumorigenic and metastatic potential in castrated hosts (Rhee *et al.* 2001). The derivative LNCaP sublines were observed to undergo further chromosomal alterations, demonstrated by comparative genomic hybridization (CGH), which mimicked the genetic changes found in clinical human prostate cancer specimens (Rhee *et al.* 2001, Hyytinen *et al.* 1997). These observations demonstrate the importance of cell–cell contact and soluble and insoluble factors in the microenvironment, which together could induce and permanently alter the genetics and behaviors of tumor epithelial cells.

Thirdly, to gain access to distant anatomical sites, metastatic prostate cancer cells must fulfill a number of conditions, including local cell proliferation, invasion through basement membranes, attachment to basolateral surfaces of endothelial cells, migration and invasion through intercellular space between endothelium or the lining cells in the lymphatic channels, intravasation to the blood circulation to form and survive as circulating tumor emboli, attachment to endothelial cells residing at metastatic sites and, finally, invasion, migration and extravasation at the metastatic sites, such as the lymph node or skeleton. Once tumor cells arrive at these distant sites, they may re-establish their proliferative potential and enhance their interaction with local stromal cells and further invade, migrate and metastasize to form additional soft tissue deposits.

Using co-cultured prostate cancer epithelial cells with either prostate or bone stromal cells, we have demonstrated permanent nonrandom genotypic and phenotypic changes in prostate stromal cells subsequent to cell–cell interaction under 3-D growth conditions (Rhee *et al.* 2001). We used a rotary wall vessel (RWV) invented by the NASA Bioengineering Group to establish prostate organoids by co-culturing human prostate cancer cells with either human prostate or bone stromal cells under low shearing forces. After these cell cultures, prostate cancer and bone stromal cells were further isolated from the prostate organoid and tested extensively for their growth and gene expression capabilities. Table 9.1 summarizes a study in which we demonstrated that LNCaP derivative RWV1, 2 and 3 cells have undergone permanent genetic and phenotypic alterations when co-cultured with collagen-coated microcarrier beads (RWV1), with human prostate fibroblasts (RWV2) or with human bone stromal cells (RWV3) *in vitro*. As shown in Table 9.1, the derivative RWV1, 2, and 3 cells, unlike their parental LNCaP cells, have acquired the ability to grow in castrated hosts and express varying degree of metastatic potential *in vivo*. These results are further supported by

Table 9.1 Tumorigenicity and metastatic potentials of parental LNCaP and its derivative RWV sublines in castrated hosts with tumor cells administered orthotopically

Cell lines	Incidence of tumorigenicity* (%)	Incidence of metastasis† (%)			
		Lymph node	Lung	Liver	Bone
LNCaP	0/5 (0)	0/5 (0)	0/5 (0)	0/5 (0)	0/5 (0)
RWV1	7/8 (87.5)	7/8 (87.5)	1/8 (12.5)	0/8 (0)	5/8 (62.5)
RWV2	7/8 (87.5)	7/8 (87.5)	1/8 (12.5)	1/8 (12.5)	7/8 (87.5)
RWV3	8/8 (100)	7/8 (87.5)	2/8 (25)	2/8 (25)	5/8 (62.5)

*Incidence is defined as numbers of tumors/numbers of animals. Percentage of tumor formation and metastasis are calculated directly from the observed incidence.
†All metastases, including bones, were observed in animals with primary tumor.

chromosomal changes in prostate cancer cells, as demonstrated by both cytogenetic and CGH analyzes (Rhee *et al.* 2001). In a reciprocal manner, we have also co-cultured the human bone stromal cell line MG63 with an androgen-independent and metastatic C4-2 cell line (a lineage-derived LNCaP subline) under 3-D conditions in the RWV system. We observed similar permanent genetic and phenotypic changes in MG63 cells subsequent to cell–cell interaction with C4-2 cells. MG63 cells have been observed to undergo nonrandom genetic alterations, demonstrated by conventional cytogenetic and CGH analyzes (unpublished results). The altered MG63 cells after *in-vitro* cell–cell interaction with C4-2 cells in RWV condition appeared to be less well-differentiated (decreased OC and alkaline phosphatase expression) and to be more inductive in stimulating growth and PSA expression when co-cultured with LNCaP cells under 3-D conditions (Figure 9.1). These results raise the possibility that an intercellular communication cascade could trigger permanent genetic and phenotypic changes in prostate stromal and epithelial cells, culminating in the increased malignant potential of tumor epithelium. Figure 9.2 proposes the hypothesis of a 'ping-pong' mechanism where tumor epithelial cells could interact with tumor associated stromal cells in the following manner. First, tumor epithelial cells, with either inherited or acquired genetic changes, could induce a desmoplastic response in tumor-associated stromal cells in the prostate gland. Initially, the tumor and stroma responses may involve a fundamental change in gene expression rather than genetic modifications. Secondly, after prolonged interaction between tumor epithelium and surrounding stromal cells under *in-vivo* growth conditions, the behaviorally altered prostate stromal cells could signal epithelial cells to undergo additional genetic and behavior changes characterized by the ability of prostate cancer cells to secrete soluble and insoluble factors, further modifying the adjacent tumor stroma microenvironment. Thirdly, in response to inductive influence from tumor epithelium, tumor-associated stroma could become receptive and undergo permanent genetic and phenotypic changes so that they become more inductive and instructive

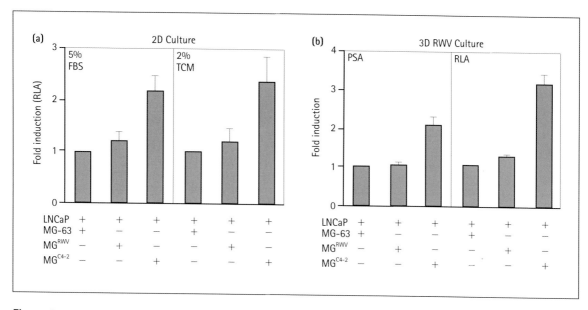

Figure 9.1

Increased cell growth and PSA production by LNCaP cells (stably transfected with luciferase gene) treated with conditioned media collected from MG^C4-2 cells. Luciferase activity was found to correlate linearly with total cell number as analyzed by both cell count and MTT assay. (a) MG^C4-2 CM, either collected with 2% FBS or without 2% TCM serum, stimulated the growth of LNCaP cells cultured under 2-D conditions (growth of LNCaP cells was measured by RLA or relative luciferase activity); comparatively, CMs obtained from either MG63 or MG^RMV, stimulated to a lesser extent, LNCaP cell growth *in vitro*. (b) Similar growth and PSA stimulatory activities were observed in LNCaP cells when cultured under 3-D conditions exposed to CM prepared from MG^C4-2, but not from MG63 or MG^RMV cells (prepared in 2% serum-free TCM). These results support the conclusion that permanent changes have been introduced in MG63 cells after co-culture with human prostate cancer C4-2.

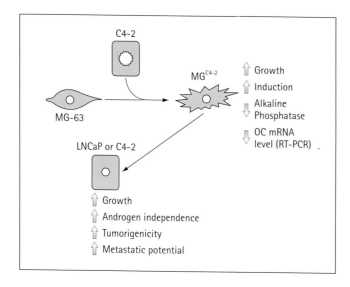

Figure 9.2

A proposed 'ping-pong' mechanism indicating the close interplay between tumor and stroma. Co-culture of MG-63 with C4-2 cells induced permanent genetic and phenotypic changes of parental MG-63 cells to express enhanced growth and inductive activity; the altered MG-63 cells, or MG^C4-2, appear to be less well differentiated (decreased expression of alkaline phosphatase and OC mRNA). Altered MG-63 C4-2 appeared to induce LNCaP cells to progress to androgen-independence and expressed higher growth and metastatic potentials (Rhee *et al.* 2001).

and modify the behaviors of prostate cancer epithelial cells in the direction of further increasing their androgen-independent and malignant potentials. It is also likely that cancer cells in the skeleton may serve as a 'reservoir' for further metastatic dissemination to soft tissues. The increasing malignant potential of prostate cancer cells in the skeleton following tumor–bone stroma interaction could further metastasize to liver, lung, brain and kidney. Alternatively, the enhanced malignant potential of prostate cancer cells subsequent to cell–cell interaction with osteoblasts could result in the ability of prostate cancer cells to synthesize and secrete highly active cachectic factors into circulation, with lethal consequences to patients.

Osteomimetic properties of prostate cancer cells

Localized metastatic prostate cancer cells acquire the ability to synthesize and deposit 'bone-like' proteins, such as osteopontin, osteocalcin, osteonectin and bone sialo-protein. The ability of prostate cancer cells to synthesize and deposit these bone matrix proteins parallels the enhanced differentiation of osteoblasts from their immature to mature states, where these bone matrix proteins are synthesized and deposited by the maturing osteoblasts. The molecular mechanism by which prostate cancer cells express 'bone-like' proteins is not fully known, but clearly a switching of intracellular transcription factors with the regulatory role of the promoter regions of these bone matrix proteins must play a role in instructing the transformed prostatic epithelial cells to behave and function effectively in the bone microenvironment. We

recently hypothesized that the osteomimetic property of prostate cancer cells underlies the predilection of prostate cancer for metastasis and growth in the bone microenvironment (Koeneman *et al.* 1999). Several major factors need to come into play to determine the ultimate osteoblastic and osteolytic responses by prostate cancer cells in bone. We propose an initial implantation of prostate cancer cells in the bone with growth factor cascade predominance, stimulated by urinary plasminogen activator (uPA) and endothelin-1 (ET1) production by the prostate carcinoma. We propose three stages of prostate cancer growth: implantation state, activation state and blastic state. Each of these states involves specific changes in the soluble growth factor and matrix milieu, resulting in the initial exponential growth of the prostate cancer cells in the implantation state, osteolytic response induced by the secondary action of uPA and parathyroid hormone-related peptide (PTHrP) and low PSA. At the activation state, TGFβ may stimulate the activity of bone morphogenic proteins (BMPs), increase prostatic adenocarcinoma cell mass in the bone and initiate neovascularization. At the blastic state, a series of bone transcription activators and the general transcriptional machinery are activated, culminating in the phenotypic expression of prostate cancer cells from a preosteoblast to an osteoblastic-like phenotype. This is made possible through coupled increase of PSA production that inactivates PTHrP, a factor that may be required for bone pitting via enhanced interaction between RANK ligand (RANKL) and RANK. The increased and unopposed action of BMPs may further activate the blastic phenotype in prostate cancer cells in the late stage of prostate growth and osteoblastic reactions seen in the bone (Koeneman *et al.* 1999).

It should be emphasized that a number of common growth factors in bone and prostate cancer cells could be responsible for the trophism of prostate cancer to bone. For example, the IGF axis can be enhanced by ET1 and uPA, resulting in the overall stimulation of osteoblast and prostate growth and differentiation, enhanced prostate cancer invasion and androgen-independent growth and survival. Basic FGF secretion and action can be enhanced by ET1, resulting in strong stimulation of prostate and bone cell growth and osteoclastic activity. TGFβ, on the other hand, could be regulated by various proteases and uPA, stimulating extracellular matrix protein turnover, inhibiting prostate tumor growth, suppressing host immune response and stimulating the production of BMPs (Koeneman *et al.* 1999). A paracrine growth factor such as hepatocyte growth factor/scatter factor (HGF/SF) may be induced through androgen ablation (Humphrey *et al.* 1995, Matsumoto 1994). HGF/SF could induce cell motility, migration and invasion, and also could be responsible for stimulating osteoblast growth and recruitment of osteoclasts that could change the balance between prostate cancer and bone stroma (Koeneman *et al.* 1999).

Stroma–epithelium interaction: possible co-targeting using gene therapy

Gene therapy holds a promise for treatment of metabolic diseases and cancer. However, this form of therapy is still in its infancy because of the inefficiency of gene delivery to target cells, and the difficulties encountered with delivery of viral vectors, expression of therapeutic genes specifically at tumor sites without damaging normal organs and the viral protein-elicited host immune responses that prevent repeated and long-term application of therapeutic viruses to hosts with an intact immune system.

In this chapter we describe our efforts in developing a co-targeting strategy for both prostate epithelial and stromal compartments to increase cell kill. Several studies have shown that such an approach is justified at the pre-clinical and the clinical levels. First, Hsieh *et al.* (2004) observed that when prostate cancer cells were co-cultured with bone stromal cells transduced with *hsv*TK (herpes simplex virus thymidine kinase) gene, the growth of prostate cancer was enhanced 2- to 3-fold. Upon the destruction of bone stromal cells in the presence of a prodrug ganciclovir (GCV), marked prostate cancer cell death has been induced. This study is also supported by *in-vivo* results where the growth of prostate cancer chimera with bone stroma was markedly inhibited upon the treatment of animals with systemic GCV. Secondly, in a co-culture study where an adenoviral vector Ad-OC-*hsv*TK, when infected both prostatic epithelial and stromal cell compartments resulted in increased prostate tumor cell death *in vitro*. These results further substantiated the concept that co-targeting both prostate cancer and bone stromal compartments with Ad-OC-*hsv*TK in the presence of prodrug GCV could induce more effective tumor cell killing. The effectiveness of this strategy relies on the expression of the *hsv*TK gene in both tumor epithelium and bone stroma compartments. Thirdly, in a series of studies using either Ad-OC-*hsv*TK/GCV (toxic gene approach) or replication-competent or oncolytic adenovirus approach with early viral gene E1a driven by OC promoter (Ad-OC-E1a), we demonstrated that administration either intratumorally (Ad-OC-*hsv*TK) or systemically (Ad-OC-E1a) could effectively induce either local tumor cell death or eradicate pre-existing tumors at metastatic sites, respectively (Matsubara *et al.* 2001, Gardner *et al.* 1998). A series of preclinical studies also demonstrated that both Ad-OC-*hsv*TK and Ad-OC-E1a are of low toxicity, have no adverse effect on liver or kidney function and do not damage normal bone (Koeneman *et al.* 2000). The effectiveness of this form of adenoviral therapy can be explained by the uniqueness of OC promoter, which presumably drives the expression of toxic gene or oncolysis in at least three cellular compartments – tumor epithelium, bone stroma and vascular endothelial pericytes – because all three of these cellular compartments were shown to express OC protein (Matsubara *et al.* 2001, Chung & Zhau 2001). Fourthly, the rationale for co-targeting bone stroma and prostate cancer epithelial cells was supported in a recent clinical study where Tu *et al.* (2001) demonstrated that bone targeting of metastatic prostate cancer in the bone with chemoinduction plus strontium 89 (Sr89) significantly improved patient survival in comparison to Sr89 or chemoinduction alone. The improved survival of patients subjected to co-targeting of bone stroma and prostate tumor epithelium using chemoinduction and Sr89 dramatizes the additional advantages of co-targeting, and supports our strategy of co-targeting tumor epithelium and bone stroma by gene therapy, which could eventually result in the improved survival of patients with metastatic prostate cancer in the bone.

In our laboratory, we have recently conducted additional studies to enhance gene delivery and tumor cell kill. Egawa *et al.* (unpublished data) demonstrated that a bifunctional PSMA (prostate-specific membrane antigen) antibody conjugated to antiviral fiber antibody resulted in improved specificity of viral delivery to target epithelial cells that express PSMA cell surface antigen. Park *et al.* (unpublished data) observed that IL12 and IL2 tumor vaccines could also improve the efficiency of adenoviruses to exert systemic anti-tumor effects mediated by cytokines against the growth of prostate tumor cells tagged with a luciferase marker. These approaches could further enhance both the specificity and the immunogenicity of adenoviral targeting to improve tumor cell kill and decrease tumor cell survival at metastatic sites.

Summary and conclusion

Reciprocal interaction between tumor ('seed') and stroma ('soil') has been recognized clinically by Paget (1889) and is further defined and characterized in this chapter using prostate tumor cell models. We provide evidence to support the concept that:

1. permanent genetic and phenotypic alterations of prostate cancer and bone stromal cells can be achieved by co-culturing these cell types under 3-D conditions
2. co-targeting tumor growth using adenoviral vectors with therapeutic gene expression driven by tissue-specific and tumor-restrictive bone matrix protein promoters can yield improved tumor cell kill, reduce the ability of tumor cells to evolve and decrease their subsequent invasive and metastatic potentials.

Co-targeting has been applied successfully in various preclinical *in-vitro* and *in-vivo* models. We have observed that animals with pre-existing prostate tumor growth in the bone respond favorably to this type of therapy, with some animals 'cured' of prostate tumors grown in the skeleton (Matsubara *et al.* 2001).

Based on recent data from patient studies (Tu *et al.* 2001), we hypothesize that co-targeting prostate tumor and bone stroma could result in increased survival and an improved quality of life for patients with prostate cancer bony metastasis.

Acknowledgement

The authors want to express their deep appreciation for financial support from the Kluge and CaPCURE Foundations, NIH CA-85555 and CA-76620 NASA-NC88-171 and Direct Gene, Incorporated to LWKC. The editorial and secretarial assistance provided by Gary Mawyer, Lynna Chung, Angela Sherman, Rob Mawyer and Lindsay Walker and the artwork by Bekir Cinar are also gratefully appreciated.

References

Anastasiadis PZ, Reynolds AB (2000) The p120 catenin family: complex roles in adhesion, signaling and Cancer. *J Cell Sci* **113**:1319–1334.

Baker SJ, Markowitz S, Fearon ER, Wilson JK, Vogelstein B (1990) Suppression of human colorectal carcinoma cell growth by wild-type p53. *Science* **249**:912–915.

Baylin SB, Herman JG, Graff JR, Vertino PM, Issa JP (1998) Alterations in DNA methylation: A fundamental aspect of neoplasia. *Adv Cancer Res* **72**:141–196.

Bayne CW, Donnelly F, Chapman K, Bollina P, Habib FK (1998) A novel co-culture model for benign prostatic hyperplasia expressing both isoforms of 5α-reductase. *J Clin Endocrinol Metab* **83**:206–213.

Chang SM, Chung LWK (1989) Interaction between prostatic fibroblast and epithelial cells in culture: role of androgen. *Endocrinology* **125**:2719–2727.

Chen T, Wang LH, Farrar WL (2000) Interleukin 6 activates androgen receptor-mediated gene expression through a signal transducer and activator of transcription 3-dependent pathway in LNCaP prostate cancer cells. *Cancer Res* **60**:2132–2135.

Chung LWK, Davies R (1996) Prostate epithelial differentiation is dictated by its surrounding stroma. *Mol Biol Rep* **23**:13–19.

Chung LWK, Zhau HE (2001) Stromal–epithelial interaction from bench to bedside. In Chung LWK, Isaacs WB, Simons JW, eds. *Prostate Cancer Biology, Genetics, and the New Therapeutics* Totowa, NJ: Humana Press, pp.341–362.

Chung LWK, Anderson NG, Neubauer BL, *et al.* (1981) Tissue interactions in prostate development: roles of sex steroids. In Alan R, *Prostatic Cells: Structure and Function* Liss, pp.177–203.

Culig Z, Hobisch A, Cronauer MV, *et al.* (1994) Androgen receptor activation in prostatic tumor cell lines by insulin-like growth factor-1, keratinocyte growth factor and epidermal growth factor. *Cancer Res* **54**:5474–5478.

Cunha GR, Chung LWK (1981) Stromal–epithelial interactions I. Introduction of prostatic phenotype in urothelium of testicular feminized (Tfm/y) mice. *J Steroid Biochem* **14**:1317–1324.

Compagni A, Christofori G (2000) Recent advances in research on multistage tumorigenesis. *Br J Cancer* **83**:1–5.

Fusenig NE, Boukamp P (1998) Multiple stages and genetic alterations in immortalization, malignant transformation and tumor progression of human skin keratinocytes. *Mol Carcinog* **23**:144–158.

Gao J, Isaacs JT (1998) Development of an androgen receptor-null model for identifying the initiation site for androgen stimulation of proliferation and suppression of programmed (apoptotic) death of PC-82 human prostate cancer cells. *Cancer Res* **58**:3299–3306.

Gardner TA, Ko SC, Kao C, *et al.* (1998) Exploiting stromal–epithelial interaction for model development and new strategies of prostate cancer and osteosarcoma metastases. *Gene Therapy Mol Biol* **2**:41–58.

Gleave ME, Hsieh JT, von Eschenbach AC, Chung LWK (1992) Prostate and bone fibroblasts induce human prostate cancer growth in vivo: Implications for bidirectional tumor–stromal cell interaction in prostate carcinoma growth and metastasis. *J Urol* **147**:1151–1159.

Grant ES, Batchelor KW, Habib FK (1996) Androgen-independence of primary epithelial cultures of the prostate is associated with a down-regulation of androgen receptor gene expression. *Prostate* **29**:339–349.

Hanahan D, Weinberg RA (2000) The hallmarks of cancer. *Cell* **100**:57–70.

Hsieh CL, Gardner TA, Miao L, Balian G, Chung LW (2004) Cotargeting tumor and stroma in a novel chimeric tumor model involving the growth of both human prostate cancer and bone stromal cells. *Cancer Gene Ther* (in press).

Humphrey PA, Zhu X, Zarnegar R, *et al.* (1995) Hepatocyte growth factor and its receptor (c-met) in prostatic carcinoma. *Am J Pathol* **147**:386–396.

Hyytinen ER, Thalmann GN, Zhau HYE, *et al.* (1997) Genetic changes associated with the acquisition of androgen-independent growth, tumorigenicity and metastatic potential in a prostate cancer model. *Br J Cancer* **75**:190–195.

Kinzler KW, Vogelstein B (1997) Cancer susceptibility genes. Gatekeepers and caretakers. *Nature* **386**: 761–763.

Koeneman KS, Yeung F, Chung LWK (1999) Osteomimetic properties of prostate cancer cells: A hypothesis supporting the predilection of prostate cancer metastasis and growth in the bone environment. *Prostate* **39**:246–261.

Koeneman KS, Kao C, Ko SC, *et al.* (2000) Osteocalcin directed gene therapy for prostate cancer bone metastasis. *World J Urol* **18**:102–110.

Kokontis JM, Liao S (1999) Molecular action of androgen in the normal and neoplastic prostate. *Vitamins and Hormones* **55**:219–307.

Levine MD, Liotta LA, Stracke ML (1995) Stimulation and regulation of the tumor cell motility in invasion of metastasis. *EXS* **74**:157–179.

McCawley L, Matrisian LM (2000) Matrix metalloproteinases: Multifunctional contributors to tumor progression. *Mol Med Today* **6**:149–156.

Matsumoto K, Nakamura T, Kramer RH (1994) Hepatocyte growth factor 1 scatter factor induces tyrosin phosphorylation of focal adhesion kinase (p125[FAK]) and promotes migration and invasion by oral squamous carcinoma cells. *J Biol Chem* **269**:31807–31813.

Matsubara S, Wada Y, Gardner TA, *et al.* (2001) A conditional replication-competent adenoviral vector, Ad-OC-E1a, to co-target prostate cancer and bone stroma in an experimental model of androgen-independent prostate cancer bone metastasis. *Cancer Res* **61**: 6012–6019.

Ni Z, Lou W, Leman ES, Gao AC (2000) Inhibition of constitutively activated Stat3 signaling pathway suppresses growth of prostate cancer cells. *Cancer Res* **60**: 1225–1228.

Nowell PC (1976) The clonal evolution of tumor cell populations. *Science* **194**:23–28.

Paget S (1889) The distribution of secondary growths in cancer of the breast. *Lancet* **1**:571–573.

Qiu Y, Ravi L, Kung HJ (1998) Requirement of ErbB2 for signaling by interleukin 6 in prostate carcinoma cells. *Nature* **393**:83–85.

Rhee HW, Zhau HE, Pathak S, *et al.* (2001) Permanent phenotypic and genotypic changes of prostate cancer cells cultured in a three-dimensional rotating-wall vessel. *In Vitro Cell Dev Biol Animal* **37**:127–140.

Song Z, Powell WC, Kasahara N, *et al.* (2000) The effect of fibroblast growth factor 8, isoform b, on the biology of prostate carcinoma cells and their interaction with stromal cells. *Cancer Res* **60**:6730–6736.

Tu SM, Millikan RE, Mengistu B, *et al.* (2001) Bone-targeted therapy for advanced androgen-independent carcinoma of the prostate: a randomized phase II trial. *Lancet* **357**:336–341.

Wen Y, Hu MCT, Makino K, *et al.* (2000) HER-2/neu promotes androgen-independent survival and growth of prostate cancer cells through the Akt pathway. *Cancer Res* **60**:6841–6845.

Wu TT, Sikes RA, Cui Q, *et al.* (1998) Establishing human prostate cancer cells xenografts in bone: induction of osteoblastic reaction by prostate-specific antigen-producing tumors in athymic and SCID/bg mice using LNCaP and lineage-derived metastatic sublines. *Int J Cancer* **77**:887–894.

10 Pathological angiogenesis: molecular aspects and therapeutic approaches

Dieter Marmé

Introduction

Growth of solid tumors and the formation of metastases are dependent on the formation of new blood vessels. This hypothesis was proposed by Judah Folkman more than 25 years ago and has been substantially supported by recent discoveries which unraveled the molecular and cellular processes involved in tumor angiogenesis. Clinical data clearly indicate the correlation between vascularization and aggressive tumor growth and metastases formation. Many of the angiogenic factors produced by tumors have been identified and their roles in the formation of new blood vessels have been elucidated (Folkman 1995).

According to our present understanding of cancerogenesis, each tumor originates from a single cell which has been transformed by one or more genetic events. This includes the activation of oncogenes as well as the inactivation of tumor suppressor genes. These cells can grow out to form a cell clone of only a few millimeters in size before the supply of nutrients becomes limited. The tumor clones can remain at this stage for months or years, unless they are eliminated by the immune system or the so-called angiogenic switch is turned on. At the cellular level, the angiogenic switch is defined by the onset of expression and secretion of angiogenic factors. If sufficient of the secreted angiogenic factors reach the neighboring capillaries of the vasculature by diffusion they initiate the sprouting of new blood vessels from pre-existing ones.

Among the angiogenic factors, the vascular endothelial growth factor (VEGF) plays a pivotal role. Most solid tumors express high levels of VEGF and the VEGF receptors appear predominantly in endothelial cells of vessels surrounding or penetrating the malignant tissue (Marmé 1996, Ferrara & Davis-Smyth 1997). Thus, VEGF-mediated tumor angiogenesis requiring both the ligand and its receptors to be in place seems to be an ideal therapeutic target for cancer therapy. One might expect that the effect of any compound designed to block the VEGF signaling cascade will most likely be restricted to the diseased area. However, the possibility that the presence of other angiogenic mechanisms and/or the loss of anti-angiogenic processes should not be neglected. Also, the combination of anti-angiogenic strategies with more conventional therapies such as cytotoxic chemotherapy should be considered.

This chapter will briefly summarize what we know about the various factors and mechanisms underlying the expression of VEGF in tumors and of the VEGF receptors in tumor endothelial cells. Furthermore, the various experimental approaches undertaken to disrupt the VEGF signaling cascade will be discussed.

Mechanisms of VEGF expression

Expression of VEGF is induced by a variety of factors and growth conditions in normal cells and tumor cells, as well as by genetic changes in tumor cells. Regulation of VEGF expression has been reported to occur at the level of gene transcription, at the level of mRNA stabilization and at the level of mRNA translation. Transcription of the VEGF gene is enhanced by a variety of growth factors and cytokines, including platelet-derived growth factor (PDGF)BB, basic fibroblast growth factor (bFGF), insulin-like growth factor-1, keratinocyte growth factor, epidermal growth factor, tumor necrosis factor (TNF)α, transforming growth factor (TGF)α, TGFβ1, interleukin-1β and interleukin 6 in a variety of cultured cells (Finkenzeller et al. 1992, Brogi et al. 1994, Detmar et al. 1994, Petovaara et al. 1994, Frank et al. 1995, Li et al. 1995, Cohen et al. 1996, Warren et al. 1996). Enhanced VEGF expression has been reported upon activation of protein kinase C by tumor promoters (Finkenzeller et al. 1992, Tischer et al. 1991) and in cells harboring activated oncogenes, such as ras, raf and src (Grugel et al. 1995, Rak et al. 1995, Mukhopadhyay et al. 1995a), as well as in cells carrying inactivating mutations or deletions of p53, and of von Hippel–Lindau (VHL) tumor suppressor genes, respectively (Mukhopadhyay et al. 1995a, Kieser et al. 1994, Siemeister et al. 1996). In addition, VEGF expression is markedly elevated in cultured cells by hypoxic conditions and in regions of tumors located near necrotic areas (Shweiki et al. 1992, Plate et al. 1992).

Recent work has shed some light on the diverse molecular mechanisms involved in enhanced VEGF expression. Sequence analysis of the human VEGF gene promoter (Tischer et al. 1991) revealed several potential binding sites for transcription factors AP-1, AP-2 and Sp-1 which are candidate mediators of VEGF promoter activation. Detailed promoter analyzes using reporter gene assays, electrophoretic mobility shift assays and mutagenesis of promoter elements resulted in the identification of a G+C-rich region at −50 to −96 relative to the single transcriptional start site to be essential for induction of VEGF by TNFα (Ryoto et al. 1996), TGFα (Gille et al. 1997), and PDGF-BB (Finkenzeller et al. 1997), respectively. This promoter region contains four consensus binding sites for transcription factors Sp-1 and/or Sp-3, two putative binding sites for Egr-1 which are overlapping with the second, third and fourth Sp-1/Sp-3 sites, respectively, and one AP-2 binding site which is identical to the 5′ Egr-1 site. Ryuto et al. (1996) have shown that the four Sp-1/Sp-3 binding sites are essential for basal transcription of the VEGF gene and for TNFα-dependent promoter activation in a human glioma cell line. Deletion of the most 5′ Sp-1/Sp-3 binding site reduced basal transcription and abolished TNFα responsiveness. Stimulation of the cells with TNFα or bFGF resulted in increased binding of Sp-1 to the promoter element, whereas addition of mithramycin, an inhibitor of Sp-1, inhibited activation of the VEGF gene promoter suggesting Sp-1 as a downstream mediator of TNFα-induced VEGF gene expression. Finkenzeller et al. (1997) and Gille et al. (1997) found a promoter element covering the second to fourth Sp-1 consensus binding sites necessary and sufficient for VEGF gene promoter activation in PDGF-BB-stimulated NIH3T3 fibroblasts and in TGFα-stimulated A431 human epidermoid carcinoma cells. Sp-1 and Sp-3 were shown to bind in a constitutive manner to this promoter region. In A431 cells the formation of TGFα-inducible DNA binding complex containing AP-2 and Egr-l transcription factors was observed on this DNA fragment. Transfection of AP-2 and Egr-1 expression vectors revealed AP-2, but not Egr-1, as a transcription factor which activates VEGF gene expression. In NIH3T3 cells, mutations within the VEGF promoter element which abolished binding of AP-2 and Egr-1 had no effect on PDGF-responsiveness, whereas mutations which eliminated binding of Sp-1 and Sp-3 impaired PDGF-stimulated transcription of the VEGF gene promoter. Although TNFα, TGFα and PDGF-BB signaling pathways address different transcription factors or use different modes of their activation, they converge at the proximal promoter region.

Further evidence for the important role of the proximal promoter region for control of VEGF gene expression came from recent findings of Mukhopadhyay *et al.* (1997) who identified the −50 and −144 region to mediate transcriptional repression of the VEGF promoter by the VHL gene product. Renal carcinoma cells that either lacked wild-type VHL gene or were transfected with an inactive mutant VHL gene showed deregulated expression of VEGF that was reverted by introduction of wild-type VHL gene (Siemeister *et al.* 1996). Mukhopadhyay *et al.* (1997) showed that wild-type VHL protein binds to Sp-1 transcription factor and represses Sp-1-mediated activation of the VEGF gene promoter, indicating that VHL regulation of VEGF occurs at least partly at the transcriptional level. Moreover, their results suggest that loss of Sp-1 inhibition may be important in the pathogenesis of VHL disease. Originally, VHL protein was discovered as a negative regulator of the transcriptional elongation factor elongin (Duan *et al.* 1995, Aso *et al.* 1995, Kibel *et al.* 1995). By binding to the regulatory elongin subunits B and C VHL protein disrupts elongin function. Whether VHL protein is involved in regulation of transcriptional elongation of

the VEGF gene remains open so far. Instead, increased VEGF mRNA stabilization, a mechanism that is also driven by hypoxia, has been observed in cells lacking VHL function (Iliopoulos *et al.* 1996). Short-time hypoxia (3 h) initially induced VEGF mRNA transcription 3–4-fold, whereas continued hypoxia (15 h) resulted in an 8–10-fold VEGF induction that was the product of both enhanced transcription and an approximately 3-fold increased mRNA stability (Ikeda *et al.* 1995). Both mechanisms have been shown to work *in vivo* in a rat C6 glioma model (Damert *et al.* 1997a). Upon subjection of cells to hypoxia, formation of RNA–protein complexes on three adenylate–uridylate-rich elements (AREs) in the 3′-untranslated region of the VEGF mRNA was observed, which mediates mRNA stabilization (Levy *et al.* 1996a, 1996b). AREs destabilize mRNAs and stabilization of labile mRNA is thought to be mediated by specific binding of proteins to AREs that mask the ARE-destabilizing motifs. Formation of these hypoxia-inducible RNA–protein complexes on the VEGF mRNA is constitutively elevated in cells lacking functional VHL protein (Levy *et al.* 1996b). As no direct interaction between VHL protein and the hypoxia-inducible complex has been observed to date the molecular mechanism by which the VHL protein mediates constitutive formation of the complex remains to be clarified.

Hypoxia-inducible factor 1 (HIF-1), a heterodimeric basic helix–loop–helix protein that activates transcription of the human erythropoietin gene in hypoxic cells, was shown to be involved in hypoxia-induced VEGF gene transcription and an HIF-1 binding site was identified at −975 of the human gene promoter (Forsythe *et al.* 1996). An AP-1 transcription factor binding site at −1129 cooperates with the HIF-1 site in the way that this site is unable to confer hypoxia responsiveness on its own, but potentiates hypoxia induction of the human VEGF gene via HIF-1 approximately 2-fold (Damert *et al.* 1997b). The H-*ras* oncogene enhances the induction of VEGF by hypoxia via the HIF-1 promoter element (Mazure *et al.* 1996). The signaling pathway of H-Ras in induction of VEGF expression involves the phosphatidylinositol 3-kinase/Akt pathway, whereas the c-Raf/mitogen-activated kinase and the stress-activated kinase pathways appear to be dispensable (Mazure *et al.* 1997, Arbiser *et al.* 1997). c-Src or Src-like kinases have conversely been reported to be involved (Mukhopadhyay *et al.* 1995b) or not involved (Gleadle & Ratcliffe 1997) in hypoxia-induced VEGF expression.

Recent work of Kevil *et al.* (1996) revealed translational regulation as an important factor for enhanced VEGF expression. Transfection of Chinese hamster ovary cells to overexpress the protein synthesis factor eukaryotic initiation factor 4E increased VEGF secretion up to 130-fold. Eukaryotic initiation factor 4E is a 25 kDa polypeptide that recruits mRNAs for translation by binding to the 7-methylguanosine-containing cap of mRNA. Its overexpression has been observed in metastatic breast carcinomas (Kerekatte *et al.* 1995) and transformed cell lines (Miyagi *et al.* 1995), suggesting a contribution to carcinoma progression and survival.

Mechanisms of VEGF receptor expression

In contrast to our knowledge about the regulation of VEGF expression, only little is known about the mechanisms which control VEGF receptor expression. A striking observation had been made even before the VEGF receptor

genes had been identified: the distribution of high-affinity VEGF binding sites revealed a pattern restricted to endothelial cells which had been interpreted as the consequence of cell-specific receptor expression (Olander *et al.* 1991). After the identification of the VEGF receptor-1 (FLT-1) gene and VEGF receptor-2 (KDR/FLK-1) gene, *in-situ* hybridization confirmed that the expression of both genes was tightly restricted to endothelial cells and its progenitors (Quinn *et al.* 1993, Peters *et al.* 1993, Millauer *et al.* 1993). Moreover, receptor expression is not only endothelial cell-specific but is also downregulated in quiescent endothelial cells. Upregulation of both receptors occurs when angiogenesis takes place, as in the case of tumor growth. Two main questions arise from these findings:

- Which mechanisms are responsible for the endothelial cell-specific expression of both receptors?
- Which mechanisms are responsible for the downregulation of receptor expression in quiescent endothelial cells and the upregulation in proliferating endothelial cells?

Whereas almost nothing is known about the molecular basis of endothelial cell-specific expression, there is growing evidence for paracrine mechanisms which are involved in the regulation of VEGF receptor expression.

A number of growth factors and cytokines can regulate angiogenesis positively or negatively (Klagsbrun & D'Amore 1991).

Conflicting results have been reported for TNFα, an inflammatory and neoplasia-associated cytokine. TNFα promotes angiogenesis *in vivo* and stimulates the migration of endothelial cells (Frater-Schroder *et al.* 1987) although it has been described as a potent inhibitor of endothelial cell growth *in vitro* (Leibovich *et al.* 1987). In a recent publication Patterson *et al.* (1996) demonstrated the interference of TNFα with the VEGF signaling system of endothelial cells. TNFα blocks the VEGF-stimulated DNA synthesis by significantly lowering the mRNA levels of both VEGF receptors. The underlying molecular mechanisms are not yet fully understood. However, it is likely that transcription is affected, since mRNA stability was not influenced by TNFα. TGFβ1 has been reported to downregulate VEGF receptor-2 (KDR/FLK-1) expression of endothelial cells *in vitro* (Mandriota *et al.* 1996). Receptor downregulation has been observed at the mRNA and protein level but the molecular basis is still unclear. An elegant experimental setup for studying the regulation of VEGF receptor expression has been reported by Kremer *et al.* (1997). By using cultured cerebral tissue slices, Kremer *et al.* (1997) could demonstrate hypoxia-induced VEGF receptor-2 expression. Further analysis revealed that hypoxia-induced VEGF expression in these tissue slices was responsible for enhanced VEGF receptor-2 expression. In other terms, VEGF itself can stimulate the expression of its VEGF receptor-2. Experiments addressing the question of how VEGF receptor-1 expression can be stimulated were published by Barleon *et al.* (1997). Incubation of cultured human umbilical vein endothelial cells (HUVECs) with conditioned medium of various tumor cell lines led to an increase of VEGF receptor-1 expression. As in the case of VEGF receptor-2 upregulation in brain slices, VEGF itself was identified as the soluble factor produced by the tumor cells and responsible for enhanced VEGF receptor-1 expression. Thus, evidence accumulates that VEGF itself is an important paracrine factor which upregulates the expression of its own receptors *in vivo*.

Hypoxia

The growth of malignant tumors is associated with tissue hypoxia and hypoxia has been described to be a major mechanism leading to the upregulation of VEGF and its receptors *in vivo*. However, this is not restricted to growing tumors (Plate *et al.* 1992), but also occurs in the vasculature of hypoxic lung (Tudor *et al.* 1995) or skin explants (Detmar *et al.* 1997). Conflicting results were coming from experiments where cultured endothelial cells had been exposed to hypoxia. Thieme *et al.* (1995) showed an increase in the number of VEGF receptors of bovine retinal and aortic endothelial cells. Studying VEGF receptor expression in hypoxia-treated HUVECs we and others failed to demonstrate upregulation of both VEGF receptors (Kremer *et al.* 1997, Brogi *et al.* 1996, Barleon & Marmé unpublished work). Detmar *et al.* (1997) described the upregulation of VEGF receptor-1 mRNA and the downregulation of VEGF receptor-2 mRNA in dermal microvascular endothelial cells. Meanwhile, the promoter regions of both VEGF receptor genes have been cloned (Morishita *et al.* 1995, Patterson *et al.* 1995, Ronicke *et al.* 1996). Transient transfection of promoter reporter constructs showed a strong transcriptional activation of the VEGF receptor-1 gene under hypoxic conditions, while the VEGF receptor-2 activity remained unchanged (Gerber *et al.* 1997). The authors could identify the element mediating the hypoxic response as a heptamer sequence matching the consensus sequence of the hypoxia inducible factor-1 (HIF). This element acts like an enhancer, and mutation within this HIF consensus binding site led to impaired activation by hypoxia (Gerber *et al.* 1997). Thus, the observed hypoxia-mediated expression of both VEGF receptors *in vivo* seems to be regulated by different molecular mechanisms.

While direct transcriptional activation mediated by HIF and can upregulate only VEGF receptor-1 expression, hypoxia-induced paracrine factors like VEGF are able to activate the expression of both VEGF receptors.

Therapeutic opportunities

Inhibition of the VEGF-mediated signaling cascade has already been shown in various experimental animal models to effectively interfere with tumor vascularization, tumor growth and metastases formation.

Functional inhibition of the mouse VEGF receptor, FLK-1, the mouse homologue of human KDR, by the use of a dominant-negative mutant lacking protein tyrosine kinase, leads to significant inhibition of tumor growth and vascularization. This effect was obtained either by co-injecting a cell line producing retroviruses encoding the dominant-negative mutant together with the glioblastoma cell line, C6, or by local injection of retroviral supernatants (Millauer *et al.* 1994).

The availability of specific monoclonal antibodies against VEGF made it possible to investigate the role of VEGF in tumor angiogenesis. Nude mice injected subcutaneously with a large variety of human cancer cell lines were treated with anti-VEGF antibodies. In all cases significant reduction of tumor growth was observed (Ferrara & Davis-Smyth 1997, Millauer *et al.* 1994). In agreement with the hypothesis that inhibition of tumor growth is due to the inhibition of tumor vascularization, it could be shown that tumors from treated animals had a reduced density of blood vessels (Kim *et al.* 1993). Intravital videomicroscopy techniques revealed almost complete suppression of tumor

angiogenesis in tumor-bearing nude mice treated with anti-VEGF antibodies (Borgström *et al.* 1996). In an orthotopic nude mouse model of liver metastasis, after inoculation with human colon carcinoma, the systemic application of VEGF antibodies resulted in a dramatic decrease in the number and size of metastases (Warren *et al.* 1995). Combination treatment with anti-VEGF monoclonal antibodies and doxorubicin results in a signficant enhancement of the efficacy of either agent alone and led in some cases to a complete regression of tumors derived from MCF-7 breast carcinoma cells in nude mice (Ferrara & Davis-Smyth 1997).

VEGF antisense technology was used to explore whether a reduction of VEGF secretion by the tumor cells leads to inhibition of vascularization and tumor growth. In this case, rat C6 glioma cells, secreting VEGF, were stably transfected with a eukaryotic expression vector bearing an antisense-VEGF cDNA. Cell lines with reduced VEGF production were transplanted into nude mice. Substantial reduction of tumor growth, tumor vascularization and significant increase of necrosis was observed (Saleh *et al.* 1996). Lowering VEGF expression in tumor cells has also been achieved by blocking EGF-stimulated expression of VEGF in A431 human epidermoid carcinoma cells using an anti-EGF receptor neutralizing antibody. Similar results were reported with an anti-ErbB2/neu monoclonal antibody for SKBR-3 human breast cancer cells (Petit *et al.* 1997). This implicates the potential use of antibodies against growth factor receptors different from VEGF receptors but involved in the control of VEGF expression in tumor cells.

Recently, it was shown that angiogenesis and tumor invasion of malignant human keratinocytes in surface transplants on nude mice could be prevented by using a monoclonal antibody which inhibits the activation of the VEGF receptor-2 (Skobe *et al.* 1997). This again demonstrates that interfering with VEGF signaling results in the disruption of the sequence of events involved in tumor progression.

Assuming a substantial redundancy in tumor angiogenesis – i.e. the involvement of several angiogenic factors in the same process, as has been demonstrated for primary breast cancer (Relf *et al.* 1997) – one might suggest that blocking signaling by one angiogenic factor will not be sufficient. As it will be difficult to estimate in each individual case which angiogenic factors are involved, a cytotoxic approach for endothelial cells involved in tumor angiogenesis might be a therapeutic alternative. By using VEGF-diphtheria toxin conjugates, it could be shown that VEGF receptor-2 expressing endothelial cells were affected, whereas receptor-negative ovarian cells were not. Furthermore, the conjugate blocked neovascularization in the chick chorioallantoic membrane assay (Ramakrishnan *et al.* 1996).

Inhibition of the tyrosine kinase activity of VEGF receptors by small molecule compounds is another promising approach to treating tumor angiogenesis. A joint project of Novartis Pharma AG (Basel), Schering AG (Berlin), and Tumor Biology Center (Freiburg), succeeded in developing a potent and orally active inhibitor of VEGF receptor tyrosine kinases (Wood *et al.* 2000, Drevs *et al.* 2000). PTK787/ZK222584, a phtalazine derivative, represents a novel class of protein tyrosine kinase inhibitors. PTK787/ZK222584 inhibits KDR, Flk-1 and human Flt-1 tyrosine kinase activities *in vitro* with IC_{50} values of 0.1, 0.3 and 0.5 µmol, respectively. It also inhibits PDGF receptor tyrosine kinase but is not active against kinases from other receptor families (EGF, FGF) and non-receptor kinases (c-Src, v-Abl, PKC). Using KDR-overexpressing Chinese hamster ovary cells, human microvascular endothelial cells

and HUVEC, PTK787/ZK222584 inhibited VEGF-stimulated KDR autophosphorylation with an IC_{50} value of 0.02 µmol (Siemeister *et al.* 2000). Growth factor-induced activation of MAP kinases was used as a measure for receptor downstream signaling. PTK787/ZK222584 inhibited selectively VEGF-induced but not basic FGF-induced MAP kinase activation in HUVEC. Proliferation and migration of HUVEC and of human microvascular endothelial cells induced by VEGF were selectively inhibited by PTK787/ZK222584, whereas the response to basic FGF was not affected. In accordance with its anti-angiogenic activity, PTK787/ZK222584 dose-dependently inhibited the growth of A431 human epithelial carcinoma xenografts on nude mice. Tumor growth was initiated by subcutaneous injection of a tumor cell suspension, and daily oral treatment was started when palpable primary tumors reached a size of about 25 mm². Administration of doses of 50 and 75 mg/kg reduced tumor size by 50%. In addition, PTK787/ZK222584 showed antitumor and antimetastatic activity against a panel of human nude mouse xenografts and syngenic mouse and rat tumor models. (Siemeister *et al.* 2000). Phase I clinical trials are ongoing. Preliminary data were highly encouraging.

References

Arbiser JL, Moses MA, Fernandez CA, *et al.* (1997) Oncogenic H-ras stimulates tumor angiogenesis by two distinct pathways. *Proc Natl Acad Sci USA* 94:861–866.

Aso T, Lane WS, Conaway JW, Conaway RC (1995) Elongin (SI-II): A multisubunit regulator of elongation by RNA polymerase 11. *Science* 269:1439–1443.

Barleon B, Siemeister G, Martiny-Baron G, *et al.* (1997) Vascular endothelial growth factor up-regulates its receptor fms-like tyrosine kinase 1 (FLT-1) and a soluble variant of FLT-1 in human vascular endothelial cells. *Cancer Res* 57:5421–5425.

Borgström P, Hillan KJ, Sriramarao P, Ferrara N (1996) Complete inhibition of angiogenesis and growth of microtumors by anti-vascular endothelial growth factor neutralizing antibodies. Novel concepts of angiostatic therapy from intravital videomicroscopy. *Cancer Res* **56**:4032–4039.

Brogi E, Wu T, Namiki A, Isner JM (1994) Indirect angiogenic cytokines upregulate VEGF and bFGF gene expression in vascular smooth muscle cells, whereas hypoxia upregulates VEGF expression only. *Circulation* 90:649–652.

Brogi E, Schatteman G, Wu T, *et al.* (1996) Hypoxia-induced paracrine regulation of vascular endothelial growth factor receptor expression. *J Clin Invest* **97**: 469–476.

Cohen T, Nahari D, Cerem LW, Neufeld G, Levi BZ (1996) Interleukin 6 induces the expression of vascular endothelial growth factor. *J Biol Chem* **271**:736–741.

Damert A, Machein M, Breier G, *et al.* (1997a) Up-regulation of vascular endothelial growth factor expression in a rat glioma is conferred by two distinct hypoxia-driven mechanisms. *Cancer Res* 57:3860–3864.

Damert A, Ikeda E, Risau W (1997b) Activator-protein-I binding potentiates the hypoxia-inducible factor-1-mediated hypoxia-induced transcriptional activation of vascular endothelial growth factor expression in C6 glioma cells. *Biochem* J 327: 419–423.

Detmar M, Brown LF, Berse B, *et al.* (1997) Hypoxia regulates the expression of vascular permeability factor/vascular endothelial growth factor (VPF/VEGF) and its receptor in human skin. *J Invest Dermatol* 108:263–268.

Detmar M, Brown LE, Claffey KP, *et al.* (1994) Overexpression of vascular permeability factor/vascular endothelial growth factor and its receptors in psoriasis. *J Exp Med* **180**:1141–1146.

Drevs J, Hofmann I, Hugenschmidt H, *et al.* (2000) Effects of PTK787/ZK222584, a specific vascular endothelial growth factor (VEGF)–receptor tyrosine kinase inhibitor, on primary tumor, metastasis, vessel density and blood flow in a murine renal cell carcinoma. *Cancer Res* 60:4819–4824.

Duan DR, Pause A, Burgess WH, *et al.* (1995) Inhibition of transcription elongation by the VHL tumor suppressor protein. *Science* **269**:1402–1406.

Ferrara N, Davis-Smyth T (1997) The biology of vascular endothelial growth factor. *Endocr Rev* 18:4–25.

Finkenzeller G, Marmé D, Weich HA, Hug H (1992) Platelet-derived growth factor-induced transcription of the vascular endothelial growth factor gene is mediated by protein kinase C. *Cancer Res* 52:4821–4823.

Finkenzeller G, Sparacio A, Technau A, Marmé D, Siemeister G (1997) Sp1 recognition sites in the proximal promoter of the human vascular endothelial growth factor gene are essential for platelet-derived growth factor-induced gene expression. *Oncogene* 15:669–676.

Folkman J (1995) Angiogenesis in cancer, vascular, rheumatoid, and other disease. *Nat Med* **1**:27–31.

Forsythe JA, Jiang BH, Iyer NV, *et al.* (1996) Activation of vascular endothelial growth factor gene transcription by hypoxia-inducible factor 1. *Mol Cell Biol* **16**: 4604–4613.

Frank S, Hubner G, Breier G, *et al.* (1995) Regulation of vascular endothelial growth factor expression in cultured keratinocytes. Implications for normal and impaired wound healing. *J Biol Chem* 270:12607–12613.

Frater-Schroder M, Risau W, Hallmann R, Gautsch P (1987) Tumor necrosis factor type α, a potent inhibitor of endothelial cell growth *in vitro*, is angiogenic *in vivo*. *Proc Natl Acad Sci USA* 84:5277–5281.

Gerber H-P, Condorelli F, Park J, Ferrara N (1997) Differential transcriptional regulation of the two vascular endothelial growth factor receptor genes. *J Biol Chem* 272:23659–23667.

Gille J, Swerlick RA, Caughman SW (1997) Transforming growth factor-α-induced transcriptional activation of the vascular permeability factor (VPF/VEGF) gene requires AP-2-dependent DNA binding and transactivation. *EMBO J* 16:750–759.

Gleadle JM, Ratcliffe PJ (1997) Induction of hypoxia-inducible factor-1, erythropoietin, vascular endothelial growth factor, and glucose transporter-1 by hypoxia: evidence against a regulatory role for src kinase. *Blood* 89:503–509.

Grugel S, Finkenzeller G, Weindel K, Barleon B, Marmé D (1995) Both v-Ha-Ras and v-Raf stimulate expression of the vascular enclothelial growth factor in NIH 3T3 cells. *J Biol Chem* 270:25915–25919.

Ikeda E, Achen MG, Breier G, Risau W (1995) Hypoxia-induced transcriptional activation and increased mRNA stability of vascular endothelial growth factor in C6 glioma cells. *J Biol Chem* 270:19761–19766.

Iliopoulos O, Levy AP, Jiang C, Kaelin WG Jr, Goldberg MA (1996) Negative regulation of hypoxia-inducible genes by the von Hippel–Lindau protein. *Proc Natl Acad Sci USA* 93:10595–10599.

Kerekatte V, Smiley K, Hu B, *et al*. The proto-oncogene/translation factor eIF4E: a survey of its expression in breast carcinomas. *Int J Cancer* **64**:27–31.

Kevil CG, De Benedetti A, Payne DK, *et al*. (1996) Translational regulation of vascular permeability factor by eukaryotic initiation factor 4E: implications for tumor angiogenesis. *Int J Cancer* **65**:785–790.

Kibel A, Iliopoulos O, DeCaprio JA, Kaelin WG Jr (1995) Binding of the von Hippel–Lindau tumor suppressor protein to Elongin B and C. *Science* **269**:1444–1446.

Kieser A, Weich HA, Brandner G, Marmé D, Kölch W (1994) Mutant p53 potentiates protein kinase C induction of vascular endothelial growth factor expression. *Oncogene* **9**:963–969.

Kim KJ, Li B, Winer J, *et al*. (1993) Inhibition of vascular endothelial growth factor-induced angiogenesis suppresses tumour growth *in vivo*. *Nature* **362**:841–844.

Klagsbrun M, D'Amore PA (1991) Regulators of angiogenesis. *Ann Rev Physiol* **53**:217–239.

Kremer C, Breier G, Risau W, Plate KH (1997) Up-regulation of flk-1/vascular endothelial growth factor receptor 2 by its ligand in a cerebral slice culture system. *Cancer Res* **57**:3852–3859.

Leibovich S, Polverini P, Shepard H, *et al*. (1987) Macrophage-induced angiogenesis is mediated by tumour necrosis factor-α. *Nature* **329**:630–632.

Levy AP, Levy NS, Goldberg MA (1996a) Post-transcriptional regulation of vascular endothelial growth factor by hypoxia. *J Biol Chem* **271**:2746–2753.

Levy AP, Levy NS, Goldberg MA (1996b) Hypoxia-inducible protein binding to vascular endothelial growth factor mRNA and its modulation by the von Hippel–Lindau protein. *J Biol Chem* **271**: 25492–25497.

Li J, Perrella MA, Tsai JC, *et al*. (1995) Induction of vascular endothelial growth factor gene expression by interleukin-1 beta in rat aortic smooth muscle cells. *J Biol Chem* **270**:308–312.

Mandriota SJ, Menoud P-A, Pepper MS (1996) Transforming growth factor-β1 down-regulates vascular endothelial growth factor receptor 2/flk-1 expression in vascular endothelial cells. *J Biol Chem* **271**:11500–11505.

Marmé D (1996) Tumor angiogenesis: The pivotal role of vascular endothelial growth factor (VEGF). *World J Urol* **14**:166–174.

Mazure NM, Chen EY, Yeh P, Laderoute KR, Giaccia AJ (1996) Oncogenic transformation and hypoxia synergistically act to modulate vascular endothelial growth factor expression. *Cancer Res* **56**:3436–3440.

Mazure NM, Chen EY, Laderoute KR, Giaccia AJ (1997) Induction of vascular endothelial growth factor by hypoxia is modulated by a phosphatidylinositol 3-kinase/Akt signaling pathway in Ha-ras-transformed cells through a hypoxia inducible element. *Blood* **90**:3322–3331.

Millauer B, Wizigmann-Voos S, Schnirch H, *et al*. (1993) High affinity VEGF binding and developmental expression suggest Flk-1 as a major regulator of vasculogenesis and angiogenesis. *Cell* **72**:835–846.

Millauer B, Shawver KL, Plate KH, Risau W, Ullrich A (1994) Glioblastoma growth inhibited *in vivo* by a dominant-negative Flk-1 mutant. *Nature* **367**:576–579.

Miyagi Y, Sugiyama A, Asai A, *et al*. (1995) Elevated levels of eukaryotic translation initiation factor eIF-4E mRNA in a broad spectrum of transformed cell lines. *Cancer* Lett **91**:247–252.

Morishita K, Johnson DE, Williams LT (1995) A novel promoter for vascular endothelial growth factor (flt-1) that confers endothelial-specific gene expression. *J Biol Chem* **270**:27948–27953.

Mukhopadhyay D, Tsiokas L, Sukhatme VP (1995a) Wild-type p53 and v-Src exert opposing influences on human vascular endothelial growth factor gene expression. *Cancer Res* **55**:6161–6165.

Mukhopadhyay D, Tsiokas L, Zhou XM, *et al*. (1995b) Hypoxic induction of human vascular endothelial growth factor expression through c-Src activation. *Nature* **375**:577–581.

Mukhopadhyay D, Knebelmann B, Cohen HT, Ananth S, Sukhatme VP (1997) The von Hippel–Lindau tumor suppressor gene product interacts with Spl to repress vascular endothelial growth factor promoter activity. *Mol Cell Biol* **17**:5629–5639.

Olander JV, Connolly DT, DeLarco JE (1991) Specific binding of vascular permeability factor to endothelial cells. *Biochem Biophys Res Comm* **175**:68–76.

Patterson C, Perrella MA, Hsieh C-M, *et al*. (1995) Cloning and functional analysis of the promoter for KDR/flk-1, a receptor for vascular endothelial growth factor. *J Biol Chem* **270**:23111–23118.

Patterson C, Perrella MA, Endege WO, *et al*. (1996) Downregulation of vascular endothelial growth factor by tumor necrosis factor-α in cultured human vascular endothelial cells. *J Clin Invest* **98**:490–496.

Pertovaara L, Kaipainen A, Mustonen T, *et al*. (1994) Vascular endothelial growth factor is induced in response to transforming growth factor-beta in fibroblastic and epithelial cells. *J Biol Chem* **269**: 6271–6274.

Peters KG, De Vries C, Williams LT (1993) Vascular endo-thelial growth factor expression during embryogenesis and tissue repair suggests a role in endothelial differentiation and blood vessel growth. *Proc Natl Acad Sci USA* **90**:8915–8919.

Petit AMV, Rak J, Hung M-C, *et al.* (1997) Neutralizing antibodies against epidermal growth factor and ErbB-2/neu receptor tyrosine kinases down-regulate vascular endothelial growth factor production by tumor cells *in vitro* and *in vivo:* Angiogenic implications for signal transduction therapy of solid tumors. *Am J Pathol* **151**: 1523–1530.

Plate KH, Breier G, Weich HA, Risau W (1992) Vascular endothelial growth factor is a potential turnout angiogenesis factor in human gliomas *in vivo*. *Nature* **359**: 845–848.

Quinn TP, Peters KG, De Vries C, Ferrara N (1993) Fetal liver kinase I is a receptor for vascular endothelial growth factor and is selectively expressed in vascular endothelium. *Proc Natl Acad Sci USA* **90**: 7533–7537.

Rak J, Mitsuhashi Y, Bayko L, *et al.* (1995) oncogenes upregulate VEGF/VPF expression: implications for induction and inhibition of tumor angiogenesis. *Cancer Res* 55:4575–4580.

Ramakrishnan S, Olson TA, Bautch VL, Mohanraj D (1996) Vascular endothelial growth factor-toxin conjugate specifically inhibits KDR/flk-1-positive endothelial cell proliferation *in vitro* and angiogenesis *in vivo*. *Cancer Res* 56:1324–1330.

Relf M, LeJeune S, Scott PAE, *et al.* (1997) Expression of the angiogenic factors vascular endothelial growth factor, acidic and basic fibroblast growth factor, tumor growth factor P-1, platelet-derived endothelial cell growth factor, placenta growth factor, and pleiotrophin in human primary breast cancer and its relation to angiogenesis. *Cancer Res* 57:963–969.

Ronicke V, Risau W, Breier G (1996) Characterization of the endothelium-specific murine vascular endothelial growth factor receptor-2 (Flk-1) promoter. *Cite Res* 79:277–285.

Ryuto M, Ono M, Izumi H, *et al.* (1996) Induction of vascular endothelial growth factor by tumor necrosis factor α in human glioma cells: possible roles of Sp-l. *J Biol Chem* 271:28220–28228.

Saleh M, Stacker SA, Wilks AF (1996) Inhibition of growth of C6 glioma cells *in vivo* by expression of antisense vascular endothelial growth factor sequence. *Cancer Res* **56**:393–401.

Shweiki D, Itin A, Soffer D, Keshet E (1992) Vascular endothelial growth factor induced by hypoxia may mediate hypoxia-initiated angiogenesis. *Nature* **359**: 843–845.

Siemeister G, Weindel K, Mohrs K, *et al.* (1996) Reversion of deregulated expression of vascular endothelial growth factor in human renal carcinoma cells by von Hippel–Lindau tumor suppressor protein. *Cancer Res* **56**:2299–2301.

Siemeister G, Menrad A, Schirner M, *et al.* (2000) Inhibition of VEGF receptor tyrosine kinase. In: Rubanyi GM, ed, *Angiogenesis in Health and Disease. Basic Mechanisms and Clinical Applications* (Marcel Dekker: New York).

Skobe M, Rockwell P, Goldstein N, Vosseler S, Fusenig NE (1997) Halting angiogenesis suppresses carcinoma cell invasion. *Nature Med* **3**:1222–1227.

Thieme H, Aiello LP, Takagi H, Ferrara N, King GL (1995) Comparative analysis of vascular endothelial growth factor receptors on retinal and aortic vascular endothelial cells. *Diabetes* **44**:98–103.

Tischer F, Mitchell R, Hartman T, *et al.* (1991) The human gene for vascular endothelial growth factor. Multiple protein forms are encoded through alternative exon splicing. *J Biol Chem* **266**: 11947–11954.

Tuder RM, Flook BE, Voelkel NF (1995) Increased gene expression for VEGF and the VEGF receptors KDR/Flk and Flt in lungs exposed to acute or to chronic hypoxia. *J Clin Invest* **95**:1798–1807.

Warren RA, Yuan H, Math MR, Gillett NA, Ferrara N (1995) Regulation by vascular endothelial growth factor of human colon cancer tumorigeneses in a mouse model of experimental liver metastasis. *J Clin Invest* **95**:1789–1797.

Warren RS, Yuan H, Math MR, Ferrara N, Donner DB (1996) Induction of vascular endothelial growth factor by insulin-like growth factor I in colorectal carcinoma. *J Biol Chem* **271**:29483–29488.

Wood JM, Bold G, Buchdunger E, *et al.* (2000) PTK787/ZK 222584, a novel and potent inhibitor of VEGF receptor tyrosine kinases, impairs VEGF-induced responses and tumor growth after oral administration. *Cancer Res* **60**:2178–2189.

11 Protein kinases as targets for cancer therapy

Giampaolo Tortora and Fortunato Ciardiello

Introduction

Innovative anticancer strategies are based on the integration of conventional drugs with novel agents selectively targeting molecules directly involved in cell proliferation, angiogenesis and apoptosis. Several tyrosine and serine–threonine kinases have been implicated in the development and progression of the majority of human cancers, becoming potentially relevant therapeutic targets (Gibbs 2000, Levitzki 1999). Different approaches have been developed to block signaling protein kinases activation and/or function in cancer cells, including the generation of monoclonal antibodies, small molecules and second-generation antisense oligonucleotides. Many of these compounds have shown a potent antitumor activity in preclinical models, ability to cooperate with selected class of conventional cytotoxic drugs and activity following oral administration, inhibiting angiogenesis and inducing apoptosis. Such properties may increase therapeutic efficacy and reduce the toxicity, allowing long-term treatment and control of cancer growth. Several of these novel agents are currently under clinical evaluation in cancer patients in early clinical trials or in phase III trials in combination with standard therapeutic regimens. The kinases most extensively studied and exploited for therapeutic purposes are those of the erbB family (epidermal growth factor receptor, EGFR, and erbB-2), as tyrosine kinases, and the cAMP-dependent protein kinase (PKA), as serine–threonine kinase (Tortora & Ciardiello 2000). For these reasons they will be the main object of this chapter.

ErbB receptors family

Epidermal growth factor receptor (EGFR)

The EGF is the prototype of a large family of closely related growth factors which includes the transforming growth factor α (TGFα), amphiregulin, heparin-binding-EGF and betacellulin (Salomon *et al.* 1995). TGFα is a key modulator of cell proliferation in both normal and malignant epithelial cells. TGFα binds to the EGF receptor (EGFR), activating its tyrosine kinase that, in turn, triggers several intracellular transducers, including the ras/raf and mitogen-activated protein kinase (MAPK) pathway. The EGFR is part of a subfamily of four closely related receptors: EGFR (or erbB-1), erbB-2 (Her2/neu), erbB-3 (Her3) and erbB-4 (Her4). The receptors exist as inactive monomers which dimerize following ligand activation and cause homodimerization or heterodimerization of EGFR and another member of the erb family of receptors (Klapper *et al.* 2000).

TGFα and/or EGFR are overexpressed in many different solid human cancers, including prostate, non-small cell lung (NSCL), breast, head and neck, gastric, bladder, ovarian, colorectal carcinomas and glioblastomas, in which it is generally associated with advanced disease and poor prognosis (Salomon *et al.* 1995, Woodburn 1999, Ciardiello 2000). Overexpression of EGFR has also been associated with resistance to hormonal therapy, cytotoxic agents and radiotherapy (Woodburn 1999, Ciardiello 2000). More recently, it has been shown that EGFR is directly involved in other processes, including angiogenesis, metastatic spread and inhibition of apoptosis. For instance, TGFα is a positive regulator of angiogenesis, as it is secreted by cancer cells to stimulate normal endothelial cell growth through paracrine mechanisms, inducing expression and secretion of vascular endothelial growth factor (VEGF) and basic fibroblast growth factor (bFGF). Moreover, EGF and TGFα can upregulate the production of VEGF in human cancer cells at the transcriptional level (Gille *et al.* 1997, Schmitt & Soares, 1999).

The identification and development of selective and potent inhibitors of EGFR activation has been a successful area of translational research in cancer treatment (Woodburn 1999, Mendelsohn 2000, Ciardiello 2000). Among the different approaches used to target the EGFR, the most promising are the monoclonal antibodies, which prevent ligand binding, and the 'small molecules', which inhibit the tyrosine kinase enzymatic activity and downstream intracellular signaling. Other approaches include recombinant proteins containing TGFα or EGF fused to toxins, such as *Pseudomonas aeruginosa* toxin, EGFR-directed vaccines (Gonzalez *et al.*

1998) and the use of antisense oligonucleotides to the EGFR (Ciardiello and Tortora 1996).

Monoclonal antibodies

Several blocking monoclonal antibodies have been developed against the EGFR. Among these, IMC-225 is a chimeric human–mouse monoclonal IgG$_1$ antibody that has been the first anti-EGFR targeted therapy to enter clinical evaluation in cancer patients in phase II–III studies alone and in combination with conventional therapies such as radiotherapy and chemotherapy. IMC-C225 induces a G1 arrest and increases the levels of the p27^{kip1} inhibitor of cyclin-dependent kinases. In nude mice IMC-C225 significantly inhibits the growth of prostate, epidermoid, colon and renal cell carcinoma xenografts and this effect is generally accompanied by a significant increase in mice survival (Mendelsohn 2000, Prewett *et al.* 1996, Ciardiello 2000). Moreover, studies in nude mice have demonstrated that IMC-C225 inhibits several angiogenic factors, including TGFα, VEGF, bFGF and interleukin-8 (IL-8) and tumor-induced angiogenesis (Ciardiello *et al.* 1996, Ciardiello and Tortora 1996, Perrotte *et al.* 1999). IMC-C225 has shown an additive or cooperative growth inhibitory effect with various cytotoxic agents, including doxorubicin, cisplatin, paclitaxel, gemcitabine or topotecan *in vitro* and *in vivo* (Mendelsohn 2000, Ciardiello *et al.* 1999). Moreover, several studies have also shown an enhancement of tumor radioresponse by IMC-C225 in human epidermoid, head and neck and colon cancer xenografts (Milas *et al.* 2000; Huang *et al.* 1999, Bianco *et al.* 2000). We have also demonstrated a marked cooperative effect of this antibody in combination with an antisense targeted to human VEGF (AS-VEGF). The combination treatment caused antitumor activity in nude mice xenografts, suppressing VEGF expression and neovessel formation in tumor specimens (Ciardiello *et al.* 2000a).

Three phase I clinical trials were carried out with IMC-C225 intravenously, alone or in combination with cisplatin. IMC-C225 toxicity was minimal and the maximum tolerated dose was not reached in any of the studies, while objective responses were observed (Baselga *et al.* 2000). In phase II studies IMC-C225 determined partial response and disease stabilization in patients with metastatic renal cell carcinoma, while, in combination with radiotherapy, caused a complete response in 87% of patients with locally advanced head and neck cancer (Mendelsohn 2000, Bonner *et al.* 2000).

Small molecule inhibitors of the EGFR tyrosine kinase

Several tyrosine kinase inhibitors, which reversibly compete with ATP for binding to the intracellular catalytic domain of the EGFR tyrosine kinase, have been synthesized and evaluated for potential preclinical activity. ZD1839 (Iressa™) and OSI-774 are currently in phase II–III development. ZD1839 is a low-molecular-weight, synthetic anilinoquinazoline, reversible selective inhibitor of EGFR tyrosine kinase, with oral activity. A growth-inhibiting activity of ZD1839 has been demonstrated in a wide range of human cancer cell lines that express functional EGFRs, including prostate, breast, ovarian, colon, epidermoid, small cell lung (SCL) and NSCL associated with a dose-related increase in apoptosis *in vitro* (Ciardiello 2000). Moreover, daily oral administration of ZD1839 to athymic nude mice caused marked reductions in tumor growth in a variety of human cancer xenografts, including hormone-resistant prostate, ovarian, ductal carcinoma *in situ* (DCIS) of the breast, colon, vulval, SCL and NSCL (Ciardiello 2000b). Enhancement of cell growth inhibition, induction of apoptosis and increased antitumor activity, *in vitro* and *in vivo*, were observed when ZD1839 was combined with cisplatin, carboplatin, oxaliplatin, paclitaxel, docetaxel, doxorubicin, etoposide, topotecan and raltitrexed (Ciardiello 2000). ZD1839 has entered clinical evaluation, showing promising activity. Antitumor activity has been observed in patients with hormone-resistant prostate, colorectal, ovarian, NSCL, head and neck and renal cancers (Baselga & Averbuch, 2000). In particular, ZD1839 has shown encouraging results in patients with NSCL cancer, in which it is currently under evaluation in combination with chemotherapy in phase III studies.

OSI-774 is another quinazoline derivative; it is an irreversible inhibitor of the EGFR that shows activity against various human tumor xenografts *in vivo*. OSI-774 in combination with cisplatin produced substantial growth inhibition of human cancer xenografts in mice (Pollack *et al.* 1999). Moreover, it has been reported to have drug activity in phase I studies. OSI-774 is currently in phase II development in advanced head and neck, NSCL and ovarian cancer.

ErbB-2

ErbB-2 (HER-2/neu) has no known ligand and can act either by heterodimerization with other receptors of the EGFR family or by homodimerization with other erbB-2 molecules (Klapper *et al.* 2000). Therefore, it is generally conceived that the downstream signal transduction pathway of erbB-2 is mostly the same used by EGFR. ErbB-2 is overexpressed in several cancer types compared with normal tissues and its overexpression is often related to worse prognosis. Moreover, laboratory and clinical data have demonstrated that erbB-2 overexpression results in resistance to hormonal therapy.

A high-affinity, humanized monoclonal antibody directed against the extracellular domain of erbB-2, trastuzumab (Herceptin), has been generated. Trastuzumab acts in different ways: accelerating erbB-2 degradation, inducing cyclin-dependent kinase inhibitors, such as p27, and, finally, increasing immune-mediated effects, such as ADCC. Trastuzumab has been shown to be effective against different cancer types, *in vitro* and *in vivo* (Hung & Lau 1999). Moreover, it is able to enhance the activity of different cytotoxic drugs such as doxorubicin, taxanes and cisplatin in nude mice xenografted with human tumors. Clinical studies have shown a relevant activity of trastuzumab alone and in combination with doxorubicin or taxol (Baselga 2001). For these reasons it is a commonly used agent in breast cancer patients overexpressing erbB-2.

A reversible inhibitor of both EGFR and erbB-2 tyrosine kinases, PKI166 has demonstrated antitumor activity in several EGFR-expressing tumor xenograft models in nude mice and has entered phase I trials in patients (Traxler & Furet 1999).

It has also been shown that a novel small molecule, PD158780, can selectively inhibit heregulin-dependent tyrosine phosphorylation and cellular signaling through erbB-2, erbB-3 and erbB-4 (Sherwood *et al.* 1999)

cAMP-dependent protein kinase (PKA)

The cAMP-dependent protein kinase (PKA) is a serine–threonine kinase that plays a major role in the control of cellular growth and homeostasis in mammalian cells through two isoforms defined PKAI and PKAII. They share a similar catalytic subunit (C), while differing in the regulatory subunits (termed RI in PKAI and RII in PKAII, respectively), which affect the subcellular distribution and the function of the isoforms (Cho-Chung 1999). Differential expression of PKAI and PKAII has been correlated with cell differentiation and neoplastic transformation. In fact, preferential expression of PKAII is found in normal nonproliferating tissues and in growth-arrested cells, while PKAI and/or its regulatory subunit RIα are generally overexpressed in human cancer cell lines and primary tumors and are induced following transformation by certain GFs, such as TGFα, or oncogenes, such as ras and erbB-2 (Tortora & Ciardiello 2000). Moreover, RIα/PKAI overexpression is associated with a worse prognosis in cancer patients affected by different neoplasia, and PKAI has been directly implicated in the acquisition of the multidrug resistant (MDR) phenotype (Cho-Chung 1999, Tortora & Ciardiello 2000). Increased RIα/PKAI levels are induced in normal cells by mitogenic stimuli of different hormones and GFs, including EGF and TGFα, and are necessary for G1>S phase traverse. Moreover, PKAI directly participates in the transduction of mitogenic signaling through a structural interaction with EGFR, via the binding of PKA subunit RIα to Grb2 at the site of the ligand-activated EGFR. This has been the first demonstration of a direct interaction between a tyrosine kinase receptor, such as EGFR, and a serine kinase, such as PKAI (Tortora *et al.* 1997a). PKAI has also been implicated in the mechanism of neoangiogenesis and apoptosis (Bianco *et al.* 1997).

For all the above reasons, PKAI has been proposed as a potentially relevant target for cancer therapy. In this regard, two classes of selective downregulators of RIα/PKAI expression have been developed: the site-selective cAMP analogs, the most potent of which is 8-Cl-cAMP, and a novel class of antisense oligonucleotides targeting the RIα regulatory subunit of PKAI (AS-PKAI), defined mixed backbone oligonucleotides (MBOs) (Cho-Chung 1999, Nesterova & Cho-Chung 1995, Tortora & Ciardiello 2000). MBOs exhibit a significant improvement of pharmacokinetic properties and antitumor activity *in vivo*. The most recent and potent among them, a DNA/RNA hybrid MBO AS-PKAI, also defined as GEM231, has shown potent antitumor activity *in vivo* also following oral administration (Tortora *et al.* 2000). Both 8-Cl-cAMP and AS-PKAI have completed phase I trials in cancer patients.

These agents determine growth inhibition in a wide variety of cancer cell types *in vitro* and *in vivo*, associated to inhibition of the expression of different oncogenes, such as *myc*, *ras* and erbB-2, and of GFs of the EGF family. Moreover, both PKAI inhibitors, 8-Cl-cAMP and AS-PKAI, are able to cooperate with selected anticancer drugs, such as taxanes, topoisomerase II inhibitors and platinum derivatives, causing a synergistic antitumor activity associated with increased apoptosis in a wide variety of human cancer types *in vitro* and *in vivo*. Finally, they affect angiogenesis and metastatic spread, inhibiting the production of VEGF and bFGF as well as vessels formation, and inhibit cancer cell ability to invade the basement membrane matrix. Interestingly, AS-PKAI is able to produce all these effects also following oral administration (Tortora *et al.* 1997b, 1997c, 2000, Tortora & Ciardiello 2000; Bianco *et al.* 1997). It has also been shown that PKAI is implicated in bcl-2-dependent apoptotic pathway and that downregulation of PKAI induces bcl-2 phosphorylation (Tortora & Ciardiello 2000).

The functional and structural interactions between the EGFR and the PKAI pathways have potential therapeutic implications. In fact, we have shown a cooperative antitumor effect, *in vitro* and *in vivo*, of either 8-Cl-cAMP or AS-PKAI in combination with the anti-EGFR antibody IMC-C225 in several human cancer types provided with an active TGFα-EGFR autocrine pathway. The combination of low doses of these agents significantly prolongs mice survival, with no signs of toxicity. These effects are accompanied by inhibition of autocrine GFs, such as TGFα, AR and CRIPTO, and angiogenic GFs, such as VEGF and bFGF, with marked inhibition of vessels formation (Ciardiello *et al.* 1996, 1998).

Furthermore, specific classes of cytotoxic drugs, such as taxanes, or ionizing radiations, can be added to the combination of EGFR and PKAI inhibitors, achieving maximal antitumor effect with suboptimal doses of each agent (Tortora *et al.* 1999, Bianco *et al.* 2000).

Other protein kinases

Among the protein kinases, raf-1, protein kinase C (PKC) and Jun kinase (JNK) have attracted attention for development of selective inhibitors, mostly of the antisense oligonucleotides class.

c-raf-1

Key steps of the signaling cascade triggered by tyrosine kinase receptors involve activation of ras, raf and MAP kinase. A member of a family of serine–threonine kinases, c-*raf*-1 is recruited to plasma membrane where it binds ras-GTP and activates a cascade of downstream events phosphorylating MEK1. In addition to *ras*, c-*raf*-1 can also be activated by other kinases such as src, PKC and JAK1

(Gibbs 2000). An effective strategy to inhibit c-*raf*-1 expression and function has been the use of antisense oligonucleotides. ISIS 5132 has shown activity against a variety of tumor types *in vitro* and in nude mice bearing cancer xenografts (Monia *et al.* 1996). It has successfully completed phase I trials in cancer patients, demonstrating the ability to down-regulate c-raf-1 expression in peripheral blood mononuclear cells collected from advanced cancer patients following treatment. The time course of c-*raf*-1 depletion in mononuclear cells following ISIS 5132 treatment paralleled the clinical benefit in treated patients (O'Dwyer *et al.* 1999).

PKC

Protein kinase C is a family of at least 12 closely related isozymes with serine–threonine functions, acting as intracellular transducers of growth factors and hormones (Nishizuka 1992). PKC has been implicated in inflammation and carcinogenesis (Yuspa 1994). The existence of several isoforms and the cooperation of some of them in mediating intracellular signaling have complicated the development of PKC inhibitors. The most successful approach has been the targeting of PKCα, the most relevant isoform, by specific antisense oligonucleotides (AS-PKCα). One of them, ISIS3251 has shown marked activity in different human cancer lines *in vitro* and *in vivo* in nude mice xenografts (Dean *et al.* 1996). This compound has completed phase I clinical evaluation in cancer patients affected by different cancer types (Nemunaitis *et al.* 1999) and is under evaluation in phase II trials.

JNK

Jun kinase (JNK) is an amino-terminal kinase existing in at least 10 isoforms, and is a downstream target of the so-called JNK pathway. It has been shown that JNK may be an important effector of EGFR-triggered signaling and may play a role in bcl-2 phosphorylation, affecting cell proliferation and apoptosis. Antisense oligonucleotides targeting JNK1, JNK2 and JNK3 kinases have proven effective *in vitro* against human cancer cells (Bost *et al.* 1999).

Conclusion

In conclusion, the most recent and innovative therapeutic strategies are based on the integration of conventional treatments, with selective inhibitors of molecules playing a key role in the mechanisms of cell proliferation, apoptosis and angiogenesis. Several protein kinases have such characteristics and have been regarded as potentially relevant therapeutic targets. The past few years have witnessed a rapid development of novel agents, blocking selected protein kinases, that have entered clinical evaluation alone and in combination with chemotherapy or radiotherapy. It can be easily foreseen that, in the next years, protein kinase inhibitors will become widely used therapeutic drugs, providing the opportunity to design novel anticancer strategies that are less toxic and more selective.

References

Baselga J (2001) Clinical trials of Herceptin (trastuzumab). *Eur J Cancer* **37**(suppl 1):18–24.

Baselga J, Averbuch S (2000) ZD1839 (Iressa) as an anticancer agent. *Drugs* **60**:33–40.

Baselga J, Pfister D, Cooper MR, *et al.* (2000) Phase I studies of anti-epidermal growth factor receptor chimeric antibody C225 alone and in combination with cisplatin. *J Clin Oncol* **18**:904–914.

Bianco C, Tortora G, Baldassarre G, *et al.* (1997) 8-chloro-cAMP inhibits autocrine and angiogenic growth factors production in human colorectal and breast cancer. *Clin Cancer Res* **3**:439–448.

Bianco C, Bianco R, Tortora G, *et al.* (2000) Antitumor activity of combined treatment of human cancer cells with ionizing radiations and anti-epidermal growth factor receptor monoclonal antibody C225 plus type I protein kinase A antisense oligonucleotide. *Clin Cancer Res* **6**:4343–4350.

Bonner JA, Ezekiel MP, Robert F, *et al.* (2000) Continued response following treatment with IMC-225, an EGFr MoAb, combined with RT in advanced head and neck malignancies. *Proc Am Soc Clin Oncol* **19**:4,5F [Abstract].

Bost F, McKay R, Bost M, *et al.* (1999) The Jun kinase 2 isoform is preferentially required for epidermal growth factor-induced transformation of human A549 lung carcinoma cells. *Mol Cell Biol* **19**:1938–1949.

Cho-Chung YS (1999) Antisense oligonucleoide inhibition of serine/threonine kinase: An innovative approach to cancer treatment. The regulatory subunit of cAMP-dependent protein kinase as a target for chemotherapy of cancer and other cellular dysfunctional-related diseases. *Pharmacol Therap* **60**:265–288.

Ciardiello F (2000) Epidermal growth factor receptor tyrosine kinase inhibitors as anticancer agents. *Drugs* **60**:25–32.

Ciardiello F, Damiano V, Bianco R, *et al.* (1996) Antitumor activity of combined blockade of epidermal growth factor receptor and protein kinase A. *J Natl Cancer Inst* **88**:1770–1776.

Ciardiello F, Caputo R, Bianco R, *et al.* (1998) Cooperative inhibition of renal cancer growth by anti-EGF receptor antibody and protein kinase A antisense oligonucleotide. *J Natl Cancer Inst* **90**:1087–1094.

Ciardiello F, Bianco R, Damiano V, *et al.* (1999) Antitumor activity of sequential treatment with topotecan and anti-epidermal growth factor receptor monoclonal antibody C225. *Clin Cancer Res* **5**: 909–916.

Ciardiello F, Bianco R, Damiano V, *et al.* (2000a) Antiangiogenic and antitumor activity of anti-EGFR C225 monoclonal antibody in combination with Vascular Endothelial Growth Factor antisense oligonucleotide in human GEO colon cancer cells. *Clin Cancer Res* **6**:3739–3747.

Ciardiello F, Caputo R, Bianco R, *et al.* (2000b) Antitumor effect and potentiation of cytotoxic drugs activity in human cancer cells by ZD-1839 (Iressa), an EGFR-selective tyrosine kinase inhibitor. *Clin Cancer Res* **6**:2053–2063.

Ciardiello F, Caputo R, Troiani T, *et al.* (2001) Antisense oligonucleotides targeting the epidermal growth factor receptor inhibit proliferation, induce apoptosis, and cooperate with cytotoxic drugs in human cancer cell lines. *Int J Cancer* **93**:172–178.

Ciardiello F, Tortora G (1996) A novel approach in the treatment of cancer: targeting the epidermal growth factor receptor. *Clin Canc Res* **7**:2958–2970.

Dean NM, McKay R, Miraglia L, *et al.* (1996) Inhibition of growth of human tumor cell lines in nude mice by an antisense oligonucleotide inhibitor of protein kinase C-alpha expression. *Cancer Res* **56**: 3499–3507.

Fan Z, Mendelsohn J (1998) Therapeutic application of anti-growth factor receptor antibodies. *Curr Opin Oncol* **10**:67–73.

Gibbs JB (2000) Anticancer drug targets: growth factors and growth factor signalling. *J Clin Invest* **105**:9–13.

Gille J, Swerlick RA, Caughman SW (1997) Transforming growth factor alpha-induced transcriptional activation of the vascular permeability factor (VPF/VEGF) gene requires AP2-dependent DNA binding and transactivation. *EMBO J* **16**:750–759.

Gonzalez G, Crombet T, Catala M, *et al.* (1998) A novel vaccine composed of human-recombinant epidermal growth factor linked to a carrier protein: report of a pilot clinical trial. *Ann Oncol* **9**:431–435.

Hung MC, Lau YK (1999) Basic science of HER-2/neu: a review. *Semin Oncol* **26**:51–59.

Huang SM, Bock JM, Harari PM (1999) Epidermal growth factor receptor blockade with C225 modulates proliferation, apoptosis, and radiosensitivity in squamous cell carcinomas of the head and neck. *Cancer Res* **15**:1935–1940.

Klapper LN, Kirshbaum MH, Sela M, Yarden Y (2000) Biochemical and clinical implications of the ErbB/HER signaling network of growth factor receptors. *Adv Cancer Res* **77**:25–79.

Levitzki A (1999) Protein tyrosine kinase inhibitors as novel therapeutic agents. *Pharmacol Ther* **82**:231–239.

Mendelsohn J (2000) Blockade of receptors for growth factors: an anticancer therapy. *Clin Cancer Res* **6**: 747–753.

Milas L, Mason K, Hunter N, *et al.* (2000) In vivo enhancement of tumor radioresponse by C225 antiepidermal growth factor receptor antibody. *Clin Cancer Res* 6:701–708.

Monia BP, Johnston JF, Geiger T, Muller M, Fabbro D (1996) Antitumor activity of a phosphorothioate antisense oligodeoxynucleotide targeted against *C-raf* kinase. *Nature Medicine* 2:668–675.

Nemunaitis J, Holmlund JT, Kraynak M, *et al.* (1999) Phase I evaluation of ISIS 3521, an antisense oligodeoxynucleotide to protein kinase C-alpha in patients with advanced cancer. *J Clin Oncol* 17:3586–3595.

Nesterova M, Cho-Chung YS (1995) A single-injection protein kinase A-directed antisense treatment to inhibit tumour growth. *Nature Medicine* 1:528–533.

Nishizuka Y (1992) Intracellular signaling by hydrolysis of phospholipids and activation of protein kinase C. *Science* 258:607–608.

O' Dwyer PJ, Stevenson JP, Gallagher M, *et al.* (1999) c-raf-1 depletion and tumor responses in patients treated with the c-raf-1 antisense oligodeoxynucleotide ISIS 5132 (CGP 69846A). *Clin Cancer Res* 5: 3977–3982.

Perrotte P, Matsumoto T, Inoue K, *et al.* (1999) Antiepidermal growth factor receptor antibody C225 inhibits angiogenesis in human transitional cell carcinoma growing orthotopically in nude mice. *Clin Cancer Res* 5:257–264.

Pollack VA, Savage DM, Baker DA, *et al.* (1999) Inhibition of epidermal growth factor receptor-associated tyrosine phosphorylation in human carcinomas with CP-358,774: dynamics of receptor inhibition in situ and antitumour effects in athymic mice. *J Pharmacol Exp Ther* 291:739–748.

Prewett M, Rockwell P, Rockwell RF, *et al.* (1996) The biological effects of C225, a chimeric monoclonal antibody to the EGFR, on human prostate carcinoma. *J Immunother Emphasis Tumor Immunol* 19:419–427.

Salomon DS, Brandt R, Ciardiello F, Normanno N (1995) Epidermal growth factor-related peptides and their receptors in human malignancies. *Crit Rev Oncol/ Haematol* 19:183–232.

Schmitt FC, Soares R (1999) TGFα and angiogenesis. *Am J Surg Pathol* 23:358–359.

Sherwood V, Bridges AJ, Denny WA, *et al.* (1999) Selective inhibition of heregulin-dependent tyrosine phosphorylation and cellular signaling through erbB2, erbB3 and erbB4 by PD 158780 and a new irreversible inhibitor, PD 183805. *Proc Am Assoc Cancer Res* 40:4778 [Abstract].

Tortora G, Ciardiello F (2000) Targeting of epidermal growth factor receptor and protein kinase A: Molecular basis and therapeutic applications. *Ann Oncol* 11: 777–783.

Tortora G, Damiano V, Bianco C, *et al.* (1997a) The RIα subunit of protein kinase A (PKA) binds to Grb2 and allows PKA interaction with the activated EGF-receptor. *Oncogene* 14:923–928.

Tortora G, di Isernia G, Sandomenico C, *et al.* (1997b) Synergistic inhibition of growth and induction of apoptosis by 8-Chloro-cAMP and paclitaxel or cisplatin in human cancer cells. *Cancer Res* 57: 5107–5111.

Tortora G, Caputo R, Damiano V, *et al.* (1997c) Synergistic inhibition of human cancer cell growth by cytotoxic drugs and mixed backbone antisense oligonucleotide targeting protein kinase A. *Proc Natl Acad Sci USA* 94:12586–12591.

Tortora G, Caputo R, Pomatico G, *et al.* (1999) Cooperative inhibitory effect of novel mixed backbone oligonucleotide targeting protein kinase A in combination with docetaxel and anti-epidermal growth factor-receptor antibody on human breast cancer cell growth. *Clin Cancer Res* 5:875–881.

Tortora G, Bianco R, Damiano V, *et al.* (2000) Oral antisense targeting protein kinase A cooperates with taxol and inhibits tumor growth, angiogenesis and growth factor production. *Clin Cancer Res* 6:2506–2512.

Traxler P, Furet P (1999) Strategies toward the design of novel and selective protein tyrosine kinase inhibitors. *Pharmacol Ther* 82:195–206.

Woodburn JR (1999) The epidermal growth factor receptor and its inhibition in cancer therapy. *Pharmacol Ther* 82:241–250.

Yuspa SH (1994) The pathogenesis of squamous cell cancer: lessons learned from studies of skin carcinogenesis. *Cancer Res* 54:1178–1189.

12 Monoclonal antibodies in the management of prostate cancer: an update

Menuhin I Lampe, Egbert Oosterwijk and Peter FA Mulders

Introduction

Almost 100 years ago, Ehrlich had already suggested that tumors expressed specific antigens that could be targeted with antibodies, the so-called magic bullet concept (Ehrlich 1957). In the 1950s, polyclonal antisera were used as therapeutic agents, but except for some casuistic reports of tumor regression, these antisera proved unsuitable. The inherent heterogeneity, batch-to-batch variation and undefined specificity appeared to be major obstacles, precluding successful clinical application.

In the 1970s, Kohler & Milstein (1975) developed the hybridoma technology whereby production of monoclonal antibodies (mAbs) became feasible. The availability of unlimited supplies of mAbs with predefined specificity was seen as a major breakthrough for antibody-guided therapy. Actually, this technology had a profound impact on all aspects of immunological investigation and on the development of, for example, diagnostic assays.

Epidemiology

Prostate cancer (PCa) is the most common non-cutaneous cancer in US males and the second leading cause of cancer death after lung cancer in the USA and many European countries. The American Cancer Society estimates that within the USA 198 100 men will be diagnosed with PCa and 31 500 men will die from this disease in 2001 (Greenlee *et al.* 2001). Evidently, PCa is a significant health problem and the costs accompanying are considerable.

Developments in the management of prostate cancer

In the last decades of the 20th century, great progress was made in the diagnosis and management of localized disease:

- the introduction of prostate-specific antigen (PSA) as a marker for diagnosis and progression
- the clinical application of transrectal ultrasound (TRUS) coupled to the introduction of a spring-loaded biopsy gun allowing for transrectal biopsies
- the development of nerve-sparing prostatectomy, reducing morbidity and mortality
- innovations in radiotherapy and brachytherapy, reducing morbidity and increasing efficacy.

All these developments have dramatically changed the way we manage PCa. Thirty years ago, most patients would present to the clinic with advanced disease. Today, the majority of patients present with early-stage localized disease. However, these developments have created new questions and challenges. Does the shift to early-stage disease at the time of diagnosis significantly reduce mortality? Are the small PCa lesions detected of clinical relevancy? How can we distinguish between indolent and aggressive tumors? In the years ahead of us, these will be important issues to resolve.

In contrast to the developments in the management of localized disease, not much has changed since hormonal therapy was introduced about 50 years ago for the management of advanced disease. Approximately 50% of patients in the United States and Western Europe will develop metastases (Pienta 1998). These patients are usually treated with androgen deprivation therapy. Despite initial response to this therapy, all patients will eventually relapse with androgen-independent disease. No current standard therapy consistently confers a significant survival benefit to patients who develop androgen-independent prostate cancer. The 2.5-year survival for this group of patients is still only 50% (Denis *et al.* 1993).

Metastatic PCa can remain sensitive to radiation therapy, but dissemination of the cancer precludes external beam radiotherapy to all disease sites. Several chemotherapeutic agents have been evaluated in clinical trials, but with little success to date. Evidently, there is a need for new treatment modalities and additional diagnostic tools to select the right patients for the right therapy.

Basic principles of mAb-based strategies

Antigens can be defined as components of cells or other substances that can be recognized by the immune system. In general, tumor cells have a decreased ability to induce an immune response. This is not surprising, since the vast majority of the expressed antigens are normal differentiation antigens, against which tolerance exists. Additionally, tumor cells employ several strategies by which they can escape immuno-surveillance, even if tumor-specific antigens are expressed.

Antibodies (immunoglobulins) are produced by B lymphocytes in response to antigenic stimuli. They are composed of two different domains: the Fab domain conferring specificity and the Fc domain determining the effector functions of the antibody. Antibody-directed strategies attempt to exploit the specificity of the antibody–antigen reaction.

In oncology, the main target for mAb-based diagnostics and therapeutics has been the tumor. Tumor cells can be targeted using mAbs directed against tumor-specific antigens, tumor-associated antigens or tissue-specific antigens. In addition, various (differentially expressed) antigens/receptors or growth factors can be targeted with mAbs.

When expression patterns are correlated with disease stage and/or progression, mAbs can be useful in diagnosis and prognosis. In pathology, immunohistochemical staining of biopsies or surgical specimens using mAbs is daily routine. Immunoassays have been developed, whereby it is possible to screen body fluids for the presence of the antigen of interest. Moreover, with quantification analysis, useful tools for follow-up have been developed. In the field of imaging, immunoscintigraphy can aid in staging, with potential additional value over conventional imaging techniques. Conventional imaging modalities (CT, MRI, ultrasound) mainly rely on anatomical abnormalities (enlargements) for the detecting of lymph node metastases, with a detection minimum of about 1 cm. In contrast, immunoscintigraphy is based on the presence of antigen – thus, on histological characteristics revealing the tumor. Using optimal scanning techniques, it is possible to detect smaller lesions with consistent sensitivity.

For therapeutic purposes, mAbs can be used to trigger the host immune system eliciting cell lysis by complement-dependent cytotoxicity (CDC) or antibody-dependent cellular cytotoxicity (ADCC). MAbs can also be used as targeting tools in conjunction with, for example, toxins, cytotoxic drugs or radionuclides, using the mAb as a 'magic bullet' to specifically direct the conjugate to the tumor, possibly with less systemic side effects.

The potential benefits of immunotoxins include their high potency, catalytic action and the well-defined biology and chemistry. However, toxins elicit a potent human anti-toxin immune response, which precludes multiple therapy cycles. Improved toxin design together with a better selection of the targeted tumor antigens may lead to clinically applicable toxin conjugates with considerable therapeutic impact.

Radioimmunoconjugates have comparable advantages as immunotoxins. In addition, the radius of action is wider by virtue of the emission characteristics of many of the commonly used radionuclides. This results in irradiation of antigen-negative tumor cells, thus preventing escape of these cells. Radioimmunotherapy (RIT) has been the most extensively studied immunoconjugate treatment strategy. In particular, in the treatment of hematologic neoplasms, there has been considerable success with radioimmunoconjugates. In patients with chemotherapy-refractory B-cell lymphoma, treatment with ^{131}I-labeled anti-CD20 mAb resulted in complete response rates of 40% (low-dose) and 84% for high-dose treatment with autologous bone marrow support (as reviewed in Weiner 1999). Success in solid tumors has been limited, which may be due to the intrinsic differences between hematological malignancies and solid tumors. In solid tumors, various factors influencing mAb accrual have been identified, including antigen expression, affinity, mAb format (IgG, F (ab') 2, Fab', single chain mAb), interstitial fluid pressures, and perfusion. Overcoming these obstacles will be necessary for the development of successful mAb-based approaches in solid tumors.

Recently, the role of neovascularization in the growth of primary and metastatic tumor has been appreciated (van Hinsbergh *et al.* 1999). In particular, vascular endothelial growth factor (VEGF) has received much attention, as it is a potent angiogenic factor that has been identified as a key regulatory paracrine growth factor for endothelial cells. Whereas VEGF is expressed at low levels in quiescent vasculature of normal tissue, it is expressed at high levels in a broad spectrum of malignancies, thus making it a suitable target for mAb therapy. The use of mAbs as anti-angiogenic agents may be a new promising avenue in cancer therapy.

Monoclonal antibodies in prostate cancer

The characteristics of prostate cancer are well suited for mAb-directed strategies. Metastases of PCa predominantly involve the bone marrow compartment and lymph nodes, sites that theoretically can accumulate high amounts of mAb. The individual metastatic tumor sites tend to be small in volume, which is ideal for antibody penetration. Furthermore, organ specificity should suffice, since any specific uptake outside the prostate itself would represent metastatic disease, thus obviating the need for tumor specificity versus prostate tissue specificity.

Prostate-specific antigen

One of the most useful markers in oncology is prostate-specific antigen. PSA was identified in 1979 (at that time denoted prostate antigen) by rabbit antiserum raised against crude extracts of normal human prostatic tissue using an immunoprecipitation technique (Wang *et al.* 1979). Subsequently, it was shown that this antigen could be detected in the sera obtained from patients with advanced prostatic cancer, while it was undetectable in sera from patients harboring non-prostatic tumor (Papsidero *et al.* 1980). Soon thereafter, a sensitive enzyme immunoassay became available (Kuriyama *et al.* 1980) and it was possible to quantify serum PSA levels. The potential prognostic value of serum PSA levels in monitoring prostate cancer was already recognized in 1981 (Kuriyama *et al.* 1981). Furthermore, in immunohisto-chemistry the value of PSA as an immuno-histochemical diagnostic marker for prostate cancer was established (Nadji *et al.* 1981). In 1982 and 1983, the first monoclonal antibodies were developed using hybridoma technology (Frankel *et al.* 1982, Papsidero *et al.* 1983), con-firming the specificity of PSA and representing adequate probes for detection and differential diagnosis of metastatic PCa in immunohisto-chemistry.

However, it was not until the early 1990s that the use of PSA as a serum marker for detection and monitoring of disease progression became relatively common. The immunoassays, based on anti-PSA monoclonal antibodies, have since become very sensitive, with detection limits of 0.1–0.5 ng/ml. Today, PSA plays a central role in screening and early detection of prostate cancer. It is the only serum marker approved for

diagnostic purposes by the US Food and Drug Administration. Nevertheless, PSA is not the ideal tumor marker, as elevated PSA levels can be related to various other conditions. Especially in the gray zone of 4–10 ng/ml PSA performance is limited, mainly due to BPH. Several modalities have been introduced to enhance PSA performance: PSA velocity, PSA density and transition zone density, and age-adjusted PSA. In addition, it was discovered that PSA circulates in serum in several molecu-lar forms: as non-complexed, free PSA and as complexed PSA, i.e. complexed to a number of protease inhibitors. MAbs have been developed and characterized, whereby sensitive immuno-assays have been developed for the detection of serum free PSA (Black *et al.* 1999, Matsumoto *et al.* 1999). It was demonstrated that the free PSA/total PSA ratio is lower for patients with PCa compared to those without the disease. Calculating this ratio enhanced specificity as compared with total PSA alone (as reviewed in Brawer 1999). The precise role of these various modalities in improving the diagnostic poten-tial of PSA in daily clinical practice remains to be determined.

Meanwhile, research on PSA continues and it is now recognized that PSA is not strictly prostate specific, as expression has been shown in various other cell types. PSA was shown to belong to the family of the so-called human kallikreins. MAbs that recognize other mem-bers of this family, including human kallikrein 1 and human kallikrein 2, have been devel-oped. Human kallikrein 2 (hK2) is closely related to PSA (Hk3) and prostate specific (Young *et al.* 1996). Functionally, it probably plays a role in the activation of PSA (Lovgren *et al.* 1997, Takayama *et al.* 1997). Immuno-histochemical analysis revealed that the inten-sity and extent of hK2 expression was greater in lymph node metastases than in primary cancer. Furthermore, hK2 expression in primary cancer was greater than in benign epithelium. In contrast, PSA expression was higher in primary cancer than in lymph node tissue. These findings suggest that tissue expression of hK2 may be regulated independently of PSA (Darson *et al.* 1997, 1999). Serum assays were also developed for the detection of hK2. The additional value of hK2 levels in serum is currently under investigation. Studies are accumulating that indicate that it could be a helpful marker to identify the patients with PCa in the gray zone of PSA (Becker *et al.* 2000, Nam *et al.* 2000). Additionally, it may even discriminate between organ-confined versus non-organ-confined prostate cancer (Haese *et al.* 2000, Recker *et al.* 2000).

Interestingly, to our knowledge, there were no reports of anti-PSA mAbs for therapeutic purposes in the literature. Probably due to the presence of PSA in the blood circulation, attempts to target PCa using mAbs have either not been carried out or the results have not been published. Only recently one study was published in which the authors describe the construction and evaluation of a bispecific antibody (BsAb), recognizing both PSA and the T-cell-associated CD3 antigen (anti-PSA × anti-CD3) (Katzenwadel *et al.* 2000). The anti-PSA × anti-CD3 BsAb was tested *in vitro* and *in vivo*. Using the LNCaP cell line and human effector cells, it was possible to elicit specific tumor lysis *in vitro*. For *in-vivo* evaluation a nude mice model was used, with mice bearing LNCaP tumors treated with the BsAb together with human effector cells. Control mice received either no therapy or only effector cells. In the treated group, there was a significant reduction in tumor growth as compared to the control groups. This study shows that it is feasible to target PCa, using anti-PSA antibody. Furthermore, this approach has the advantage of specifically activating the cellular immunoresponse, by retargeting T cells to prostate carcinoma. Such an approach may provide a new tool for immunotherapy for PCa.

PSMA

MAb 7E11-C5, developed by immunizing mice with the human prostate cell line LNCaP, is the most extensively studied monoclonal antibody for clinical applications in prostate cancer (Horoszewicz *et al.* 1987). This mAb recognizes a prostate glycoprotein, denoted prostate-specific membrane antigen (PSMA). PSMA is a 750 amino acid type-2 transmembrane glycoprotein consisting of three domains: an intracellular domain, a transmembrane region and a large extracellular domain. PSMA is expressed in normal and malignant prostate epithelium. Extraprostatic PSMA expression appears to be restricted to duodenal mucosa, a subset of proximal renal tubules, and a subpopulation of colonic neuroendocrine cells and to tumor-associated neovasculature of a wide spectrum of malignancies (Silver *et al.* 1997). This latter finding was confirmed using various newly developed anti-PSMA mAbs (Chang *et al.* 1999). In prostate tissue, expression increases incrementally from benign epithelium to high-grade PIN or adenocarcinoma (Bostwick *et al.* 1998). Most lymph node metastases also express PSMA, albeit with lower intensity than primary cancer (Sweat *et al.* 1998). Whereas short-term (3 months) neoadjuvant androgen deprivation therapy did not affect PSMA expression in benign epithelium, high-grade PIN or PCa (Chang *et al.* 2000), it was previously shown that expression is enhanced in tissue, both primary and metastatic and LNCaP cells after androgen deprivation (Wright *et al.* 1996). PSMA may therefore be an attractive target for mAb-directed modalities in the management of patients with hormone-escaped disease.

Currently, the clinical application of anti-PSMA mAb is confined to radioimmunodetection for staging. CYT-356 (mAb 7E11-C5 conjugated with linker-chelator GYK-DTPA), also designated capromab pendetide, was linked to indium 111, employing it as diagnostic marker for detection of prostate cancer metastasis and recurrence *in vivo*. This diagnostic imaging test is marketed under the name ProstaScint® (Cytogen Corp., Princeton, NJ). In 1997, the US Food and Drug Administration gave approval for the use of ProstaScint for preoperative staging of patients at high risk for metastatic disease and for the detection of recurrence for patients with biochemical relapse after prostatectomy for localized disease. Several trails have evaluated the potential of radioimmunodetection using ProstaScint (Elgamal *et al.* 1998, Haseman *et al.* 1996, Hinkle *et al.* 1998, Kahn *et al.* 1994, 1998a, 1998b, Manyak *et al.* 1999, Murphy *et al.* 2000, Petronis *et al.* 1998, Polascik *et al.* 1999, Seltzer *et al.* 1999, Texter & Neal 1998). Most of these studies demonstrate that both metastatic and recurrent PCa can be detected and that the scan has an additional value over conventional imaging modalities. In some of these studies, biopsies were performed in a number of patients. If biopsy was considered the gold standard for metastasis or recurrence of disease, the overall sensitivity rate was found to be 49–86% and the specificity 43–86% (Table 12.1). Only one study thus far has not been able to show the additional value of ProstaScint (Seltzer *et al.* 1999), where they directly compared helical CT, PET scan and ProstaScint. The data suggested that the mAb scan had a lower detection rate compared to CT or PET. However, due to the study design, biopsies were performed only in patients with abnormal CT findings, thus introducing an inherent bias favoring CT. Overall, the majority of evidence indicates that the ProstaScint scan may be a useful adjunct for the early detection and localization of metastatic or recurrent PCa. It is a safe and non-invasive test, although the cost of the scan is considerable (approx. $2000). Technically, it is a demanding procedure which is best performed and interpreted at institutions that have gained sufficient experience and expertise. Therefore, it is not likely that this scan will become an integral part of daily clinical practice in urology in the next few years. Further studies are warranted to determine the precise role of ProstaScint in the management of patients with prostate

Table 12.1 Comparative analysis between results of studies of ProstaScint scan.

References	Sensitivity (%)	Specificity (%)	PPV (%)	NPV (%)
Elgamal *et al.* 1998	89	67	89	NA
Haseman *et al.* 1996	86	43	60	75
Hinkle *et al.* 1998	75	86	81	NA
Kahn *et al.* 1998b	49	71	50	70
Manyak *et al.* 1999	62	72	62	72
Polascik *et al.* 1999	62	80	67	76
Texter and Neal, 1998	63	72	62	72

PPV, positive predictive value; NPV, negative predictive value.

cancer. Meanwhile, it can be a valuable tool, especially in clinical trials for follow-up of disease response, to complement PSA.

The potential of CYT-356 for therapeutic purposes is under investigation. In a phase I dose-escalation study using ^{90}Y-CYT-356 in 12 patients with hormone-refractory PCa none of the patients attained a complete or partial response based on PSA measurements and/or radiological criteria (Deb *et al.* 1996). Three patients had transient subjective improvements in the symptomatology of their disease. The maximal tolerated dose was established at 9 mCi/m^2, resulting in grade 1–2 myelosuppression. Moreover, myelosuppression was the dose-limiting toxicity and occurred at 12 mCi/m^2 ^{90}Y-CYT-356. Recently, the results of a phase II study of ^{90}Y-Capromab (9 mCi/m^2) treatment in men with biochemical recurrence after radical prostatectomy were published (Kahn *et al.* 1999). In addition to a progressively rising level of PSA (>0.2 ng/ml), each of the patients had at least one lesion outside the prostatic fossa, as documented on a diagnostic ^{111}indium capromab scan, while no evidence of disease on bone scan or conventional imaging was found. Initially, the trial was designed for 14 patients, but it was terminated due to the lack of objective responses and considerable toxicity after analysis of the first eight subjects. There were no complete or partial responses, as evaluated by PSA serum levels or by imaging criteria. Four patients had stable disease, while the other four had progression, based on PSA. Toxicity was considerable: two patients had grade 3 leukopenia and neutropenia, one had grade 4 neutropenia and 3 patients had grade 3 thrombocytopenia. The last two patients received co-infusions of edetate calcium disodium to decrease bone marrow suppression and they only developed grade 1 toxicity. It is unclear why toxicity was more severe than in patients in the previous phase I trial receiving the same doses.

The 7E11-C5 epitope is located on the intracellular domain of PSMA (Troyer *et al.* 1995), which may in part account for the disappointing results in the clinical trials: targeting of intracellular epitopes is dependent upon occurrence of dead/necrotic cells. PCa tumors are usually rather small and vital, with little necrosis occurring; thus, little antigen would be available. Surprisingly, antigen-specific mAb CYT-356 uptake has been demonstrated using viable LNCaP cells *in vitro* (Barren *et al.* 1997). The mechanism driving CYT-356 uptake in view of the extracellular absence of the epitope is unclear. Currently, a clinical trial is ongoing to investigate an mAb that recognizes the extracellular domain of PSMA (NH Bander *et al.* pers. comm.), which may show improved targeting and may possibly be a better tool for therapeutic interventions.

CC49

MAb CC49 recognizes TAG-72, a high-molecular-weight mucin antigen expressed by many adenocarcinomas, including PCa. In a phase II trial, 75 mCi/m^2 ^{131}I-CC49 was administered to 15 patients with hormone-resistant metastatic prostate cancer. Although six of 10 symptomatic patients had bone pain relief, none of the patients showed an objective response by PSA measurements and/or radiological criteria (Meredith *et al.* 1994). Slovin *et al.* (1998) pretreated 14 androgen-independent PCa patients with IFN-γ for 7 days, based on the observation that IFN-γ increases TAG-72 expression in several tumor systems. Subsequently, the patients received 75 mCi/m^2 of ^{131}I-labeled CC49. Despite successful targeting of tumor in 12 of the 14 patients, no objective responses were observed, based on PSA criteria. Two patients had a stabilization of PSA for 5 and 6 months, respectively, and three patients had pain relief, which suggested some anti-tumor effect (Slovin *et al.* 1998). In a similar phase II trial, 14 patients received four doses IFN-γ from day −5 to day +1 on alternate days and 75 mCi/m^2 ^{131}I-CC49 treatment. In eight patients radioimmunoscintigraphy was positive, with positive lesions consistent with known metastatic disease. Two patients had a minor radiographic objective response, and three had PSA reductions by >50%. Compared to the group treated without IFN (Meredith *et al.* 1994), mean tumor dose, dose/mCi, and tumor:whole body ratios were all significantly higher for the patients receiving IFN, suggesting enhancement of CC49 targeting. No differences were seen in immunogenicity or bone marrow suppression (Meredith *et al.* 1999). The cause for the difference in response outcome between the two IFN adjuvant studies is unclear. The only apparent difference in study protocol was the scheme of IFN injection, e.g. 7 vs 4 days. The use of humanized or chimerized CC49 (Kashmiri *et al.* 1995, Slavin Chiorini *et al.* 1995), allowing for multiple treatment cycles, should be evaluated; in combination with IFN-γ pretreatment, this approach may lead to enhanced anti-tumor efficacy.

Prostate stem cell antigen

Recently, prostate stem cell antigen (PSCA) was identified (Reiter *et al.* 1998). PSCA is a 123 amino acid glycoprotein with 30% identity to stem cell antigen 2 (Sca 2), a cell surface marker of immature thymic lymphocytes. It belongs to the Thy-1/Ly-6 family of glycosylphosphatidylinositol (GPI)-anchored cell surface antigens. PSCA mRNA was expressed predominantly in prostate and placenta. MRNA in-situ hybridization localized PSCA expression in normal prostate to the basal cell compartment. PSCA mRNA was also detected in more than

80% of primary prostate tumors by in-situ analysis. Moreover, mRNA expression often appeared to be stronger in malignant epithelium than in adjacent normal glands, suggesting that PSCA might have some tumor specificity. Several mAbs were isolated and characterized, recognizing the PSCA–GTS fusion protein. Expression of PSCA protein was detectable on the cell surface using these antibodies. Furthermore, it was demonstrated that PSCA expression increases in more advanced stages and grades of prostate cancer. In addition, PSCA expression was strong in all cases of PCa bone metastasis examined (Gu *et al.* 2000). These results indicate that PSCA might be a potential target for mAb-based strategies, both diagnostic and therapeutic, in prostate cancer. Further studies are warranted to evaluate the suitability of anti-PSCA mAbs to target prostate cancer *in vivo*.

Miscellaneous mAbs

Various monoclonal antibodies have been evaluated *in vitro* and in animal studies for their potential use in the treatment of PCa. **MAb L6** reacts with a cell-surface, tumor-associated antigen expressed on several adenocarcinomas, including PCa. Unconjugated L6 possesses tumoricidal capacity, manifested by ADCC and CDC. Furthermore, L6 targets human prostate cancer xenografts in nude mice and has a low–normal organ uptake, making it a good candidate for use in PCa (O'Donnell *et al.* 1998). L6 has been used in RIT for breast cancer patients, resulting in clinically measurable tumor responses (DeNardo *et al.* 1997), that emphasize its potential.

MAb E4 identifies a human prostatic cell-surface specific antigen expressed in normal prostate tissue and malignant prostate tissue of all Gleason grades, albeit to somewhat lesser extent in poorly differentiated PCa. RIT studies in DU-145 spheroids with ^{131}I-labeled E4 demonstrated that this immunoconjugate induced significant reduction of spheroid size (Essand *et al.* 1995). In a recent animal study, the anti-tumor effect of ^{131}I-labeled E4 was assessed in nude mice xenografted with DU-145. Mice were treated with either single or repeated injections of radiolabeled mAb, or with non-labeled mAb. Although the tumor volumes between treatment groups did not differ, tumors of ^{131}I-E4 treated animals consisted of significantly lower numbers of viable tumor cells, suggesting an anti-tumor effect of the immunoconjugate (Rydh *et al.* 1999). In-vitro studies established that E4 could be internalized into the cell (Essand *et al.* 1996), which opens the way for immunotoxin-based therapy. E4–*Pseudomonas* exotoxin constructs demonstrated antigen-specific cytotoxicity of E4-positive prostate cell lines, making this immunotoxin a potential candidate for the treatment of prostate cancer (Essand & Pastan 1998).

The effects of **mAb A4.6.1**, raised against human VEGF, on angiogenesis and growth of primary tumors were studied in a dorsal skinfold chamber animal model. Treatment with A4.6.1 completely inhibited neovascularization and prevented tumor growth beyond the prevascular growth phase (Borgstrom *et al.* 1998). In a subsequent animal model, Melnyk *et al.* (1999) demonstrated that A4.6.1 treatment led to significant tumor growth inhibition and impaired establishment of metastases. These promising results appear to justify clinical evaluation of this mAb.

Recently, a recombinant humanized **huKS1/4-interleukin 2** (IL2) fusion-protein was constructed to evaluate its potential in immunocytokine therapy. This antibody recognizes a human epithelial cell adhesion molecule, KSA.

Targeting with huKS1/4-IL2 effectively inhibited both growth and dissemination of lung and bone marrow metastases of human prostate carcinoma in severe combined immunodeficient mice and significantly prolonged the life span of these mice. This antitumor effect was specific for the immunocytokine and dependent on the targeting of the tumor (Dolman *et al.* 1998). Currently, a phase I clinical trial is ongoing to evaluate the potential of huKS1/4-IL2 in PCa.

MAb 730 was developed by immunization of mice with DU145 cells, an androgen-independent human prostatic cancer cell line. This mAb was selected for both immunoreactivity and cytotoxicity *in vitro*. It was demonstrated that approximately 80% of the DU145 cells bound the antibody and were susceptible to lysis at saturating levels of mAb 730 in the presence of complement. MAb 730 was also cytotoxic to PC3, another androgen-independent cell line. Immunofluorescence analysis revealed reactivity with prostate cancer tissue but not with benign glandular tissue. Furthermore, no reactivity with various normal human tissues was seen (Talwar *et al.* 2001). These data suggest that the antigen recognized by mAb 730 is prostate cancer specific.

MAb 3.10 was recently isolated in our laboratory, after immunization of mice with primary prostate tumor homogenates. MAb 3.10 reacts with both normal and malignant prostate epithelium. Expression is retained in lymph node metastasis, both hormone responsive and unresponsive. Furthermore, a unique series of primary PCa samples obtained from hormone-pretreated patient (3 or 6 months) revealed consistent expression. Exhaustive screening revealed no cross reactivity with non-prostate tissue (unpublished data). Currently, characterization of the antigen recognized by mAb 3.10 is in progress.

Conclusions

Since the introduction of hybridoma technology, mAbs have become indispensable tools in the fields of both basic and applied immunology. Immunohistochemistry, immunoassays and immunoscintigraphy are all techniques that are now an integral part of the diagnostic armamentarium. Using mAb technology, numerous markers were identified; this has been pivotal in increasing our understanding in the fields of (tumor) cell biology and tumor immunology, among others.

Although initial expectations of mAb-based therapy in the late 1970s and early 1980s were high, results of the early clinical trials did not live up to these high expectations. Most of these initial trials focused on unconjugated antibodies and the majority of these were lacking anti-tumor efficacy. However, considerable progress has been made and continuous effort is being invested in improving clinical efficacy of mAb therapy. Currently, eight mAbs are approved by the FDA for a variety of diseases. In oncology, mAbs are approved for imaging (PCa) and for treatment (non-Hodgkin's lymphoma and breast cancer). In Germany, an mAb has been approved for the treatment of colon cancer.

PCa is one of the cancers that has profited tremendously from the surge of mAb technology, mainly in the field of diagnostics. Today, PSA as a marker to diagnose PCa and to follow disease progression after treatment is central in the management of patients with prostate cancer. PSMA-based scintigraphy (ProstaScint) has been approved by the FDA for the detection of lymph node metastasis preoperatively and for recurrence. More research is warranted to determine the additional value in daily clinical practice. It may take some time before clinical decision-making will be changed, but it is not unconceivable that detection tests such as ProstaScint will eventually significantly affect the management of PCa patients.

Currently, due to the success of mAb-based therapy in several cancers, the focus is once again directed at the therapeutic potential of mAbs. Prostate cancer has favorable characteristics for mAb-based treatment modalities. Several PCa-related antigens have been identified that provide potential targets for mAb therapy. Despite the increasing efforts and the growing number of mAbs used in clinical trials in PCa patients, to date no major objective responses have been attained. One aspect to consider is the group of patients involved in most trials: patients with advanced metastatic disease. Although no major objective responses were obtained, some minor objective responses and symptomatic relief was reported, indicating modest anti-tumor effect, which is a remarkable finding in this group of patients. It is not probable that any single therapy will be successful in advanced metastatic disease. Combining several different treatment modalities may prove more effective. In view of the relatively low-toxicity profile of mAb-directed therapy, combination with other treatment approaches such as endocrine therapy or chemotherapy seems feasible. To date, only one study has evaluated the role of mAb therapy (anti-PSMA) in patients treated with radical prostatectomy for localized disease with biochemical recurrence. Results were disappointing, while toxicity was considerable. The increased toxicity was not in concordance with previous reports and the reason remains unclear.

It is evident that several hurdles have yet to be taken before effective mAb-based therapy becomes available. Selection of adequate mAbs conjugates to enhance anti-tumor efficacy should be pursued, while strategies to reduce toxicity should be developed. It is expected that patients with biochemical recurrence after radical prostatectomy without evidence of significant tumor load would benefit most from an effective mAb therapy. The tools needed to detect such patients are already available and continued efforts should be directed towards the enhancement of specific and effective mAb-based therapies.

References

Barren RJ3, Holmes EH, Boynton AL, Misrock SL and Murphy GP (1997) Monoclonal antibody 7E11.C5 staining of viable LNCaP cells. *Prostate* 30:65–68.

Becker C, Piironen T, Pettersson K, *et al.* (2000) Discrimination of men with prostate cancer from those with benign disease by measurements of human glandular kallikrein 2 (HK2) in serum. *J Urol* **163**: 311–316.

Black MH, Grass CL, Leinonen J, Stenman UH, Diamandis EP (1999) Characterization of monoclonal antibodies for prostate-specific antigen and development of highly sensitive free prostate-specific antigen assays. *Clin Chem* 45:347–354.

Borgstrom P, Bourdon MA, Hillan KJ, Sriramarao P, Ferrara N (1998) Neutralizing anti-vascular endothelial growth factor antibody completely inhibits angiogenesis and growth of human prostate carcinoma micro tumors in vivo. *Prostate* 35:1–10.

Bostwick DG, Pacelli A, Blute M, Roche P, Murphy GP (1998) Prostate specific membrane antigen expression in prostatic intraepithelial neoplasia and adenocarcinoma: a study of 184 cases. Cancer 82:2256–2261.

Brawer MK (1999) Prostate-specific antigen: current status. *CA Cancer J Clin* 49:264–281.

Chang SS, Reuter VE, Heston WD, *et al.* (1999) Five different anti-prostate-specific membrane antigen (PSMA) antibodies confirm PSMA expression in tumor-associated neovasculature. *Cancer Res* 59:3192–3198.

Chang SS, Reuter VE, Heston WD, *et al.* (2000) Short term neoadjuvant androgen deprivation therapy does not affect prostate specific membrane antigen expression in prostate tissues. Cancer 88:407–415.

Darson MF, Pacelli A, Roche P, *et al.* (1997) Human glandular kallikrein 2 (hK2) expression in prostatic intraepithelial neoplasia and adenocarcinoma: a novel prostate cancer marker. *Urology* 49:857–862.

Darson MF, Pacelli A, Roche P, *et al.* (1999) Human glandular kallikrein 2 expression in prostate adenocarcinoma and lymph node metastases. *Urology* 53: 939–944.

Deb N, Goris M, Trisler K, *et al.* (1996) Treatment of hormone-refractory prostate cancer with 90Y-CYT-356 monoclonal antibody. *Clin Cancer Res* 2:1289–1297.

DeNardo SJ, O'Grady LF, Richman CM, *et al.* (1997) Radioimmunotherapy for advanced breast cancer using I-131-ChL6 antibody. *Anticancer Res* 17:1745–1751.

Denis LJ, Carnelro de Moura JL, Bono A, *et al.* (1993) Goserelin acetate and flutamide versus bilateral orchiectomy: a phase III EORTC trial (30853). EORTC GU Group and EORTC Data Center. *Urology* 42:119–129.

Dolman CS, Mueller BM, Lode HN, *et al.* (1998) Suppression of human prostate carcinoma metastases in severe combined immunodeficient mice by interleukin 2 immunocytokine therapy. *Clin Cancer Res* 4:2551–2557.

Ehrlich P (1957) On immunity with special reference to cell life. In: Himmelweit F, Marquardt M, and Dale H, eds, *The Collected Papers of Paul Ehrlich, Volume II: Immunology and Cancer Research* (Pergamon Press: London).

Elgamal AA, Troychak MJ, Murphy GP (1998) ProstaScint scan may enhance identification of prostate cancer recurrences after prostatectomy, radiation, or hormone therapy: analysis of 136 scans of 100 patients. *Prostate* 37:261–269.

Essand M, Pastan I (1998) Anti-prostate immunotoxins: cytotoxicity of E4 antibody–Pseudomonas exotoxin constructs. *Int J Cancer* 77:123–127.

Essand M, Gronvik C, Hartman T, Carlsson J (1995) Radioimmunotherapy of prostatic adenocarcinomas: effects of ^{131}I-labelled E4 antibodies on cells at different depth in DU 145 spheroids. *Int J Cancer* 63: 387–394.

Essand M, Logdahl P, Nilsson S, *et al.* (1996) Retention and processing of the monoclonal anti-prostate E4 antibody after binding to prostatic adenocarcinoma DU 145 cells. *Cancer Immunol Immunother* 43:39–43.

Frankel AE, Rouse RV, Wang MC, Chu TM, Herzenberg LA (1982) Monoclonal antibodies to a human prostate antigen. *Cancer Res* 42:3714–3718.

Greenlee RT, Hill-Hamon MB, Murray T, Thun M (2001) Cancer statistics, 2001. *CA Cancer J Clin* 51:15–36.

Gu Z, Thomas G, Yamashiro J, *et al.* (2000) Prostate stem cell antigen (PSCA) expression increases with high Gleason score, advanced stage and bone metastasis in prostate cancer. *Oncogene* 19:1288–1296.

Haese A, Becker C, Noldus J, *et al.* (2000) Human glandular kallikrein 2: a potential serum marker for predicting the organ confined versus non-organ confined growth of prostate cancer. *J Urol* 163:1491–1497.

Haseman MK, Reed NL, Rosenthal SA (1996) Monoclonal antibody imaging of occult prostate cancer in patients with elevated prostate-specific antigen. Positron emission tomography and biopsy correlation. *Clin Nucl Med* 21:704–713.

Hinkle GH, Burgers JK, Neal CE, *et al.* (1998) Multicenter radioimmunoscintigraphic evaluation of patients with prostate carcinoma using indium-111 capromab pendetide. *Cancer* 83:739–747.

Horoszewicz JS, Kawinski E, Murphy GP (1987) Monoclonal antibodies to a new antigenic marker in epithelial prostatic cells and serum of prostatic cancer patients. *Anticancer Res* 7:927–935.

Kahn D, Austin JC, Maguire RT, *et al.* (1999) A phase II study of [90Y] yttrium-capromab pendetide in the treatment of men with prostate cancer recurrence following radical prostatectomy. *Cancer Biother Radiopharm* 14:99–111.

Kahn D, Williams RD, Haseman MK, *et al.* (1998a) Radioimmunoscintigraphy with In-111-labeled capromab pendetide predicts prostate cancer response to salvage radiotherapy after failed radical prostatectomy. *J Clin Oncol* 16:284–289.

Kahn D, Williams RD, Manyak MJ, *et al.* (1998b) [111]Indium-capromab pendetide in the evaluation of patients with residual or recurrent prostate cancer after radical prostatectomy. The ProstaScint Study Group. *J Urol* 159:2041–2046.

Kahn D, Williams RD, Seldin DW, *et al.* (1994) Radioimmunoscintigraphy with [111]indium labeled CYT-356 for the detection of occult prostate cancer recurrence. *J Urol* 152:1490–1495.

Kashmiri SV, Shu L, Padlan EA, *et al.* (1995) Generation, characterization, and in vivo studies of humanized anticarcinoma antibody CC49. *Hybridoma* 14:461–473.

Katzenwadel A, Schleer H, Gierschner D, Wetterauer U, Elsasser BU (2000) Construction and in vivo evaluation of an anti-PSA × anti-CD3 bispecific antibody for the immunotherapy of prostate cancer. *Anticancer Res* 20:1551–1555.

Kohler G, Milstein C (1975) Continuous cultures of fused cells secreting antibody of predefined specificity. *Nature* 256:495–497.

Kuriyama M, Wang MC, Lee CI, *et al.* (1981) Use of human prostate-specific antigen in monitoring prostate cancer. *Cancer Res* 41:3874–3876.

Kuriyama M, Wang MC, Papsidero LD, *et al.* (1980) Quantitation of prostate-specific antigen in serum by a sensitive enzyme immunoassay. *Cancer Res* 40:4658–4662.

Lovgren J, Rajakoski K, Karp M, Lundwall A, Lilja H (1997) Activation of the zymogen form of prostate-specific antigen by human glandular kallikrein 2. *Biochem Biophys Res Comm* 238:549–555.

Manyak MJ, Hinkle GH, Olsen JO, *et al.* (1999) Immunoscintigraphy with indium-111-capromab pendetide: evaluation before definitive therapy in patients with prostate cancer. *Urology* 54:1058–1063.

Matsumoto K, Konishi N, Hiasa Y, *et al.* (1999) A highly sensitive enzyme-linked immunoassay for serum free prostate specific antigen (f-PSA). *Clin Chim Acta* 281:57–69.

Melnyk O, Zimmerman M, Kim KJ, Shuman M (1999) Neutralizing anti-vascular endothelial growth factor antibody inhibits further growth of established prostate cancer and metastases in a pre-clinical model. *J Urol* 161:960–963.

Meredith RF, Bueschen AJ, Khazaeli MB, *et al.* (1994) Treatment of metastatic prostate carcinoma with radiolabeled antibody CC49. *J Nucl Med* 35:1017–1022.

Meredith RF, Khazaeli MB, Macey DJ, *et al.* (1999) Phase II study of interferon-enhanced ^{131}I-labeled high affinity CC49 monoclonal antibody therapy in patients with metastatic prostate cancer. *Clin Cancer Res* 5:3254s–3258s.

Murphy GP, Elgamal AA, Troychak MJ, Kenny GM (2000) Follow-up ProstaScint scans verify detection of occult soft-tissue recurrence after failure of primary prostate cancer therapy. *Prostate* 42:315–317.

Nadji M, Tabei SZ, Castro A, *et al.* (1981) Prostatic-specific antigen: an immunohistologic marker for prostatic neoplasms. *Cancer* 48:1229–1232.

Nam RK, Diamandis EP, Toi A, *et al.* (2000) Serum human glandular kallikrein-2 protease levels predict the presence of prostate cancer among men with elevated prostate-specific antigen. *J Clin Oncol* 18:1036–1042.

O'Donnell RT, DeNardo SJ, Shi XB, *et al.* (1998) L6 monoclonal antibody binds prostate cancer. *Prostate* 37:91–97.

Papsidero LD, Croghan GA, Wang MC, *et al.* (1983) Monoclonal antibody (F5) to human prostate antigen. *Hybridoma* 2:139–147.

Papsidero LD, Wang MC, Valenzuela LA, Murphy GP, Chu TM (1980) A prostate antigen in sera of prostatic cancer patients. *Cancer Res* 40:2428–2432.

Petronis JD, Regan F, Lin K (1998) Indium-111 capromab pendetide (ProstaScint) imaging to detect recurrent and metastatic prostate cancer. *Clin Nucl Med* 23:672–677.

Pienta K (1998) Etiology, epidemiology, and prevention of carcinoma of the prostate. In: Walsh P, Retik A, Vaughan E, Wein A, eds, *Campbell's Urology*, 7 edn (WB Saunders: Philadelphia) 2489–2496.

Polascik TJ, Manyak MJ, Haseman MK, *et al.* (1999) Comparison of clinical staging algorithms and [111]indium-capromab pendetide immunoscintigraphy in the prediction of lymph node involvement in high risk prostate carcinoma patients. *Cancer* 85: 1586–1592.

Recker F, Kwiatkowski MK, Piironen T, *et al.* (2000) Human glandular kallikrein as a tool to improve discrimination of poorly differentiated and non-organ-confined prostate cancer compared with prostate-specific antigen. *Urology* 55:481–485.

Reiter RE, Gu Z, Watabe T, *et al.* (1998) Prostate stem cell antigen: a cell surface marker overexpressed in prostate cancer. *Proc Natl Acad Sci USA* 95:1735–1740.

Rydh A, Riklund Ahlstrom K, Widmark A, *et al.* (1999) Radioimmunotherapy of DU-145 tumours in nude mice – A pilot study with E4, a novel monoclonal antibody against prostate cancer. *Acta Oncologica* 38:1075–1079.

Seltzer MA, Barbaric Z, Belldegrun A, *et al.* (1999) Comparison of helical computerized tomography, positron emission tomography and monoclonal antibody scans for evaluation of lymph node metastases in patients with prostate specific antigen relapse after treatment for localized prostate cancer. *J Urol* 162: 1322–1328.

Silver DA, Pellicer I, Fair WR, Heston WD, Cordon CC (1997) Prostate-specific membrane antigen expression in normal and malignant human tissues. *Clin Cancer Res* 3:81–85.

Slavin Chiorini DC, Kashmiri SV, Schlom J, *et al.* (1995) Biological properties of chimeric domain-deleted anticarcinoma immunoglobulins. *Cancer Res* 55: 5957s–5967s.

Slovin SF, Scher HI, Divgi CR, *et al.* (1998) Interferon-gamma and monoclonal antibody ^{131}I-labeled CC49: outcomes in patients with androgen-independent prostate cancer. *Clin Cancer Res* 4:643–651.

Sweat SD, Pacelli A, Murphy GP, Bostwick DG (1998) Prostate-specific membrane antigen expression is greatest in prostate adenocarcinoma and lymph node metastases. *Urology* 52:637–640.

Takayama TK, Fujikawa K, Davie EW (1997) Characterization of the precursor of prostate-specific antigen. Activation by trypsin and by human glandular kallikrein. *J Biol Chem* 272:21582–21588.

Talwar GP, Gupta R, Gupta SK, *et al.* (2001) A monoclonal antibody cytolytic to androgen independent DU145 and PC3 human prostatic carcinoma cells. *Prostate* 46:207–213.

Texter JH Jr, Neal CE (1998) The role of monoclonal antibody in the management of prostate adenocarcinoma. *J Urol* 160:2393–2395.

Troyer J, Feng Q, Beckett M, Wright G Jr (1995) Biochemical characterization and mapping of the 7E11.C5.3 epitope of the prostate-specific membrane antigen. *Urol Oncol* 1:29–37.

van Hinsbergh VW, Collen A, Koolwijk P (1999) Angiogenesis and anti-angiogenesis: perspectives for the treatment of solid tumors. *Ann Oncol* 10(**suppl 4**): 60–63.

Wang MC, Valenzuela LA, Murphy GP, Chu TM (1979) Purification of a human prostate specific antigen. *Invest Urol* 17:159–163.

Weiner LM (1999) An overview of monoclonal antibody therapy of cancer. *Semin Oncol* 26:41–50.

Wright J, Grob BM, Haley C, *et al.* (1996) Upregulation of prostate-specific membrane antigen after androgen-deprivation therapy. *Urology* 48:326–334.

Young CY, Seay T, Hogen K, *et al.* (1996) Prostate-specific human kallikrein (hK2) as a novel marker for prostate cancer. *Prostate Suppl* 7:17–24.

13 Contemporary clinical trials of prostate cancer immunotherapy

Khaled S Hafez and Martin G Sanda

Rationale for prostate cancer immunotherapy

Prostate cancer is the second leading cause of cancer death among American men (Landis *et al*. 1999). Early detection using serum prostate-specific antigen (PSA) and digital rectal examination (DRE) have allowed for early diagnosis and treatment of disease at its earliest stages: yet, approximately 30% of these patients will fail conventional treatment measures (Jones *et al*. 1995). Metastatic prostate cancer has been routinely managed by androgen deprivation therapy. While hormone sensitive tumors tend to respond early in treatment, development of hormone refractory tumors often emerges. Systemic therapy options for prostate cancer, other than hormonal therapy, are limited: for example, the most promising novel cytotoxic chemotherapies, including regimens using estramustine in combination with taxanes, have not shown any survival benefit in prostate cancer. Alternative systemic treatment strategies for prostate cancer, such as immunotherapeutic approaches, are urgently needed.

Prostate cancer is particularly well suited to potential vaccine therapy or other immunotherapies. First, in animal models, cancer vaccines and immunotherapy have typically been most successful against microscopic tumor burden, and clinical manifestations of human prostate cancer exist in which microscopic disease burden is a hallmark. For example, post-surgical or post-radiation biochemically evident prostate cancer recurrence poses a clinical scenario of microscopic tumor burden, which, when untreated, will progress in the ensuing years. Secondly, serological markers such as serum PSA have been identified and characterized in prostate cancer, which allow such microscopic cancer burden to be continuously monitored, providing a unique avenue for gauging moderate immunotherapeutic effects (Wang, *et al*. 1979). Thirdly, tumor-associated antigens have been defined in association with prostate cancer, including PSA, PSMA and PSCA (Wang *et al*. 1979, Israeli *et al*. 1993, Reiter *et al*. 1998), which may potentially serve as specific antigenic vaccine targets.

Historical precedents in prostate cancer immunotherapy

While Ehrlich (1957) was first to suggest that the immune system could be harnessed against malignancy, Johnston (1962), was the first to conduct a prostate cancer immunotherapy trial in men, in which administration of Coley's toxin was associated with pain relief and weight gain. In 1967, Nauts used a *Pseudomonas* vaccine with the first reported immunotherapy response to prostate cancer (Guinan *et al.* 1984). Others attempted specific immunotherapy using gamma-globulin combined with autologous tumor cells, intra-prostatic levamisole or interferon without substantial responses (Czajowski *et al.* 1967, Rothange *et al.* 1981, Zamora *et al.* 1979). Guinan *et al.* (1973) and Merrin *et al.* (1975) administered BCG either intradermally (id) with a prostate preparation (Guinan *et al.* 1979) or directly into the prostate (Robinson *et al.* 1977), but this approach showed no survival benefit in advanced prostate cancer (Brosman 1977). In summary, despite having used what may now be considered as rudimentary techniques for immunotherapy, these historical trials represent pioneering efforts upon which contemporary immunotherapies for prostate cancer aim to improve.

Contemporary approaches for prostate cancer immunotherapy

Advances in tissue and genetic engineering have opened new avenues for inducing immune responses to prostate cancer as potential strategy for prostate cancer prevention and therapy. Contemporary prostate cancer immunotherapy clinical trials can be broadly characterized in three categories:

1. non-targeted, systemic cytokine administration, for non-specifically stimulating a patient's immune responsiveness;
2. prostate-targeted cytokine delivery, for stimulating inherent prostate-specific immune responses *in situ*;
3. administration of tumor antigens (via delivery systems ranging from purified antigen preparations to dendritic antigen-presenting cells to tumor cells to recombinant vectors) as cancer vaccines (Melder *et al.* 1998, Siegall 1994, Tjota *et al.* 1991, Sedlacek 1994).

Table 13.1 shows some completed trials.

The susceptibility of prostate cancer to genetic manipulation of the immune response has been demonstrated in preclinical animal models, and clinical trials based on these studies are underway (Moody *et al.* 1994, Vieweg 2000, Chen *et al.* 1998, Eder *et al.* 2000, Murphy *et al.* 1996). Initial uses of recombinant and tissue engineering for augmenting prostate cancer-specific immunity focused on ex-vivo manipulations, such as transducing tumor cells with immunostimulatory genes, or loading in-vitro differentiated dendritic cells with prostatic antigens, followed by adoptive transfer of such cells to induce prostate cancer-specific immunity in the recipients of the adoptive cell transfer (Moody *et al.* 1994, Vieweg 2000, Murphy *et al.* 1996, Kwon *et al.* 1997). These approaches, however, are limited in their potential for widespread use due to the requirement for individual in-vitro growth of patient-derived cells. For example, therapy using gene-modified autologous tumor cells is potentially limited in its applicability to patients lacking readily accessible cells for procurement, such as men with prostate cancer recurrence following radical prostatectomy. In addition, the requirement for cell culture implies potential costs that may be prohibitive to widespread use of syngeneic, patient-derived, cancer cell vaccine therapies.

Alternative recombinant vaccine therapies have been developed to circumvent these

Table 13.1 Completed contemporary prostate cancer immunotherapy clinical trials

Treatment modality	Site of trial (Reference)	Agent	Patient number	Toxicity	PSA response	Clinical response
Immunostimulatory cytokines administered systemically or regionally to augment immune responses *in situ*						
Systemic	UCSF (Small et al. 1999)	GM-CSF (subcutaneous)	36	Injection site erythema	3%	NR
Intra-prostatic	Thomas Jefferson (Harris et al. 1999)	IL-2 (leukocyte interleukin)	5	'Mild' dysuria, frequency	0	0
	UCLA (Pantuck et al. 2001)	IL-2 (plasmid-DNA-liposome)	24	NR	38%	NR
Prostatic antigen vaccination: purified antigen administered directly or delivered by dendritic cells or recombinant vectors						
Purified antigen	Memorial Sloan–Kettering (Slovin & Scher 1999)	MUC1 glycoprotein	18	Erythema, fever, myalgia	0%	0%
	Memorial Sloan–Kettering (Slovin & Scher 1999)	GloboH carbohydrate	18	Erythema, fever, myalgia	0%	0%
Dendritic cells	Stanford (Fong et al. 2001)	DC with prostatic acid phosphatase	21	Site erythema, anti-DNA Abs, transfusion reaction	NA	NA
Recombinant vectors	Multicenter (Mincheff et al. 2000)	PSMA DNA/ adenovirus	26	Rash	NA	NA
	University of Michigan (Sanda et al. 1999)	Vaccinia-PSA	6	Vaccine site erythema	NA	NA

Table 13.1 Completed contemporary prostate cancer immunotherapy clinical trials cont.

Treatment modality	Site of trial (Reference)	Agent	Patient number	Toxicity	PSA response	Clinical response
Prostatic antigen vaccination combined with immunostimulatory adjuvant						
Vaccine + systemic adjuvant	Pacific Northwest Cancer Foundation (Simmons et al. 1999)	DC with PSMA peptide ± GM-CSF	95	Site reaction, fatigue, myalgia, fever	29%	NR
Vaccine + vaccine site adjuvant	Dana Farber (Eder et al. 2000)	Vaccinia-PSA + GM-CSF	33	Vaccine site erythema	0%	0%
	Thomas Jefferson (Harris et al. 1999)	Oncovax PSA peptide + adjuvant*	40	Confusion, blurred vision, site erythema, fever	0%	NA
	Johns Hopkins (Simons et al. 1999)	GM-CSF auto CaP cells	8	Vaccine site erythema, fever, malaise	NA	NA

NA, not applicable (e.g. PSA or clinical responses in phase I study); NR, not reported (e.g. toxicity in phase I or responses in phase II).
*All patients received lipid A adjuvant (formulation = 100 μg PSA, 200 μg lipid A); in addition, 11 patients received GM-CSF into vaccine site, five patients BCG, eight patients mineral oil emulsion, and six patients received systemic IL-2 and cyclophosphamide as well as GM-CSF into vaccine site.

limitations of patient-derived, cultured cell-based vaccines. These therapies include delivery of immunostimulatory genes to primary tumors *in situ* (Lee *et al.* 1994, Kawakita *et al.* 1997) and immunization with peptide motifs or recombinant viral or plasmid vaccines encoding tumor-associated antigens as targets of therapy (Tsang *et al.* 1995, Hodge *et al.* 1995, Kantor *et al.* 1992, Bright *et al.* 1996, Disis *et al.* 1996, Rosenberg 1998). The latter has been made possible through molecular cloning of individual tumor-associated antigens (TAA), which have subsequently been targeted in clinical trials of recombinant vectors such as vaccinia or TAA-derived epitope peptide vaccine therapy with some early evidence of significant biological effects in melanoma, cervical cancer and colon cancer (Rosenberg *et al.* 1998, Tsang *et al.* 1995). Analogous clinical trials using vaccinia vectors encoding TAAs for human prostate cancer have been conducted.

Systemically administered immunostimulatory cytokines

Systemic administration of immunostimulatory cytokines – including IL-2, interferon-alpha, interferon-gamma and GM-CSF – has been broadly applied for cancers other than prostate cancer, with success largely limited to modest activity of IL-2 against advanced renal cancer. Only recently has this strategy been used in prostate cancer clinical trials, specifically in the evaluation of systemically administered GM-CSF. Granulocyte macrophage colony-stimulating factor (GM-CSF) is a hematopoietic growth and differentiation fac-

tor that, among other hematopoietic properties, promotes the differentiation of antigen-presenting cells, including dendritic cells. Early phase II trials with systemically administered GM-CSF at the NCI showed no anti-tumor activity in non-prostate cancers, and no anti-tumor activity of systemically administered GM-CSF has been seen in animal models. Nevertheless, 10 years after the preceding studies failed to show any anti-tumor effects following systemic administration of GM-CSF, Small *et al.* (1999) re-evaluated its efficacy in hormone refractory, prostate cancer patients. Thirty-six men with hormone refractory prostate cancer were enrolled; however, hormone therapy was allowed to be continued during the study, and serum testosterone levels at entry or thereafter were not monitored. Although oscillating PSA levels were noted, only one patient showed a PSA decline greater than 50%, which remained sustained for more than 6 weeks. Hormonal status of this patient was not reported. Toxicity was very mild, consisting primarily of transient constitutional symptoms and injection site reactions. Despite the study's excessive focus on oscillating PSA values, the low (<3%) objective durable response rate in this study confirmed that systemic GM-CSF lacks anti-tumor efficacy as a single agent administered systemically.

Intratumoral administration of immunostimulatory cytokines

Previous attempts at using intraprostatic, non-specific, immune modulators refer back to the era of intratumoral BCG administration.

Pulley *et al.* (1986) injected a lymphokine preparation that contained lymphotoxin and macrophage activating factor, yet devoid of interleukins, in six patients with metastatic prostate cancer. They reported some tumor necrosis and, despite marked pyrexia, the injections were well tolerated, with two patients experiencing dramatic improvement of metastatic bone pain. Harris *et al.* (1999) used transperineal intraprostatic injections of escalating doses of interleukin-2/leukocyte interleukin in five patients with hormone refractory advanced prostate cancer. Toxicity was limited to mild irritative voiding. No identifiable reduction in serum PSA was detected and needle prostate biopsy showed inflammatory reaction in only two patients. One limitation of intraprostatic injection of IL-2 or other cytokines is uncertainty regarding whether physiologically significant concentrations of cytokine can be maintained after direct injection of purified cytokine. One approach for improving the durable expression of immunostimulatory cytokine in the primary tumor is to deliver genes for the cytokine with the intent of subsequent significant gene expression. This rationale formed the basis of a phase I trial conducted at UCLA in which plasmid DNA encoding IL-2 was injected into the prostate as a liposome emulsion (the liposome serves to augment plasmid entry into prostate cells) (Pantuck *et al.* 2001, Belldegrun *et al.* 2001). A total of 24 patients were treated, 14 of whom underwent radical prostatectomy after two intraprostatic injections and 10 of whom were treated for rising PSA following radiation or cryotherapy. An objective decline in PSA after intraprostatic IL-2 therapy (greater than 50% decline in their PSA level) was noted in 38% of study subjects. Toxicity has not yet been reported and clinical responses were not monitored as an end point.

Prostatic antigen vaccination: purified antigen administered directly or delivered by dendritic cells or recombinant vectors

As an alternative to augmenting tumor responses by delivering immunostimulatory agents to in-situ tumors, purified or recombinant prostatic antigens can be administered as cancer vaccines, with the aim of inducing tumor-specific immune responses at the vaccine site. This approach does not require direct access to tumor sites and may also circumvent immunosuppression (at the tumor site) of primary immune responses. Slovin & Scher (1999) reported completed phase I studies using either biochemically purified MUC-1 glycoprotein or GloboH carbohydrate conjugated to KLH and administered as subcutaneous injection with QS21 (a saponin immune adjuvant from *Quillaija saponaria* tree bark). Eighteen patients receiving the MUC-1 formulation and 18 receiving the GloboH formulation were evaluable for responses. Induction of IgG and IgM antibodies was observed after immunization, and one-third of patients showed attenuation of PSA rise. However, no PSA responses in accordance with standard criteria (>50% decline in PSA value) were observed, and no clinical responses were seen. The impact of vaccine therapy on the PSA value and its effect on the time of radiologic progression are the focus of a phase II forthcoming trial.

Dendritic cells for prostate cancer vaccine antigen delivery

Dendritic cells (DCs) were originally identified as a cell type with highly efficient antigen-presenting capabilities (Steinman 1991), and more recent work showed that dendritic cells loaded with prostatic antigens could induce prostate-specific cytotoxic T lymphocytes *in vitro* (Tjoa *et al.* 1995, van Elsas *et al.* 1996). On the basis of these studies (and many preceding studies by others in non-prostatic models), phase I and II clinical trials have been conducted using autologous DCs as a vaccine vehicle loaded with either prostatic acid phosphatase protein (PAP) (Fong *et al.* 2001) or prostate-specific membrane antigen peptide (PSMA) (Murphy *et al.* 1996, Tjoa *et al.* 1998). Fong *et al.* (2001) treated 21 patients with dendritic cells loaded with recombinant prostatic acid phosphatase in a phase I study evaluating DC given intravenously (iv), id or via intralymphatic (il) administration. Toxicity included transfusion reaction and anti-DNA antibody induction with the iv route and vaccine site inflammation when administered id. The id route was more effective than iv or il at inducing PAP-specific T-cell responses, as measured by gamma-interferon secretion in response to PAP stimulation.

To circumvent the need for harvesting and growing dendritic cells, recombinant viruses with natural tropism for dendritic cells, such as poxviruses, have been espoused as delivery vehicles for cancer antigen vaccines. Vaccinia is the prototypical such virus: it has marked tropism for dendritic cells, is easily manipulated to introduce target antigens for in-vivo delivery and has a long-established safety record based on its prior widespread use in the eradication of smallpox and more recent use in control of animal rabies. Among several clinical trials using vaccinia-PSA as a prostate cancer vaccine, we evaluated the feasibility of interrupted androgen deprivation as a tool for modulating expression of the vaccine target antigen, as well as detecting vaccine bioactivity *in vivo* (Sanda *et al.* 1999). End points of this limited phase I study included toxicity, serum PSA rise related to testosterone restoration and immunological effects measured for anti-PSA antibody induction. Toxicity was minimal and dose-limiting toxicity was not observed. Noteworthy variability and time required for testosterone restoration was observed. One patient continued to have an undetectable serum PSA for over 8 months after testosterone restoration, an interval longer than those reported in previous deprivation interruption studies. Primary anti-PSA IgG antibody activity was induced after vaccinia-PSA immunization in one patient, although such antibodies were detectable in several patients at baseline. Although interrupted androgen deprivation might be a useful tool for modulating prostate cancer bioactivity in clinical trials developing novel biological therapies, this study showed that unexpected variance in testosterone restoration and PSA rise can complicate assessment of the PSA end point in subjects who have previously received hormone therapy.

Mincheff *et al.* (2000) conducted a phase I clinical trial for immunotherapy for prostate cancer using PSMA DNA plasmid or adenoviral vector encoding PSMA by id injection in 26 patients, some of whom underwent concurrent hormonal therapy. Immunizations were performed id at weekly intervals. Toxicity was limited to a spontaneously resolving rash in two subjects. All patients who received initial inoculation with the viral vector followed by PSMA plasmid boosts showed signs of immunization. In contrast, of the patients who received PSMA plasmid and CD86, only 50% showed signs of immunization. These findings suggest possible benefit of viral vectors as delivery vehicles over plasmid DNA vaccination, but limited sample size precludes definitive conclusions.

Prostatic antigen vaccination combined with immunostimulatory adjuvant

Immune adjuvants have long been recognized as effective agents for augmenting immunity induction by vaccines in preclinical models. To some extent, vaccine delivery vehicles, such as vaccinia virus or adenovirus, can provide indirect adjuvant, immunostimulatory effects by virtue of either pre-existing viral tropism for antigen-presenting cells or through pre-existing immunity against the viral vehicle. More direct use of immune adjuvants for prostate cancer vaccines has recently emerged whereby GM-CSF or other adjuvants are administered to patients in conjunction with a prostatic antigen vaccine.

A formulation of PSA combined with the adjuvant lipid A was used in a series of phase I trials evaluating various co-administered adjuvants given via different routes (BCG, mineral oil, cyclophosphamide, GM-CSF) (Harris *et al.* 1999, Matyas *et al.* 2001). Because the number of patients receiving any one of these adjuvants was small ($N<11$ for each), definite conclusions regarding relative efficacy of these adjuvants are not possible. However, DTH responses against PSA were rare in patients that did not receive BCG, mineral oil, cyclophosphamide, IL-2 or GM-CSF, whereas subjects who received one of these additional adjuvants showed anti-PSA DTH responses and IgG responses in $>40\%$ of cases. Clinical or PSA biochemical responses in treated patients were not reported for these phase I trials.

Simmons *et al.* (1999) evaluated subcutaneous GM-CSF administered as an adjuvant to administration of DCs pulsed with HLA-A2 specific PSMA. A total of 44 patients in a phase II clinical trial received GM-CSF, while 55 were treated without GM-CSF. Overall response rate (PSA and clinical responses combined) was 29%. One complete and eight partial responders were identified among those receiving GM-CSF. On the other hand, 2 complete and 17 partial responders were noted among those who did not receive GM-CSF. The main side effects reported were local irritation at the site of the injection, fatigue, pain and fever. Most reported side effects were of mild severity with some cases of moderate severity leading to the discontinuation of GM-CSF. The authors concluded that GM-CSF, as employed in this trial, did not enhance clinical response to DC peptide infusions or significantly enhance the measured immune response. However, as with other studies focusing on PSA responses in so-called hormone-refractory prostate cancer, the lack of data regarding serum testosterone levels preceding and following immunotherapy among the treated subjects mitigate the significance of these observed responses.

Eder *et al.* (2000) evaluated GM-CSF administered as an adjuvant with vaccinia-PSA immunization. Thirty-three patients with rising PSA after radical prostatectomy or radiation therapy or with metastatic disease at presentation were included in the study. Ten patients who received the highest dose of vaccinia-PSA also received 250 μg/m^2 GM-CSF as an immune stimulatory adjunct at the vaccine site. No patient experienced any virus-related effects beyond grade I cutaneous toxicity. Pustule formation and/or erythema occurred after the first dose in all 27 patients who received $\geq 2.65 \times 10^{-7}$ plaque-forming units. GM-CSF administration was associated with fevers and myalgias in 9 of 10 patients. Although PSA levels in 14 of the 33 patients treated with vaccinia-PSA with or without GM-CSF were stable for at least 6 months after primary immunization, no objective PSA responses ($>50\%$ decrease in serum PSA after vaccine therapy) were observed. Immunological studies demonstrated a specific T-cell immune response to PSA, and there was a trend toward greater cutaneous responses in patients who received GM-CSF.

Vaccination with irradiated autologous prostate cancer cells transduced by a retroviral vector to secrete GM-CSF was conducted in eight patients with prostate cancer who had undergone a radical prostatectomy with curative intent and were found to have metastatic prostate cancer (Simons *et al.* 1999). In this phase I trial, side effects were pruritus, erythema and swelling at the vaccination sites. Vaccine site biopsy manifested infiltrates of DCs among prostate tumor vaccine cells. Vaccination activated new T-cell and B-cell immune responses against prostate cancer antigens, demonstrating that prostate-specific immune responses to human prostate cancer can be generated by treatment with irradiated, GM-CSF prostate cancer cellular vaccine. Although the study was not designed to evaluate efficacy, all eight treated patients showed cancer progression after immunization.

Summary

Prostate cancer poses a potentially susceptible target for clinical immunotherapy, based in part on unique features of prostate cancer that include the ability to target a broad range of tissue-specific antigens for therapy and the ability to modulate minimal tumor burden responses by monitoring serum PSA. Advances in tissue and genetic engineering have heralded a renewed interest in developing prostate immunotherapies and prostate cancer vaccines. However, progress thus far must be viewed with caution. Observed responses to prostate cancer immunotherapy in several enthusiastic reports have actually been limited to marginal effects on serum PSA that either are difficult to interpret due to preceding hormonal therapy or due to the use of excessively liberal response criteria. It is not known, for example, whether stable PSA, oscillating PSA or changes in rate of PSA rise constitute a meaningful end point by any objective, widely applicable measure. Similarly, PSA response data among patients who have received prior or concurrent hormonal therapy should be accompanied, at the least, by concurrent measurement of serum testosterone to control the uncertain and irregular hormonal changes that can follow androgen deprivation. The paucity of objective PSA responses and clinical responses in clinical prostate cancer immunotherapy trials conducted thus far suggest that substantial preclinical improvement of existing prostate cancer immunotherapy is urgently needed. Finally, caution should prevail over exuberant optimism when counseling patients and interpreting clinical data regarding contemporary prostate cancer immunotherapy.

References

Belldegrun A, Naitoh J, Tso CL, *et al.* (2001) Interleukin 2 (IL-2) gene therapy for prostate cancer: phase I clinical trial and basic biology. *Hum Gene Ther* **12**:883–892.

Bright RK, Beames B, Shearer MH, Kennedy RC (1996). Protection against a lethal tumor challenge with SV40-transformed cells by the direct injection of DNA-encoding SV40 large tumor antigen. *Cancer Res* **56**:1126–1130.

Brosman S (1997) Nonspecific immunotherapy in GU cancer. In: Crispen R ed., *Neoplasm Immunity* (Franklin Institute Press: Philadelphia) 97–107.

Chen AP, Bastian A, Dahaut W, *et al.* (1998) A Phase I study of recombinant vaccinia virus (RV) that expresses prostate specific antigen (PSA) in adult patients (PTS) with adenocarcinoma of the prostate. ASCO Conference Proceedings **17**:314a.

Czajkowski NP, Rosenblatt M, Wolf PL, Vazquez J (1967) A new method of active immunisation to autologous human tumour tissue. *Lancet* **11**:905–909.

Disis ML, Gralow JR, Bernhard H, *et al.* (1996) Peptide-based, but not whole protein, vaccines elicit immunity to HER-2/neu, an oncogenic self-protein. *J Immunol* **156**:3151–3158.

Eder JP, Kantoff PW, Roper K, *et al.* (2000) A phase I trial of a recombinant vaccinia virus expressing prostate-specific antigen in advanced prostate cancer. *Clin Cancer Res* **6**:1632–1638.

Ehrlich P (1957) Immunology and cancer research. In: Himmelwiet F, ed., *The Collected Papers of Paul Ehrlich*, Vol 2. (Pergamon Press: London) 7–472.

Fong L, Brockstedt D, Benike C, Wu L, Engleman EG (2001) Dendritic cells injected via different routes induce immunity in cancer patients. *J Immunol* **166**:4254–4259.

Guinan P, Crispen R, Baumgartner G, *et al.* (1979), Adjuvant immunotherapy with Bacillus Calmette-Guerin in prostatic cancer. *Urology* **14**:561–565.

Guinan P, Bush IM, John T, Sadoughi N, Ablin RJ (1973) BCG immunotherapy in carcinoma of prostate. *Lancet* **ii**:443–444.

Guinan P, Ray P, Shaw M (1984) Immunotherapy of prostate cancer: a review. *Prostate* **5**:221–230.

Harris DT, Matyas GR, Gomella LG, *et al.* (1999) Immunologic approaches to the treatment of prostate cancer. *Semin Oncol* **26**(4):439–447.

Hodge JW, Schlom J, Donahue SJ, *et al* (1995) A recombinant vaccinia virus expressing human prostate-specific antigen (PSA): Safety and immunogenicity in a non-human primate. *Int J Cancer* **63**:231–237.

Israeli RS, Powell CT, Fair WR, Heston WD (1993) Molecular cloning of a complementary DNA encoding a prostate-specific membrane antigen. *Cancer Res* **53**:227–230.

Johnston BJ (1962) Clinical effects of Coley's toxin I. A controlled study. *Cancer Chemother Rep* **21**:19–41.

Jones GW, Mettlin C, Murphy GP, *et al.* (1995) Patterns of care for carcinoma of the prostate gland: results of a national survey of 1984 and 1990. *J Am Coll Surg* **180**: 545–554.

Kantor J, Irvine K, Abrams S, *et al.* (1992) Antitumor activity and immune responses induced by a recombinant carcinoembryonic antigen-vaccinia virus vaccine. *J Natl Cancer Inst* **84**:1084.

Kawakita M, Rao GS, Ritchey JK, *et al.* (1997) Effect of canarypox virus (ALVAC)-mediated cytokine expression on murine prostate tumor growth. *J Natl Cancer Inst* **89**:428–436.

Kwon ED, Hurwitz AA, Foster BA, *et al.* (1997) Manipulation of T cell costimulatory and inhibitory signals for immunotherapy of prostate cancer. *Proc Natl Acad Sci USA* **94**:8099–8103.

Landis SH, Murray T, Bolden S, *et al* (1999) Cancer Statistics. *CA Cancer J Clin* **49**:8–31.

Lee SS, Eisenlohr LC, McCue PA, Mastrangelo MJ, Lattime EC (1994). Intravesical gene therapy: in vivo gene transfer using recombinant vaccinia virus vectors. *Cancer Res* **54**:3325–3328.

Matyas GR, Harris DT, Alving CR, *et al.* Induction of antibodies to prostate specific antigen by OncoVaxP™, a liposome-based vaccine for therapy of prostate cancer. *Clin Cancer Res*

Melder RJ, Whiteside TL, Vujanovic NL, Hiserodt JC, Herberman RB (1988). A new approach to generating antitumor effectors for adoptive immunotherapy using human adherent lymphokine-activated killer cells. *Cancer Res* **48**:3461–3469.

Merrin C, Han T, Klein E, Wajsman Z, Murphy GP (1975) Immunotherapy of prostatic carcinoma with bacillus Calmette-Guérin. *Cancer Chemother Rep* **59**:157–163.

Mincheff M, Tchakarov S, Zoubak S, *et al.* (2000) Naked DNA and adenoviral immunizations for immunotherapy of prostate cancer: a phase I/II clinical trial. *Eur Urol* **38**:208–217.

Moody B, Lazenby A, Ewing C, Isaacs WB (1994) Interleukin-2 transfected prostate cancer cells generate a local antitumor effect in vivo. *Prostate* **24**: 244–251.

Murphy G, Tjoa B, Ragde H, Kenny G, Boynton A (1996) Phase I clinical trial: T cell therapy for prostate cancer using autologous dendritic cells pulsed with HLA-A0201-specific peptides from prostate specific membrane antigen. *Prostate* **29**:371–380.

Pantuck AJ, Zisman A, Henderson D, *et al.* (2001) Genes, vaccines, and immune-based interventions. *Urology* **57**:95–99.

Pulley MS, Nagendran V, Edwards JM, *et al.* (1986) Intravenous, intralesional and endolymphatic administration of lymphokines in human cancer. *Lymphokine Res* **5**:S157–S163(Suppl 1).

Reiter RE, Gu Z, Watabe T, *et al.* (1998) Prostate stem cell antigen: A cell surface marker overexpressed in prostate cancer. *Proc Natl Acad Sci USA* **95**: 1735–1740.

Robinson MRG, Rigby CC, Pugh RCB, Dumonde DC (1997) Adjuvant immunotherapy with BCG in carcinoma of the prostate. *Br J Urol* **49**:221–226.

Rosenberg SA, Yang JC, Schwartzentruber DJ, *et al.* (1998) Immunologic and therapeutic evaluation of a synthetic peptide vaccine for the treatment of patients, metastatic melanoma. *Nat Med* **4**:321–327.

Rothange CF, Kraushaar J, Gutschank J, Sedlacek HH (1981) Response of serum acid phosphatase to specific immunotherapy for dysfunctioning, metastasizing prostatic carcinoma. *Med Wel* **32**(2):50–53.

Sanda MG, Smith DC, Charles LG, *et al.* (1999) Recombinant vaccinia-PSA (Prostvac) can induce a prostate-specific immune response in androgen-modulated human prostate cancer. *J Urol* **53**(2): 260–266.

Sedlacek HH (1994) Vaccination for treatment of tumors: a critical comment [Review]. *Crit Rev Oncol* **5**:555–587.

Siegall CB (1994) Targeted toxins as anticancer agents [Review]. *Cancer* **74**(3 Suppl):1006–1012.

Simmons SJ, Tjoa BA, Rogers M, *et al.* (1999) GM-CSF as a systemic adjuvant in a Phase II prostate cancer vaccine trial. *Prostate* **39**:291–297.

Simons JW, Mikhak B, Chang JF, *et al.* (1999) Induction of immunity to prostate cancer antigens: results of a clinical trial of vaccination with irradiated autologous prostate tumor cells engineered to secrete granulocyte-macrophage colony stimulating factor using *ex vivo* gene transfer. *Cancer Res* **59**:5160–5168.

Slovin SF, Scher HI (1999) Peptide and carbohydrate vaccines in relapsed prostate cancer: immunogenicity of synthetic vaccines in man – clinical trials at Memorial Sloan–Kettering Cancer Center. *Semin Oncol* **26**: 448–454.

Small EJ, Reese DM, Um B, *et al.* (1999) Therapy of advanced prostate cancer with granulocyte macrophage colony-stimulating factor. *Clin Cancer Res* **5**:1738–1744.

Steinman RM (1991) The dendritic cell system and its role in immunogenicity. *Ann Rev Immunol* **9**:271–296.

Tjoa BA, Murphy GP (2000) Development of dendritic-cell based prostate cancer vaccine. *Immunol Lett* **74**(1):87–93.

Tjoa B, Erickson S, Barren III R, *et al.* (1995) In vitro propagated dendritic cells from prostate cancer patients as a component of prostate cancer immunotherapy. *Prostate* **27**:63–69.

Tjoa B, Simmons S, Bowes V, *et al.* (1998) Evaluation of phase I/II clinical trials in prostate cancer with dendritic cells and PSMA peptides. *Prostate* **36**: 39–44.

Tjota A, Zhang YQ, Piedmonte MR, Lee CL (1991) Adoptive immunotherapy using lymphokine-activated killer cells and recombinant interleukin-2 in preventing and treatment of spontaneous pulmonary metastases of syngeneic Dunning rat prostate tumor. *J Urol* **146**:177–183.

Tsang KY, Zaremba S, Nieroda CA, *et al.* (1995) Generation of human cytotoxic T cells specific for human carcinoembryonic antigen epitopes from patients immunized with recombinant vaccinia-CEA vaccine. *J Natl Cancer Inst* **87**:982–990.

Van Elsas A, van der Burgh SH, van der Minne C, *et al.* (1996) Peptide-pulsed dendritic cells induce tumoricidal cytotoxic T lymphocytes from healthy donors against stably HLA-A*0201-binding peptides from the Melan-A/MAER-1 self antigen. *Eur J Immunol* **26**: 1683.

Vieweg J (2000) The evolving role of dendritic cell therapy in urologic oncology. *Curr Opin Urol* **10**(4): 307–312.

Wang MC, Valenzuela LA, Murphy GP, Chu TM (1979) Purification of a human prostate specific antigen. *Invest Urol* **17**:159–163.

Zamora S, Bhatti RA, Ablin RJ, *et al.* (1979) In vitro stimulation of tumor-associated immunity in prostatic cancer by levamisole. *Cell Biol* **25**:57–59.

14 Autocrine and paracrine mechanisms in the development of prostate cancer

John Isaacs

Introduction

Androgens play an important role in the cellular homeostasis of the normal prostate gland, both by activating proliferative mechanisms, and thus recruiting cells into the active cell cycle, and by inhibiting apoptotic mechanisms of cell death. Moreover, they are also important in the establishment and maintenance of foci of cancerous prostate tissue, since prostate tumors, at least in their early stages, depend on androgens for survival.

How do androgens stimulate the proliferation of the prostatic epithelial cells?

It has been assumed for a long time that the action of androgens on the prostate epithelial cells was direct. Circulating testosterone would be transformed in the epithelial cells to dihydroxytestosterone by the enzyme steroid 5α-reductase. The dihydroxytestosterone would then bind to androgen receptors in the cells, promote translocation into the nucleus, binding to DNA and initiation of RNA transcription. The gene products so activated would stimulate cell proliferation and survival.

However, recent data have suggested that this simple picture may not be accurate, and, moreover, that acquisition of self-sufficiency of epithelial cell responses to androgens may be a key event in the switch from normal to cancerous cell growth. This information has come from studies in which embryonic mouse cells are grown *in vivo* and allowed to develop into prostate tissue in the presence of androgens (Cunha *et al*. 1987). If mesenchymous cells that would normally develop into the prostatic stroma are grown with prostatic epithelial stem cells, the cells organize themselves into typical prostatic acini expressing androgen receptors. Surprisingly, if the same mesenchymous cells are co-cultured with bladder epithelial cells, the latter also acquire a prostatic epithelial phenotype and express androgen receptors. Perhaps, even more surprisingly, if the bladder epithelial cells are obtained from mice in which the androgen receptor mutated to an inactive form, these cells still develop a prostatic phenotype. On the other hand, if the mesenchymal cells are obtained from the androgen receptor mutant mice, then the transformation from a bladder to a prostate phenotype does not occur. These experiments thus suggest that the primary target of the androgens is not the epithelial cell itself but the stromal cell (Cunha *et al.* 1987). Androgens would bind to receptors in the latter cells and stimulate the transcription of peptide trophic factors (Nakano *et al.* 1999). These would diffuse to the epithelial cells, bind to cell-surface receptors and trigger cell proliferation and the development of a prostatic phenotype by an MAP kinase-dependent pathway. The effects of androgens on the epithelial cells is thus an indirect paracrine one, mediated by trophic factors released from the stroma.

If androgens are removed from the medium, the epithelial cells enter an apoptotic pathway, leading to atrophy and death.

How do androgens attenuate apoptosis in prostate epithelial cells?

The anti-apoptotic actions of androgens on epithelial cells can likewise be explained by the release of trophic factors from the stromal compartment (Kurita *et al.* 2001). The same trophic factors can also inhibit apoptosis in the epithelial cells, by interfering with the phosphorylation of a protein called *Bad*, which is a cytosolic protein that can bind to the mitochondrial external envelope and interact with the apoptotic protein bcl-XL. This protein–protein interaction uncouples the protein *Bax* from the mitochondrial membrane, allowing efflux of cytochrome C from the organelle and activation of caspase 3, which is the enzyme that initiates the apoptotic cascade of DNA fragmentation, chromatin clumping and cell death. The propensity of *Bad* to bind to mitochondria is determined by its phosphorylation state, the unphosphorylated protein binding tightly and the phosphorylated one remaining cytosolic. Protein trophic factors

interact with this process by catalysing the phosphorylation of *Bad* through the receptor tyrosine kinase activity that is activated by trophic factor binding. The *Bad* protein thus remains cytosolic, and cannot trigger caspase 3 activation. By this mechanism, the trophic factors downregulate the apoptotic mechanism.

Diversity of epithelial cell responses to androgens

Although the vast majority of prostate epithelial cells are androgen-dependent, and will enter apoptosis if the hormonal stimulus is removed, there are certain exceptions. There is a population of small non-secretory basal epithelial cells that do not express androgen receptors that appear to act as a source of stem cells for regeneration of the epithelial cell layer (Isaacs & Coffey 1989). These stem cells turn over very slowly, occasionally dividing or differentiating into amplifying cells. The stem cells do not enter apoptosis when androgens are withdrawn, because their survival is not androgen-dependent. The amplifying cell population, on the other hand, can undergo rapid proliferation and differentiate into transit cells. This cell population expresses the KI67 protein, a marker of cell replication. Proliferation of amplifying cells is stimulated by androgens presumably indirectly, in response to stromal trophic factors, since these cells do not yet have androgen receptors. Because the proliferative potential of amplifying cells far exceeds their production rate from stem cells, proliferation is of a clonal nature. This mechanism probably plays a physiological role in prostate tissue repair, and also in the development of the gland in response to androgens, which occurs during puberty. The transit cells that develop from the amplifying cells start to express androgen receptors and evolve into mature secretory epithelial cells.

Trophic influence of the epithelial cells on the stroma

As well as being subjected to a trophic influence from the stromal compartment, the epithelial cells exert a reciprocal paracrine influence on the stroma. This has been demonstrated in experiments whereby human epithelial cells have been grafted into nude mice (Cunha *et al*. 1987). Initially, these cells do not proliferate (Gao *et al*. 2001). However, they co-opt nearby undifferentiated mouse mesenchymal cells and transform these into cells presenting a prostatic stromal phenotype (Hayward *et al*., 1992, 1998; Figure 14.1). The cells start to express androgen receptors, to synthesize actin, and to organize themselves around the epithelial cells. Angiogenesis from the mouse capillary bed is stimulated (Figure 14.2). This process must depend on the release of a trophic factor from the human epithelial cells that acts as a recruiting and differentiating paracrine signal on the mouse mesenchyme. The nature of this trophic factor is not known.

The stromal compartment, thus recruited, then exerts a trophic influence on the human epithelial cells (Figure 14.2). The epithelial cells proliferate and differentiate into a basal cell layer and a columnar secretory cell layer around a central lumen. Expression of the androgen receptor is upregulated and secretion of prostate-specific antigen (PSA) is initiated (Figure 14.3).

At this point, the epithelial cells stop proliferating. The signal that stops proliferation may paradoxically be a *direct* action of androgens on the epithelial cells, which are now expressing high levels of androgen receptors.

Androgens exert an autocrine effect on cancerous epithelial cells

In normal prostate cells, we have seen that androgen stimulation of epithelial cell growth is indirect, mediated by a paracrine trophic influence from the stroma. However, once the switch to a cancerous phenotype has occurred, epithelial cells seem to respond autonomously to androgens. This can be demonstrated by implantation of cancerous human epithelial cells into nude mice. Unlike what is seen with healthy tissue, described above, the cancerous cells flourish and replicate independently of a stromal component. There is no co-option of mouse mesenchymatous cells to form a host stromal matrix providing local trophic support (Cunha *et al*. 1996, Gao *et al*. 2001). Instead, the only factor required for the survival and proliferation of the cells is the host mouse's androgens. Castration of the mouse leads to apoptosis of the tumor, and castration prior to implantation prevents the survival of the transplanted cancerous cells. It thus seems that the cancerous cells respond directly to androgens to stimulate their own proliferation.

Thus, in prostate cancer, unlike normal epithelial cells, androgens play a direct autocrine role in supporting epithelial cell proliferation (Figure 14.4). This autonomous androgen response is presumably due to differences in the various intracellular signalling pathways that control DNA transcription. These changes

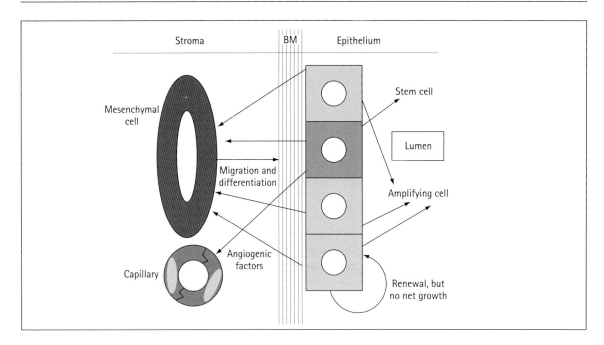

Figure 14.1
Trophic influences from the prostatic epithelium drive transformation of undifferentiated host mesenchymal tissue into a prostatic stromal phenotype. BM = basement membrane.

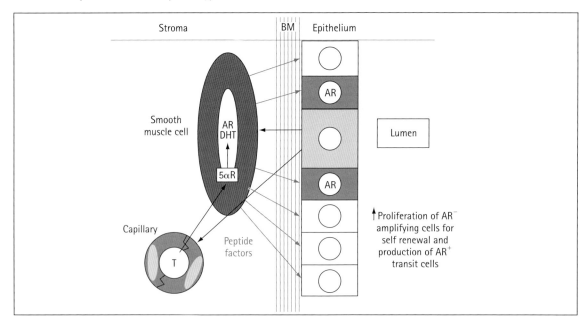

Figure 14.2
Trophic influences from the differentiated stromal compartment drive proliferation of epithelial cells and androgen receptor (AR) expression. BM = basement membrane, DHT = dihydrotestosterone, 5αR = 5α-reductase, T = testosterone.

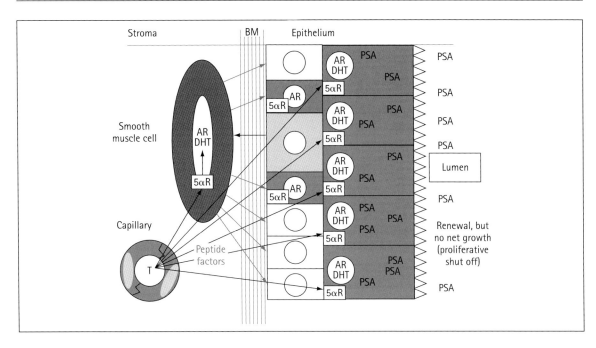

Figure 14.3
Differentiation of the prostatic epithelium, expression of androgen receptors (AR) and secretion of prostate-specific antigen (PSA). DHT = dihydrotestosterone, 5αR = 5α-reductase.

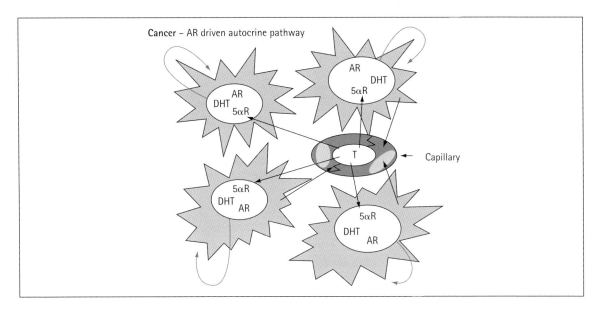

Figure 14.4
Androgen receptor (AR) activation drives epithelial cell proliferation in response to blood-borne testosterone. DHT = dihydrotestosterone, 5αR = 5α-reductase, T = testosterone.

could be associated with alterations in the nature of trophic factor stimulation, in tyrosine kinase receptor activation characteristics, in receptor cross-talk or hybridization patterns or in downstream signalling elements.

What is the trigger that switches on the cancerous phenotype and renders epithelial cells androgen-responsive?

The development of direct androgen responsiveness appears to occur early on the carcinogenetic pathway (Litvinov *et al*. 2003). A potential candidate step is the amplifying cell stage, when the cells enter into rapid clonal expansion in response to androgens. Escape from trophic control from the stroma at this stage would generate a clonal line that could develop autonomously into a rapidly proliferating focus and thus evolve into prostatic intraepithelial neoplasias, believed to be an early stage in tumor development. Normal amplifying cells are not dependent upon androgen receptor expression, while transformed amplifying cells are now directly stimulated by the occupancy of the androgen receptor. Such rapidly proliferating foci of abnormal amplifying cells are characterized by high levels of expression of the Ki67 protein. They are commonly associated with infiltration of macrophages and other markers of inflammatory responses. The inflammatory process is a defensive mechanism that leads in some cases to the atrophy of the proliferating epithelial cells and presumably to their loss (Litvinov *et al*. 2003).

One candidate for an early cancerous switch would be inactivation or loss of the enzyme glutathione-*S*-transferase. This plays an important role in the deactivation of carcinogens and in mopping up free radicals. Both carcinogens (by definition) and free radical reactive oxygen species can cause damage to nuclear DNA. Free radicals produced by macrophages in the inflammatory response may thus be an important determinant of carcinogenesis. In this respect, it is interesting to note that inhibitors of cyclo-oxygenase 2 (an enzyme induced in inflammatory responses, involved in peroxidation of free fatty acids and thus in generation of free radicals) can reduce the proliferation of prostate cancer cells in murine models. This effect may be attributable to the attenuation of free radical-induced damage to DNA (Litvinov *et al*. 2003).

Conclusions

Two factors seem to be particularly important in the development and maintenance of the healthy prostate: a dynamic interaction between stromal and epithelial compartments, mediated by local paracrine factors, and a cell- and developmental stage-specific response to circulating androgens. The development of prostate cancer is associated with deregulation of both these processes, so that the paracrine influence of the stroma is lost, and the response to androgens becomes uncontrolled. Anomalies in intercellular or intracellular signalling pathways occur following DNA damage, and those resulting in unbalanced cell growth are selected for at a stage when the epithelial cells are undergoing rapid androgen-dependent clonal proliferation. Understanding these signalling pathways will be important in the development of pharmacological agents that can reorient them appropriately and thus restore normal trophic responsiveness.

References

Cunha GR, Donjacour AA, Cooke PS, *et al.* (1987) The endocrinology and developmental biology of the prostate. *Endocr Rev* 8:338–362.

Cunha GR, Hayward SW, Dahiya R, Foster BA (1996) Smooth muscle–epithelial interactions in normal and neoplastic prostatic development. *Acta Anat* **155**: 63–72.

Gao J, Arnold JT, Isaacs JI (2001) Conversion from a paracrine to an autocrine mechanism of androgen stimulated growth during malignant transformation of prostatic epithelial cells. *Cancer Res* **61**:5038–5044.

Hayward SW, Del Buono R, Deshpande N, Hall PA (1992) A functional model of adult human prostate epithelium: the role of androgens and stroma in architectural organisation and the maintenance of differentiated secretory function. *J Cell Sci* **102**: 361–372.

Hayward SW, Haughney PC, Rosen MA, *et al.* (1998) Interactions between adult human prostatic epithelium and rat urogenital sinus mesenchyme in a tissue recombination model. *Differentiation* 63:131–140.

Isaacs JT, Coffey DS (1989) Etiology of BPH. *Prostate Suppl* 2:33–58.

Kurita, T, Wang YZ, Donjacour AA, *et al.* (2001) Paracrine regulation of apoptosis by steroid hormones in the male and female reproductive system. *Cell Death Differentiation* 8:192–200.

Litvinov IV, DeMarzo AM, Isaacs JT (2003) Is the Achilles' heel for prostate cancer therapy a gain of function in androgen receptor signalling? *J Clin Endocrinol Metab* 88:2972–2982.

Nakano K, Fukabori Y, Itoh N, *et al.* (1999) Androgen-stimulated human prostatic epithelial growth mediated by stromal-derived fibroblast growth factor-10. *Endocr J* 46:405–413.

15 Clinical uroselectivity

Michael G Wyllie

Abstract

Uroselectivity can be defined as the achievement of the desired effects on lower urinary tract symptoms in the absence of unwanted, usually cardiovascular side effects. It is well documented that classical alpha-blockers such as terazosin are effective over the same dose range in patients with benign prostatic hyperplasia as they are in the provision of effective blood pressure control in hypertensive patients. In contrast, tamsulosin has been claimed to be 'uroselective': the inference being that effective relief of BPH symptoms is achieved in the absence of blood pressure changes.

This chapter examines the existing clinical evidence for uroselectivity and presents clinical comparative data on the direct measurement of uroselectivity in volunteers. The claims of 'uroselectivity' are discussed within the context of alpha$_1$-adrencoceptor subtypes and receptor occupancy. It is concluded that the apparent differences in clinical profiles of the sulphonamide, tamsulosin, and quinazolines such as terazosin can be completely rationalized on the relative degree of receptor occupancy achieved over the therapeutic dose range. It is further concluded that 2 mg terazosin produces almost complete receptor blockade, whereas tamsulosin, 0.4 mg, is a suboptimal blocking dose. It is likely therefore that the clinical profile of all established alphablockers will be similar at doses achieving full blockade of alpha-adrenoceptors.

Further, it cannot be concluded that novel agents selectively targeting prostatic receptors or alpha$_{1A}$-receptors will offer any real clinical advantage over existing agents such as terazosin. Indeed, with respect to efficacy, such agents may have substantial limitations.

Introduction

The efficacy of alpha$_1$-adrenoceptor (AR) antagonists in improving flow rate and the lower urinary tract symptoms (LUTS) associated with benign prostatic hyperplasia (BPH) is well documented. Cardiovascular side effects may become apparent at higher doses and indeed may become dose limiting clinically. Three alpha$_1$-AR subtypes (alpha$_{1A}$, alpha$_{1B}$ and alpha$_{1D}$) are known to exist and much effort has been expended in identifying the subtypes involved in the control of periurethral stromal muscle contraction and blood pressure (Andersson *et al.* 1997). The potential theoretical attraction of selectively targeting 'the prostatic receptor' or 'uroselectivity' is the elimination of vascular side effects while maintaining the benefits arising from the intraprostatic actions.

A definition of uroselectivity agreed by the alpha-blocker subcommittee of the 5th International Consultation on BPH is the 'desired effects on obstruction and lower urinary tract symptoms (when) related to adverse effects' (Jardin *et al.* 1998). It is the opinion of the committee that a clinically relevant determination of uroselectivity can only be made in man and, further, 'none of the alpha$_1$-AR antagonists currently in common clinical use for the treatment of BPH (e.g. alfuzosin, doxazosin, prazosin, tamsulosin or terazosin) has any distinct selectivity for any one alpha$_1$-AR subtype or the prostate' (Jardin *et al.* 1998). This is supported by the receptor binding profile shown in Table 15.1. Indeed, as there is no general agreement on which alpha$_1$-receptor subtypes and locations are involved in the actions of alpha$_1$-blockers, it may be questioned as what subtype selectivity would confer an optimal clinical profile.

Despite the comprehensive analysis of the literature and unpublished data by the alpha-blocker committee, several articles at least superficially appear to support claims that tamsulosin may be 'prostate' or alpha$_{1A}$-selective, at least in comparison to other alpha-blockers (Jardin *et al.* 1998, Lee & Lee 1997,

Buzelin *et al.* 1997, Abrams *et al.* 1997). One possibility is that this is an artefact of the experimental design insofar as the drugs have not been clinically profiled over pharmacologically equivalent, parallel studies. In the absence of such studies, interpretation based on single doses is of minimal value. Equally problematical is the selection of a representative unitary equivalent dose for each drug. Tamsulosin has been variously described as being fully effective at 0.2 mg (Kawabe *et al.* 1991), producing incomplete blockade of alpha-AR (Kawabe *et al.* 1990, Lepor 1990, Wein 1990) and, in the large-scale North American studies, as providing considerably less improvement in Q_{max} than 0.8 mg (Lepor & Tamsulosin Investigator Group 1998).

An alternative approach to the determination of dose equivalence involves the construction of complete dose–response curves versus pharmacologically defined end points (Sultana *et al.* 1998, Wyllie 1999). The present study describes the direct measurement of alpha-blocker-induced changes in blood pressure (BP) and urethral pressure (P_{Ura}) in parallel. In this way a direct comparison can be made of the relative abilities to block the alpha$_1$-ARs involved in prostatic and cardiovascular con-

Table 15.1 Binding affinities (pK$_i$) for compounds at cloned human alpha$_{1A}$, alpha$_{1B}$ and alpha$_{1D}$ adrenoceptors.

Compound	alpha$_{1A}$	alpha$_{1B}$	alpha$_{1D}$
Prazosin	9.7 ± 0.20	9.6 ± 0.14	9.5 ± 0.10
Doxazosin	8.5 ± 0.20	9.0 ± 0.20	8.4 ± 0.12
Alfuzosin	8.0 ± 0.20	8.0 ± 0.20	8.5 ± 0.07
(+) Tamsulosin*	8.4 ± 0.06	7.0 ± 0.08	8.1 ± 0.04
(−) Tamsulosin	9.7 ± 0.03	8.9 ± 0.06	9.8 ± 0.09
Terazosin	10.0 ± 0.01	9.7 ± 0.01	9.8 ± 0.03

*Form used in clinical pharmacology studies.

trol. The data are then interpreted in relation to the plasma drug concentrations at therapeutic doses and the receptor occupancy calculated.

Methods

The methodology is as described in detail elsewhere (Wyllie 1999). In all studies, healthy male volunteers (age < 40 years) were evaluated over 3 or 4 study periods, separated by 1-week washout periods. The effects of a randomized single dose of placebo or an alpha-blocker on phenylephrine (PE)-induced changes in BP and P_{Ura} were evaluated in 3- or 4-way, single blind, crossover studies. In each study, attenuation of increasing doses of the agonist, PE, was used to define the dose response and hence the degree of receptor blockade (Sumner *et al.* 1998, Donnelly *et al.* 1998).

BP was measured using a Dynamp recorder. P_{Ura} was measured using customized 9Fr urethral catheters (Gaeltec Ltd) containing microtip pressure transducers. The catheters were anchored via an incorporated inflatable balloon at the bladder neck. Subsequent to insertion of the catheter, volunteers remained supine while P_{Ura} was measured continuously throughout the 5 h experimental period. During each study period, PE was infused at hourly intervals.

A series of pressor dose–response curves was obtained for each volunteer and quantified in one of two ways. The first method involved actual values and the graphical analysis of the curvilinear plots of mean arterial blood pressure (MAP) or P_{Ura} versus the log dose of the agonist PE (Sumner *et al.* 1982). The alternative method of analysis involved the extrapolation of the PE changes, from baseline, as a proportion of the 'maximum'. The maximal PE response to placebo was defined as 90% (Kenny *et al.* 1994). The degree of alpha-blockade was then calculated and compared as either ED_{25} or ED_{50}, as described in detail elsewhere (Kenny *et al.* 1994).

On this basis, ED_{50} P_{Ura} is defined as the dose of PE required to raise P_{Ura} to 50% of the maximal seen with the placebo, where the maximal placebo rise (to PE) is assigned a value of 90%. In general, ED_{50} values were obtained for the alpha-blockers, unless in the presence of the antagonist there was depression or flattening of the agonist response curves. In these cases, ED_{25} values were used for comparative purposes. Statistical comparisons were made on individual ED measurements and subsequently tabulated as mean $\pm$ SEM for treatment groups.

The selectivity of alpha$_1$-AR antagonists was determined by plotting the changes in urethral pressure versus the changes in blood pressure for each incremental dose of PE. In these plots the gradient of the line was proportional to selectivity.

Calculation of receptor occupancy was derived from the free concentration of drugs based on the following equation:

$$Y_A = [RA]/[R]_{TOT} = [A]/[A] + K_{Da}$$

Y_A = fractional receptor occupancy
$[RA]$ = concentration of receptor ligand
$[R]_{TOT}$ = concentration of total receptors
$[A]$ = concentration of free ligand
K_{Da} = equilibrium dissociation constant of ligand.

In the case of both tamsulosin and terazosin, the drugs were used in the forms commercially available in the UK and branded as Flomax and Hytrin, respectively.

Results

Baseline urethral pressure data

Over the course of the experimental period mean P_{Ura} dropped slightly (5%) in the placebo group. The magnitude of the reduction was increased by pre-treatment with alpha-blockers. In the case of terazosin the degree of reduction was dose related over the dose range 1–10 mg, reaching a maximum of about 35%. Whereas with tamsulosin, even at the highest dose (0.8 mg) only a 25% reduction in P_{Ura} observed.

The infusion of phenylephrine resulted in a dose-related increase in both BP and P_{Ura}. Although there was some degree of intersubject variability, throughout the course of the protocol the response in any one individual was relatively constant. In the studies of alpha-blockade the degree of blockade was relatively constant over the experimental period (i.e. for up to 10 h).

The effects of terazosin on BP and P_{Ura}

Pre-treatment of volunteers (1 or 2 h in advance) with terazosin produced rightward shifts in the PE blood pressure curves (Figure 15.1). The threshold for this effect was 1 mg (the lowest dose evaluated) or less.

A qualitatively and quantitatively similar profile was observed for the attenuation of PE-induced changes in urethral pressure (Figure 15.2). The doses of terazosin required to affect P_{Ura} were identical to those blocking the agonist-induced changes in BP. Thus terazosin did not show selectivity for either parameter.

The balanced profile of terazosin is also shown in Figure 15.3. In this type of plot the basic assumption is that a uroselective agent

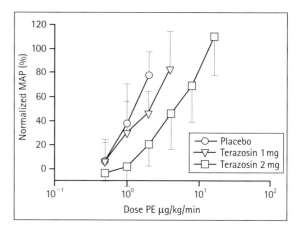

Figure 15.1
The effect of increasing doses of terazosin on PE-induced blood pressure changes. The PE dose–response curves were generated in the presence and absence of terazosin. All measurements were made at peak plasma levels in 3–8 volunteers.

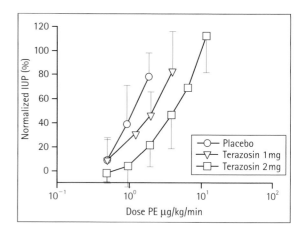

Figure 15.2
The effect of terazosin on PE-induced changes on urethral pressure (IUP). The PE dose–response curves were generated in the presence and absence of terazosin. All measurements were made at peak plasma levels in 3–8 volunteers.

will produce a greater change in the P_{Ura} response to PE than in the corresponding PE-induced change in MAP. Thus if ΔP_{Ura} is plotted versus ΔMAP for the individual PE dose,

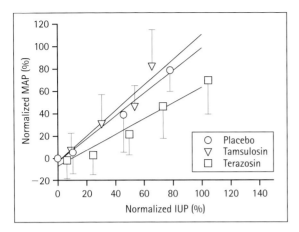

Figure 15.3
This figure utilizes the data of Figures 15.1 and 15.2 to determine relative uroselectivity. The selectivity is determined by plotting the change in urethral pressure versus the change in blood pressure for each incremental dose of PE. In this plot the gradient of the line is proportional to selectivity.

the gradient of the line will be an index of the relative selectivity. As can be seen, for terazosin, the slope is close to unity.

Attenuation of PE-induced changes by tamsulosin

Interpretation of this data was complicated by the high degree of time dependency of the response to tamsulosin, after a single dose (Figure 15.4).

At the shortest time point (2 h) there was little sign that the drug attenuated the PE-induced urethral response, even at the highest dose (0.8 mg). However, at the longest time point studied (8 h) block of the PE response was observed. The threshold for the effect was 0.4 mg tamsulosin and a much larger effect was observed at 0.8 mg. However, even at the higher dose of tamsulosin, the degree of rightward shift was only equivalent to that observed at low doses (e.g. 2 mg) of terazosin. Although only urethral pressure data is shown, the effects of tamsulosin on BP were similar. For comparative purposes the P_{Ura} responses for 0.4 mg tamsulosin and 2 mg terazosin, at the optimal time points of 8 and 2 h, respectively, are shown in Figure 15.5.

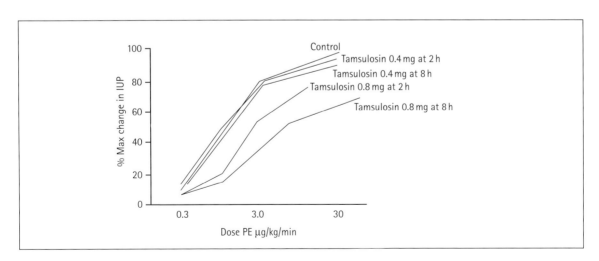

Figure 15.4
Time dependency of the urethral responses to tamsulosin. The effects of tamsulosin (0.4 and 0.8 mg) are shown at two different times. Peak tamsulosin plasma levels are achieved in the period 6–8 hours post dosing.

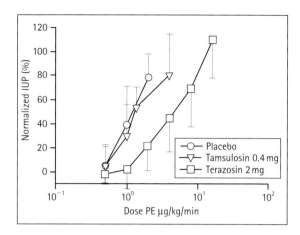

Figure 15.5
A comparison of the effects of tamsulosin and terazosin on urethral pressure. The time points chosen
reflect those at which peak plasma levels are obtained
for each drug: these are at 2 and 8 hours for terazosin
and tamsulosin, respectively.

As can be seen when the relative effects of
tamsulosin on urethral pressure and BP are
compared (Figure 15.3), there is little evidence

that the drug has any preferential effect on urethral pressure, the gradient being less than
unity (i.e. less than terazosin).

Calculation of degree of receptor occupancy and block

Based on plasma levels achieved (Taguchi *et al.*
1998) at therapeutic levels (Sekhar *et al.* 1998,
Sonders 1986, Taguchi *et al.* 1998), receptor
affinities of terazosin (Ireland *et al.* 1997) and
tamsulosin (Taguchi *et al.* 1998) (see also Table
15.1; Andersson *et al.* 2001) and the binding
isotherm described in the methods section, it
is possible to calculate receptor occupancy
(Figure 15.6).

It can be seen that, assuming 50% receptor
occupancy will constitute a reasonable pharmacological block, a dose of tamsulosin in
excess of 0.8 mg will be required. It can be likewise calculated that a dose of terazosin of
slightly greater than 1 mg, but less than 2 mg,

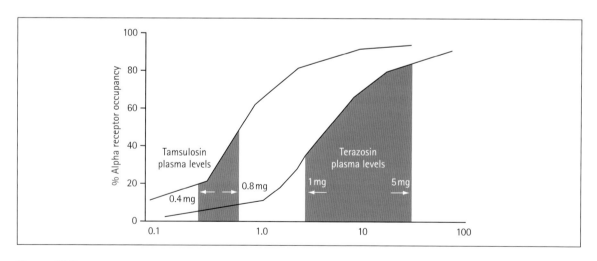

Figure 15.6
This is a theoretical plot of the predicted receptor occupancy for terazosin and tamsulosin over the therapeutic
dose ranges. The plots are derived from radioligand-binding isotherms *in vitro*. Superimposed on these are the
actual plasma drug concentrations achieved at the doses shown.

will produce an equivalent degree of blockade and hence presumably have an equivalent clinical profile.

Discussion

The prime objective of the present study was to measure simultaneously and reproducibly blood pressure (BP) and urethral pressure (P_{Ura}) in volunteers. Using attenuation of responses to the alpha-AR agonist, phenylephrine (PE), it was anticipated that clinical alpha-blocking efficacy and selectivity could be quantified. The inter-relationship between this clinical response and receptor occupancy – in effect a modified PK/PD relationship – could also be determined. This study extends previous studies using comparable methodology (Sultana et al. 1998, Wyllie 1999).

As described elsewhere (Brawer et al. 2001, Eri & Tveter 1995, Weber et al. 1991), terazosin produced slight falls in baseline BP and P_{Ura}. However, the variability and the degree of the drop made quantification difficult. On this basis, attenuation of the response to the alpha-AR agonist, PE, was used as a surrogate of the endogenous neurotransmitter, noradrenaline (norepinephrine), in the determination of the degree of alpha-blockade. Although this may not be entirely representative of normal pathophysiology, reassuringly the effective doses of terazosin versus both vascular and urethral responses were identical to the doses used in the treatment of hypertension and BPH/LUTS (Eri & Tveter 1995, Weber et al. 1991). Likewise, consistent with its therapeutic profile, there was no evidence that terazosin had selectivity for either BP or P_{Ura}. It can therefore be concluded that the profile of terazosin in this model is entirely consistent with the basic pharmacology and well-documented therapeutic profile of the drug.

Terazosin has a balanced pharmacological action (equal affinity) for all three alpha$_1$-AR subtypes (alpha$_{1A}$, alpha$_{1B}$ and alpha$_{1D}$) and the physiological functions that they subserve (Table 15.1; Andersson et al. 2001). This is reflected clinically in the drug's utility in the holistic approach to the management of the patient with BPH/LUTS. At the level of the prostate, the potent action of terazosin on the alpha$_{1A}$ subtype undoubtedly accounts for the rapid changes seen in urinary flow rate and voiding pressure, secondary to changes in urethral resistance. However, in addition to these intraprostatic actions, the extraprostatic actions of terazosin (probably alpha$_{1D}$) on the bladder, bladder neck and higher centres undoubtedly contribute to the significant impact of the drug on symptoms and bothersomeness (Andersson et al. 1997).

Tamsulosin has been claimed to have modest selectivity for the alpha$_{1A}$ subtype that has been utilized to project a perception of 'uroselectivity' or 'prostate selectivity' (e.g. Ford et al. 1996, Testa et al. 1995, Richardson et al. 1997, Yamada et al. 1994). However, the data presented here do not support the contention that tamsulosin has a selective action within the urogenital sinus. This is entirely consistent with the analysis and conclusions of the Alpha Blocker Committee of the 5th International Consultation on BPH (Jardin et al. 1998).

A major problem in the interpretation of the data is that no carefully controlled comparative studies have been completed over the full alpha-blocking range of the drugs; at best one dose of one agent may be compared with two or three of another. Although in terms of cost and complexity this is understandable, it does not form a good scientific basis for any promotional claims.

The quantification of responses on uroflow and/or symptoms is relatively straightforward.

However, this is not the case in the assessment of changes (or otherwise) in blood pressure, where it is well documented that the response is highly dependent on the haemodynamic baseline. Neither terazosin (Sonders 1986, Eri & Tveter 1995, Weber *et al.* 1991) nor tamsulosin (Buzelin *et al.* 1997, Lepor & Tamsulosin Investigator Group 1998) lower blood pressure in physiological normotensive individuals or controlled hypertensives. As would be expected, however, terazosin does lower blood pressure when sympathetic tone is high: for example, in BPH/LUTS patients who are hypertensive (see Figure 15.7; Kirby 1998, Lowe *et al.* 1999). A qualitatively similar difference between the normotensive response and hypertensive response is documented in one comparative study of tamsulosin and alfuzosin (Lee & Lee 1997) and in clinical pharmacology studies during the development of tamsulosin (Tsunoo *et al.* 1991). This dependency of the blood pressure response on the haemodynamic baseline, and thereby on the pre-drug sympathetic drive, is key to understanding the claims of physiological uroselectivity.

In any valid comparison it is essential to ensure that dose equivalency and/or optimization has been achieved. This may be a particular issue with tamsulosin, where the degree or receptor blockade is highly dependent on the time of measurement of response, post-drug administration (Figure 15.4). A more fundamental issue in assigning the label 'uroselective' is the degree of receptor blockade that is achieved at the standard 0.4 mg dose. Based on the degree of shift of the PE response, it is obvious that 0.4 mg tamsulosin is less effective than 5 and even 2 mg of terazosin. A possible explanation can be found in the studies based on relating free drug plasma levels achieved at normal therapeutic doses (Sekhar *et al.* 1998, Sonders 1986) to receptor affinities (Taguchi *et al.* 1998, Ireland *et al.* 1997, Brawer & Fitzpatrick 2001). It is almost certain that 0.4 mg is achieving less than 50% receptor

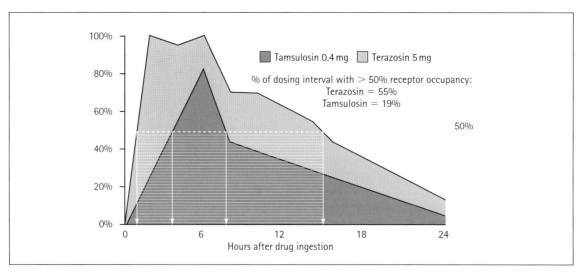

Figure 15.7

The percentage occupancy of alpha$_{1A}$-receptors achieved after single doses of tamsulosin and terazosin. As can be seen, tamsulosin 0.4 mg achieves less then optimal blockade, whereas terazosin 5 mg achieves full receptor occupancy. (Adapted from Taguchi *et al.* 1998 with permission.)

occupancy, whereas doses of > 1 mg terazosin achieve this degree of blockade. Thus, the receptor occupancy data correlate well with the degree of rightward shifts seen in the agonist response curves in the present study. This conclusion is supported by the elegant studies of Michel who showed that, compared to 5 mg terazosin, the degree of receptor occupancy with 0.4 mg tamsulosin was suboptimal (Figure 15.7; Taguchi *et al.* 1998).

Obviously it is important to relate these clinical pharmacology studies to clinical practice and reality. In an attempt to determine the clinical relevance of the predicted receptor occupancy to clinical benefit, some important clues can be found in the early literature. In one early large Japanese study, it is claimed that tamsulosin did not affect BPH symptoms or Q_{max} (Kawabe *et al.* 1991). On this basis it was concluded that only incomplete alpha-blockade was being achieved at this dose (Lepor 1990, Wein 1990). Ironically, this study has become one of the most commonly cited papers on the clinical utility of tamsulosin!

More recently, the results from a large multicentre US study have been published (Lepor & Tamsulosin Investigator Group 1998). This placebo-controlled study shows that the magnitude of the response to 0.4 mg tamsulosin is considerably less than that achieved at 0.8 mg. On the assumption that this relates to receptor occupancy that in turn relates to the degree of alpha-blockade, a reasonable assumption is that the lower dose (0.4 mg) is producing incomplete block and hence a suboptimal therapeutic response. Close scrutiny of the product information sheets on terazosin (Abbott Laboratories 1996) and tamsulosin (Boehringer Ingleheim Pharmaceuticals 1997) show increases in Q_{max} of 2–2.5 and 1–1.5 ml/s, respectively. Once again this would be consistent with incomplete blockade at 0.4 mg tamsulosin.

Although difficult, the clinical trial designer should more often follow the lead of the whole animal pharmacologist. In any study on any drug, a range of doses (bracketing the ED_{50}) should be used and measurements made at steady-state drug levels. In the absence of this level of control, studies over limited dose ranges and versus a single dose of comparative agent are of limited scientific value.

It can be concluded from the present study that a dose of terazosin of approximately 1.5 mg will achieve 50% receptor occupancy. To produce equivalent blockade a dose of tamsulosin of 0.8 mg would be required. Only clinical studies including these, or nearest equivalent doses, should be used to sustain claims relating to clinical uroselectivity.

Future perspectives

It is well documented that 'the' alpha$_1$-receptor consists of three subtypes, designated alpha$_{1A}$, alpha$_{1B}$ and alpha$_{1D}$. Until recently, based on the relative receptor density in human prostate, the alpha$_{1A}$ subtype was generally considered to be the site of action of the alpha-adrenoceptor antagonists (blockers) such as terazosin. On this basis, in an attempt to maintain efficacy and yet minimize cardiovascular side effects, the pharmaceutical industry has expended much effort over the last decade in the synthesis and development of alpha$_{1A}$-selective agents. As we enter the 21st century, only one such 'uroselective' agent, tamsulosin, is commercially available, although several others have reached clinical development.

However, evidence presented recently at the 5th International Consultation BPH (June 25–28, 2000, Paris, France) has raised major issues relating to the potential therapeutic advantage of such an approach. Before Paris there was a suspicion that selective targeting of the alpha$_{1A}$ subtype may result in less than optimal improvement in lower urinary tract symptoms (LUTS) compared to agents with a balanced action across all three subtypes, such as terazosin. These limitations with respect to the efficacy of subtype selective agents were confirmed by a presentation on a novel agent, Ro 700004 by the Roche Group. This compound is extremely selective for the alpha$_{1A}$ subtype compared to both alpha$_{1B}$ and alpha$_{1D}$ subtypes (>30 fold) *in vitro* and *in vivo*. In theory this degree of selectivity should translate well to man.

Data from a 'gold-standard, double-blind, placebo-controlled, multicentre phase II/III were presented to the alpha-blocker subcommittee. In this study of almost 300 patients, as expected, compared to placebo, there were clinically significant increases in Q_{max} in patients receiving drug (0.6–1.5 ml/s and 2–3.5 ml/s for placebo and active, respectively). Disappointingly, however, there was absolutely no evidence of an improvement in International Prostate Symptom Score (IPSS) in this 12-week study. Thus, the study would appear to confirm the anecdotal overall clinical profiles of other alpha$_{1A}$-selective agents from Recordati/SKB and Kissei that have made it into a similar stage of clinical development; the former appears to affect neither uroflow

nor symptom score (perhaps due to underdosing) whereas the latter increases uroflow yet does not affect symptoms (Table 15.2).

Should we be really surprised by these clinical profiles? Several studies in the late 1990s have already shown that there is no absolute correlation between alpha-blocker-induced changes in Q_{max} and IPSS in individual patients or across patient populations. On the basis of the literature, it is perhaps not unreasonable to conclude that alpha-blockers at the prostatic urethral level are essentially acting on bladder outlet obstruction (BOO) and that alone will not maximize the improvement of LUTS. This interpretation would be reinforced by the Roche presentation where the data would indicate that a selective action on the alpha$_{1A}$ subtype will not generate a clinically meaningful improvement in LUTS. The corollary of these clinical findings is that to optimize LUTS improvement of activity at this subtype, activity at another subtype, i.e. the alpha$_{1B}$ or alpha$_{1D}$, must be retained. Although the precise location has not been determined, preliminary evidence would indicate that, with respect to LUTS improvement, blockade of the alpha$_{1D}$ subtype is a prerequisite. The ideal clinical profile, ensuring an action on BOO and LUTS, would thus appear to be a balanced action (equal affinity or receptor blockade) at both alpha$_{1A}$ and alpha$_{1D}$ subtypes (Table 15.3).

Table 15.2 Alpha–adrenoceptor subtype involvement.

Clinical effect	*Subtype involved*
Improved uroflow (BOO)	alpha$_{1A}$
Improved symptoms (LUTS)	alpha$_{1D}$ or alpha$_{1D}$ + alpha$_{1A}$
Control of hypertension	alpha$_{1A}$ + alpha$_{1B}$ + alpha$_{1D}$

BOO, bladder outlet obstruction; LUTS, lower urinary tract symptoms.

Table 15.3 Alpha–adrenoceptor blocking affinity.

Drug effect	*Subtype affinity*
Terazosin	$alpha_{1A} = alpha_{1B} = alpha_{1D}$
Tamsulosin	$alpha_{1A} > alpha_{1D} >> alpha_{1B}$
Ro-700004	$alpha_{1A} >> alpha_{1B} = alpha_{1D}$

In summary, it cannot be concluded that novel agents selectively targeting prostatic receptors or $alpha_{1A}$ receptors will offer any real clinical advantage over existing agents such as terazosin. Indeed with respect to efficacy, such agents may have substantial limitations.

Potentially, the future could lie with the use, particularly by the specialist, of agents in combination with alpha-adrenoceptor antagonists. The most obvious candidates for inclusion as part of such a strategy would be the classical antimuscarinic, agents particularly oxybutynin and tolterodine.

References

Abbott Laboratories (1996) Patient Information. Abbott Laboratories, North Chicago, IL 60064: ref 03-4655 – R3- Rev. Oct.

Abrams P, Speakman M, Stott M, Arkell D, Pockock D (1997) A dose-ranging study of the efficacy and safety of tamsulosin the first prostate-selective $alpha_{1A}$-adrenoceptor antagonists in patients with benign prostatic obstruction (symptomatic benign prostatic hyperplasia). *Br J Urol* **80**:587–596.

Andersson K-E, Lepor H, Wyllie MG (1997) Prostatic $alpha_1$-adrenoceptors and uroselectivity. *Prostate* **30**: 202–215.

Andersson K-E, Wyllie MG (2001) Human prostatic adrenoceptors. In: Kirby RS, McConnell JD, Fitzpatrick JM, *et al.*, eds, *Textbook of Benign Prostatic Hyperplasia*, 2nd edn (Isis Medical Media: Oxford) 1–12.

Boehringer Ingleheim Pharmaceuticals (1997). Patient Information. Boehringer Ingleheim Pharmaceuticals (1997) Inc., Ridgefield, CT 06877: ref 830990 SRT02 5/97.

Brawer M, Fitzpatrick JM (2001) Terazosin in the treatment of obstruction of the lower urinary tract. In: Kirby RS, McConnell JD, Fitzpatrick JM, *et al.*, eds, *Textbook of Benign Prostatic Hyperplasia*, 2nd edn (Isis Medical Media: Oxford) 19–28.

Buzelin JM, Fonteyne E, Konturri M, Witjes WPJ, Khan A (1997) Comparison of tamsulosin with alfuzosin in the treatment of patient with lower urinary tract symptoms suggestive of bladder outlet obstruction. *Br J Urol* **80**:597–605.

Donnelly R, Meredith PA, Elliott HL (1998) Pharmacokinetic–pharmacodynamic relationships of alpha-adrenoceptor antagonists. *Clin Pharmcokinet* **17**:264–274.

Eri TM, Tveter KJ (1995) Alpha-blockade in the treatment of symptomatic benign prostatic hyperplasia. *J Urol* **154**:923–934.

Ford AP, Arrendondo NF, Blue DR, *et al.* (1996) RS-17503 (N-[2-(2-cyclopropylmethoxyphenoxy)ethyl]-5-chloro-alpha, alpha-dimethyl-1H-indole-3-ethanamine hydrochloride), a selective $alpha_{1A}$-adrenoceptor antagonist, displays low affinity for functional $alpha_1$-adrenoceptors in human prostate; implications for adrenoceptor classification. *Mol Pharmacol* **49**: 209–215.

Ireland LM, Cain JC, Rotert G, *et al.* (1997) [^{3}H]R-terazosin binds selectively to $alpha_1$-adrenoceptors over $alpha_2$-adrenoceptors – comparison with racemic [^{3}H]terazosin and [^{3}H]prazosin. *Eur J Pharmacol* **327**(1):79–86.

Jardin A, Andersson K-E, Caine M, *et al* (1998) Alpha-blockers, therapy in benign prostatic hyperplasia. In: Denis L, Griffiths K, Khoury S, *et al.*, eds, *The Fourth International Consultation on Benign Prostatic Hyperplasia (BPH)* (Scientific Communications Ltd) 599–609.

Kawabe K, Ueno A, Takimoto Y, et al. Clinical evaluation of YM 617, on bladder outlet obstruction associated with benign prostatic hypertrophy. A double-blind, multi-centre study compared with placebo. *Jpn J Urol Surg* **4**:231–242.

Kawabe K, Ueno A, Takimoto Y, et al: Use of an alph$_{a1}$-blocker, YM 617, in the treatment of benign prostatic hypertrophy. *J Urol* **144**:908–912.

Kenny BA, Naylor AM, Carter AJ, et al. (1994) Effect of alpha$_1$-adrenoceptor antagonists on prostatic pressure and blood pressure in the anaesthetised dog. *Urology* **44**:52–57.

Kirby RS (1998) Terazosin in benign prostatic hyperplasia: effects on blood pressure in normotensive and hypertensive men. *Br J Urol* **6**:1–3.

Lee E, Lee C (1997) Clinical comparison of selective and non-selective alpha$_{1A}$-adrenoceptor antagonists in benign prostatic hyperplasia: Studies on tamsulosin in a fixed dose and terazosin in increasing doses. *Br J Urol* **80**:606–611.

Lepor H (1990) Editorial comments. *J Urol* **144**:912.

Lepor H & the Tamsulosin Investigator Group (1998) Phase III multicentre, placebo-controlled study of tamsulosin in benign prostatic hyperplasia. Tamsulosin investigator group. *Urology* **51**:892–900.

Lowe FC, Olsen PJ, Padley RJ (1999) Effects of terazosin therapy on blood pressure in men with benign prostatic hyperplasia concurrently treated with other antihypertensive medications. *Urology* **54**:81–85.

Richardson CD, Conatucci CF, Page SO, et al. (1997) Pharmacology of tamsulosin: saturation-binding isotherms and competition analysis using cloned alpha$_1$-adrenergic subtypes. *Prostate* **33**:55–59.

Sekhar EC, Rao TR, Sekhar KR, et al. (1998) Determination of terazosin in human plasma, using high-performance liquid chromatography with fluorescence detection. *J Chromatogr B Biomed Sci Appl* **710**(1–2):137–142.

Sonders RC (1986) Pharmacokinetics of terazosin. *Am J Med* **80** (suppl 5B):May.

Sultana SR, Murray K, Craggs MD, Wyllie MG, Leaker R (1998) Alpha$_1$ adrenoceptor antagonist selectivity determined by simultaneous blood pressure and long-term urethral pressure monitoring in men. *Br J Clin Pharmacol* **45**:192.

Sumner DJ, Elliott HL, Reid JL (1982) Analysis of the pressor dose response. *Clin Pharmacol Ther* **32**:450–458.

Taguchi K, Schafers RF, Michel MC (1998) Radio-receptor assay analysis of tamsulosin and terazosin pharmacokinetics. *Br J Clin Pharmacol* **45**:49–55.

Testa R, Taddei C, Pogessi E, et al. (1995) REC 15/27389 (SB 216469): A novel prostate selective alpha$_1$-adrenoceptor antagonist. *Pharmacol Res Com* **6**: 79–86.

Tsunoo M, Shishito A, Soeishi Y, et al. (1991) Phase 1 clinical trial of YM 617, a new alpha$_1$-adrenoceptor antagonist – Third report: Multiple oral doses of controlled release formulation in healthy male subjects. *Rinsho Iyaku (Clin Med Pharmaceutics)* **7**: 63–93.

Weber MA, Cheung DG, Laddu AR, Luther RR (1991) Antihypertensive dose–response relationships: Studies with the selective α$_1$-blocking agent terazosin. *Am Heart J* **122**: 905–910.

Wein A (1990) Editorial comments. *J Urol* **144**:912.

Wyllie MG (1999) α$_1$-adrenoceptor selectivity: the North American experience. *Eur Urol* **36**(suppl 1):59–63.

Yamada S, Suzuki M, Tanaka C, et al. (1994) Comparative study on the alpha$_1$-adrenoceptor antagonist binding in human prostate and aorta. *Clin Exp Pharmacol Physiol* **21**:405–411.

Index